Maternal Stress during Pregnancy and Postpartum

Rafael A. Caparros-Gonzalez
Editor

Maternal Stress during Pregnancy and Postpartum

Impact on Maternal Health and Fetal Development

Springer

Editor
Rafael A. Caparros-Gonzalez
Faculty of Health Sciences,
Department of Nursing
University of Granada
Granada, Spain

Instituto de Investigacion Biosanitaria
Ibs.GRANADA
Granada, Spain

ISBN 978-3-032-09244-1 ISBN 978-3-032-09245-8 (eBook)
https://doi.org/10.1007/978-3-032-09245-8

This Springer imprint is published by the registered company Springer Nature Switzerland AG
The registered company address is: Gewerbestrasse 11, 6330 Cham, Switzerland

Prologue

Stress is a word used extensively in everyday language in many societies. In common parlance, its meaning is often linked to the psychological distress associated with difficult circumstances and events. However, the origins of the term stress in the medical field is often traced back to a physical, biological response and to the work of Hans Selye, who observed that stress could be measured by hormonal changes in the reactions we show to stressful situations. It is clear from the myriad of stress research conducted over the years that our understanding of stress can be seriously limited by lens through which we look at it. Scientific advances in the field suggest biopsychosocial models which explore the complex interplay between our physical and psychological health and our environment have much to offer to our understanding of stress and our response to it.

Pregnancy, childbirth and the postpartum are times of huge physical, psychological and social change for women and their families thus providing a unique opportunity to further our knowledge of stress, both positive and negative. Most often we see stress as distress and disease and yet eustress is a recognised concept associated with a positive stress response such as excitement. Many women have relatively uneventful, healthy pregnancies and adjust well to parenting; we need to learn more about stress from these women as well as those experiencing high levels of stress to fully comprehend maternal stress.

In addition, stress research does not always sit easily with mental health research; stress and our response to it reflects a series of events and processes rather than a condition or diagnosis. Understanding the interface of stress and mental illness is important in gaining a clear definition of stress. This is particularly evident in maternal stress research which continues to grow rapidly but has suffered from a lack of unifying definitions and theories. This book is an excellent resource for anyone interested in stress in the perinatal period. It pulls expertise and evidence about this complex subject into one space exploring the sources of stress in the perinatal period and the physical and psychological impact that high levels of stress can have on a woman and her offspring. The book also explores psychological assessment and biomarkers of stress and the brain-gut axis all of which help us to reflect, define and explore the underlying mechanisms of perinatal stressors and stress response.

By raising awareness of stress, understanding the mechanisms and finding effective ways to reduce the impact of stress on physical and mental health, we will ultimately support the agency of those who give birth and their families in managing the physical and psychological challenges of childbirth.

National Perinatal Epidemiology Unit
University of Oxford
Oxford, UK
Fiona Alderdice

Contents

1 Why Studying Maternal Stress Is Necessary: An Integrated Introduction to the Book

Rafael A. Caparros-Gonzalez

Abstract

This book is the first of its kind on maternal stress during pregnancy and postpartum. The book offers a scientific overview on the association between maternal stress and its consequences in maternal and offspring health outcomes.

Sources of maternal stress include daily-life stressors and also major stress such as natural disasters, violent conflicts, intimate partner violence, assisted reproductive technology, economic stress, the death of a relative and also birth-related stress.

Maternal stress can cross the placenta, reach the developing foetus and produce epigenetic changes which can be associated with short- and long-term health and disease outcomes in both the mother and the neonate.

Present scientific research on this topic offers some light into the complexity of this phenomenon, including the protective role of oxytocin against exposure to high levels of maternal stress.

Keywords

Maternal stress · Cortisol · Developmental origins of health and disease

R. A. Caparros-Gonzalez (✉)
Faculty of Health Sciences, Department of Nursing, University of Granada, Granada, Spain

Instituto de Investigacion Biosanitaria Ibs.GRANADA, Granada, Spain
e-mail: rcg477@ugr.es

R. A. Caparros-Gonzalez (ed.), *Maternal Stress during Pregnancy and Postpartum*, https://doi.org/10.1007/978-3-032-09245-8_1

This is the first-of-its-kind reference book on maternal stress during pregnancy and postpartum and its impact on maternal health and foetal development in human populations. This book offers an integrated approach to maternal stress and its adverse consequences in maternal and offspring outcomes from a wide variety of origins. Sources of maternal stress come from daily-life stressors (tasks of work, caring for relatives) but also from major sources of stress, such as natural disasters, armed conflicts, intimate partner violence, the death of a relative or the use of assisted reproductive technology [1].

More than 208 million pregnancies and 140 million births occur every year in the world [2]. During human life, stress is a key necessary component that supports a favourable functioning of organisms through participating in metabolism, inflammation and immunity and is in charge of an adequate adjustment to life challenges. However, maternal exposure to high levels of stress during pregnancy has been associated with adverse consequences for both the mother and the offspring [3].

Recent studies have revealed a close interplay between maternal stress and miRNA modifications through methylation of placental DNA (epigenetic changes). These epigenetic modifications can be associated with medical and psychological diseases in the mother, the foetus and future generations. Scientific advances have been made on how the prenatal environment modifies the development of the foetus in human populations since the implementation of the foetal programming hypothesis in the 1940s by David Barker [4]. The foetal programming hypothesis is a core concept belonging to a broader framework, the developmental origins of health and disease (DOHaD), which offers a reference on how the prenatal and early postnatal environment shapes our health (and disease) during our entire life [5]. And the basis of this complex procedure is maternal stress.

Maternal stress starts with a woman being exposed to high levels of stress during the perinatal period. It is known that during stressful situations, human organisms release cortisol, which is the stress hormone. Cortisol helps us deal with a stressful event through mobilization of our biological (and psychological) resources to survive. Maternal stress can be assessed using a variety of methods. In this respect, researchers and clinicians can measure psychological and physiological stress using different scientific methods. Psychological stress can be evaluated through psychological assessment using psychological instruments. Psychological assessment of stress includes instruments of general (e.g. Perceived Stress Scale, [6]) and pregnancy-specific stress (e.g. Prenatal Distress Questionnaire, [7]).

Physiological (biological) stress refers to maternal biomarkers activated while facing a stressful event (sometimes more than one) during a certain period of time that can cross the placenta from the mother to the foetus. Cortisol is one of those biomarkers, and it is possible to measure cortisol levels from a maternal blood sample but also from urine, saliva, ear wax, amniotic fluid and human milk. These matrixes are very useful for measuring maternal cortisol levels and provide accurate information of acute stress. However, measuring acute cortisol levels from these matrixes can sometimes face a few challenges. A qualified professional is needed to obtain a blood or an amniotic liquid sample, and a concrete infrastructure is required to process and store a sample. One of the most important issues when measuring cortisol from these matrixes is that acute cortisol levels can be influenced by environmental factors. This is especially relevant since levels of acute cortisol obtained may be due to the stress generated during the invasive procedure to obtain the sample and not reflecting the real state of stress of a person [8].

Hair cortisol levels offer a solution to those issues. Hair samples are easy to obtain and store and are not influenced by environmental factors. Hair cortisol levels inform of chronic stress from the last 3–6 months before collecting the sample. Hair cortisol levels are so stable through time that it has been analysed with excellent outcomes from archaeological adults from Peru that lived more than 1,000 years ago [9].

1.1 High Level of Maternal Stress Is Associated with Maternal Negative Outcomes

Maternal perinatal stress has been associated with detrimental maternal outcomes such as hypertension, pre-eclampsia, gestational diabetes, distocic delivery, post-traumatic stress disorder and a higher risk of suicide. High levels of maternal stress reduce the chances of being pregnant in women undergoing assisted reproductive techniques (ART) [10]. Besides, women using ART are reported to have high hair cortisol levels which have been found to be associated with neonatal development [11].

Maternal stress can increase the risk for preterm labour, spontaneous abortion [12], postpartum depression and suicidal and self-harm ideation [13] and has also been involved in the development of pre-eclampsia and gestational diabetes [14].

1.2 Maternal Stress and Adverse Consequences in the Offspring

High levels of maternal cortisol may reach the developing foetus through the placenta. During the gestational period, the placenta can play a twofold performance: (1) the placenta releases a hormone that increases maternal cortisol levels, placental corticotropin-releasing hormone (placental-CRH); (2) the placenta contains an enzyme named 11-b-hydroxysteroid dehydrogenase type II (11b-HSD2). The 11b-HSD2 enzyme is a natural substance that can metabolize cortisol to an inactive product, cortisone. 11b-HSD2 can protect the embryo and foetus from a potential exposure to high levels of cortisol. High levels of maternal cortisol have been reported to be associated with low levels of 11b-HSD2, which allows a high amount of cortisol to be transferred from a pregnant woman to the developing foetus through the placenta and the umbilical cord.

Additional biomarkers involved in the transmission of maternal psychological stress from the mother to the foetus through the placenta include tryptophan (associated with neurotransmitter serotonin which is involved in depression), oxidative stress (ROS), gut microbiota, adrenaline and dopamine (associated with Parkinson's disease) [15].

High levels of psychological stress have been associated with intrauterine foetal growth measured through ultrasonography (low foetal head circumference, low abdominal circumference, low foetal biparietal diameter and low birth weight). In this respect, controversial findings have been found, and high levels of pregnancy-specific stress were liked with a higher length in neonates [16]. Associations between prenatal maternal stress (including high cortisol levels) and infant's birth weight have been found. Moreover, maternal stress has been found to be a predictor of gestational age at birth. Nevertheless, the direction of this association is not always clear. In respect to neurodevelopment, some studies report a delayed neurodevelopment among neonates exposed to high levels of stress while still in womb, while other studies have informed an accelerated neurodevelopment in foetuses exposed to high cortisol levels during the third trimester. Studies on infant's gut microbiota have found an association between high levels of maternal stress during pregnancy and some potentially pathogenic neonatal gut microbiota (Clostridiaceae, *Clostridium*, *Campylobacter*, *Serratia* and *Haemophilus*) and low levels of potentially beneficial gut microbiota (*Lactobacillus*, *Actinobaculum* and *Citrobacter*). A recent systematic review reported that cortisol levels were a better predictor of adverse infant outcomes than psychological stress [17].

1.3 Sources of Maternal Stress

Sources of maternal stress throughout pregnancy that may be associated with adverse consequences on the mother and the developing foetus include a wide range of events. In this respect, highly detrimental perinatal stressors include terrorism, the death of a relative, wars, natural disasters, nuclear accidents, intimate partner violence, famines, stressful life events, work and economic stress, assisted reproductive techniques and pandemics.

Maternal exposure to a war has been associated with an increased risk of developing schizophrenia [18]. Besides, the death of a relative during pregnancy was described as one of the worst stressors a pregnant woman can face and has been liked with congenital malformations in the offspring [19]. Nuclear disasters such as the Chernobyl nuclear accident were associated with a higher risk of developing a major depression and a lower intelligence quotient [20].

Every year, more than 400 natural disasters take place in the world, causing at least 2000 homes damaged or an economic loss of over 50 million US dollars. Natural disasters include earthquakes, hurricanes, fires, volcano eruptions and floods and are sometimes considered nature experiments with a high or very high stress load. A recent systematic review based on over 1.3 million mother–child dyads concluded that natural disasters during pregnancy can have an adverse impact on cognitive and language neurodevelopment along with low performance in mathematics [21].

1.4 Maternal Stress: What Science Is Doing and Future Steps

Science is providing a number of resources and projects to minimize the detrimental effects high levels of maternal stress can have. This book provides scientific evidence on the psychological and physiological mechanisms related to maternal stress from conception to postpartum. Intimate partner violence during pregnancy and postpartum is presented as a major stress source and a problem increasing worldwide. Besides, this book pays special attention to economic stress, assisted reproductive techniques, biomarkers, the brain-gut axis, partners, foetal programming, scientific interventions to improve maternal health and neonatal development and the healing power of oxytocin as a protective factor.

Ideally, our aim is that the information contained in this book will reach the general public, clinicians, researchers, stakeholders and mainly policymakers.

References

1. Caparros-Gonzalez RA, de la Torre-Luque A, Romero-Gonzalez B, Quesada-Soto JM, Alderdice F, Peralta-Ramírez MI. Stress during pregnancy and the development of diseases in the offspring: a systematic-review and meta-analysis. Midwifery. 2021;97:102939.
2. Bearak J, Popinchalk A, Alkema L, Sedgh G. Global, regional, and subregional trends in unintended pregnancy and its outcomes from 1990 to 2014: estimates from a Bayesian hierarchical model. Lancet Glob Health. 2018;6(4):e380–9. https://doi.org/10.1016/S2214-109X(18)30029-9.
3. TREASURE: maternal perinatal stress and adverse outcomes in the offspring: maximising infants´ development. COST; COST - European Cooperation in Science and Technology. 2023. Retrieved on the 29th January 2025, from https://www.cost.eu/actions/CA22114/.
4. Barker DJ. Fetal origins of coronary heart disease. BMJ. 1995;311(6998):171–4.
5. Glover V, O'Connor TG, O'Donnell KJ. Fetal programming and public policy. J Am Acad Child Adolesc Psychiatry. 2023;62(6):618–20.
6. Cohen S, Kamarck T, Mermelstein R. A global measure of perceived stress. J Health Soc Behav. 1983;24:385–96.
7. Yali AM, Lobel M. Coping and distress in pregnancy: an investigation of medically high-risk women. J Psychosom Obstet Gynecol. 1999;20(1):39–52.
8. Wosu AC, Valdimarsdóttir U, Shields AE, Williams DR, Williams MA. Correlates of cortisol in human hair: implications for epidemiologic studies on health effects of chronic stress. Ann Epidemiol. 2013;23(12):797–811.
9. Webb EC, White CD, Van Uum S, Longstaffe FJ. Integrating cortisol and isotopic analyses of archeological hair: reconstructing individual experiences of health and stress. Am J Phys Anthropol. 2015;156(4):577–94.
10. Santa-Cruz DC, Caparros-Gonzalez RA, Romero-Gonzalez B, Peralta-Ramirez MI, Gonzalez-Perez R, García-Velasco JA. Hair cortisol concentrations as a biomarker to predict a clinical pregnancy outcome after an IVF cycle: A pilot feasibility study. Int J Environ Res and Public Health. 2020;17(9):3020.
11. Caparros-Gonzalez RA, Romero-Gonzalez B, Quesada-Soto JM, Gonzalez-Perez R, Marinas-Lirola JC, Peralta-Ramírez MI. Maternal hair cortisol levels affect neonatal development among women conceiving with assisted reproductive technology. J Reprod Infant Psychol. 2019;37(5):480–98.

12. Mulder EJ, De Medina PR, Huizink AC, Van den Bergh BR, Buitelaar JK, Visser GH. Prenatal maternal stress: effects on pregnancy and the (unborn) child. Early Hum Dev. 2002;70(1–2):3–14.
13. Reid HE, Pratt D, Edge D, Wittkowski A. Maternal suicide ideation and behaviour during pregnancy and the first postpartum year: a systematic review of psychological and psychosocial risk factors. Front Psych. 2022;13:765118.
14. Dimitriadis E, Rolnik DL, Zhou W, Estrada-Gutierrez G, Koga K, Francisco RP, et al. Pre-eclampsia. Nat Rev Dis Prim. 2023;9(1):8.
15. Rakers F, Rupprecht S, Dreiling M, Bergmeier C, Witte OW, Schwab M. Transfer of maternal psychosocial stress to the fetus. Neurosci Biobehav Rev. 2020;117:185–197.
16. Caparros-Gonzalez RA, Romero-Gonzalez B, Quesada-Soto JM, Gonzalez-Perez R, Marinas-Lirola JC, Peralta-Ramírez MI. Maternal hair cortisol levels affect neonatal development among women conceiving with assisted reproductive technology. J Reprod Infant Psychol. 2020;37(5):480–98. https://doi.org/10.1080/02646838.2019.1578949.
17. Caparros-Gonzalez RA, Lynn F, Alderdice F, Peralta-Ramirez MI. Cortisol levels versus self-report stress measures during pregnancy as predictors of adverse infant outcomes: a systematic review. Stress. 2022;25(1):189–212.
18. Malaspina D, Corcoran C, Kleinhaus KR, Perrin MC, Fennig S, Nahon D, Harlap S. Acute maternal stress in pregnancy and schizophrenia in offspring: a cohort prospective study. BMC Psychiatry. 2008;8(1):71. https://doi.org/10.1186/1471-244X-8-71.
19. Hansen D, Lou HC, Olsen J. Serious life events and congenital malformations: a national study with complete follow-up. Lancet. 2000;356(9233):875–80. https://doi.org/10.1016/S0140-6736(00)02676-3.
20. Kolominsky Y, Igumnov S, Drozdovitch V. The psychological development of children from Belarus exposed in the prenatal period to radiation from the Chernobyl atomic power plant. J Child Psychol Psychiatry Allied Discip. 1999;40(2):299–305.
21. Ünsel-Bolat G, Yıldırım S, Kılıçaslan F, Caparros-Gonzalez RA. Natural disasters as a maternal prenatal stressor and children's neurodevelopment: a systematic review. Behav Sci. 2024;14(11):1054.

From Conception to Delivery: Potential Sources of Maternal Stress

2

R. T. Amiel Castro, A. Londoño Tobón, N. Messerli-Bürgy, and S. Nazzari

Abstract

Maternal stress during pregnancy can have significant implications for both maternal health and well-being and affect pregnancy outcomes. Various sources of maternal stress may emerge throughout the gestational period. This chapter examines the psychological, obstetrical, biological, and social factors contributing to maternal stress from conception to delivery. It provides an overview of existing evidence on the diverse stressors encountered during pregnancy and investigates the mechanisms through which they affect maternal health and pregnancy outcomes. By integrating these factors, the chapter emphasizes the importance of a comprehensive understanding of maternal stress within prenatal care.

Keywords

Prenatal stressors · Pregnancy outcomes · Gestational health · Stress pathways in pregnancy · Psychological factors · Obstetrical factors · Biological mechanisms · Social determinants

R. T. Amiel Castro (✉)
Department of Clinical Psychology and Psychotherapy, University of Zurich, Zurich, Switzerland
e-mail: r.castro@psychologie.uzh.ch

A. Londoño Tobón
Department of Psychiatry, MedStar Georgetown University Hospital, Washington, DC, USA

N. Messerli-Bürgy
Family and Development Research Center, Institute of Psychology, University of Lausanne, Lausanne, Switzerland

S. Nazzari
Department of Brain and Behavioral Sciences, University of Pavia, Pavia, Italy

R. A. Caparros-Gonzalez (ed.), *Maternal Stress during Pregnancy and Postpartum*, https://doi.org/10.1007/978-3-032-09245-8_2

2.1 Introduction

Pregnancy is a multifaceted and dynamic process [1] marked by a wide range of physical, physiological, and psychological changes in a woman's life [2]. The interplay of these factors can lead to stress, a broad concept encompassing various definitions [3]. Although this concept is defined in various ways, prenatal maternal stress can be described as the emotional distress a woman experiences in response to various environmental exposures [4]. These include exposure to stressful life events, present mental health disorders (e.g., anxiety and/or depression), and emotional distress related to challenging situations but also to pregnancy-specific distress. Other psychosocial factors associated with prenatal stress include perceived racism in ethnically diverse women, personality predispositions, previous or present unhealthy behaviors, limited access to prenatal care, and a cultural background not corresponding with the present living environment [5]. Moreover, not only clinically relevant symptoms or diagnosed mental disorders can affect pregnant women; even milder stressors, such as daily hassles, can negatively impact women's well-being [3]. Many of these sources of stress are unequally distributed, with individuals in low-income settings or disadvantaged groups being at heightened risk for experiencing these stressors [6].

It is estimated that between 10% and 29% of pregnant women experience stress, with prevalence and severity varying by the timing and method of assessment [7]. Further, research indicates that higher levels of maternal stress before conception, including both recent preconception experiences (e.g., 6–12 months prior) and early childhood stress experiences, are also associated with more stressful life events and poorer mental and physical health outcomes during pregnancy [8, 9].

The timing during pregnancy when stress is most detrimental remains unclear. Some studies suggest that experiencing stress later in pregnancy, particularly in the third trimester, may have a more significant effect on pregnancy outcomes [10], with research indicating that stress-induced release of corticotropin-releasing hormone could alter the physiology of labor, potentially triggering preterm birth through uterine contractions [11, 12]. Alternatively, other evidence proposes that stress experienced earlier in pregnancy may have more profound consequences to both mothers and babies [10]. Notably, it is still unclear whether different forms of stress have different effects on mothers and babies [3]. This chapter aims to provide an overview of the diverse sources of prenatal stress and its potential impacts on women's psychological well-being (see Fig. 2.1). These have been reviewed extensively elsewhere [13–16]. In the following sections, we explore psychological and psychiatric factors, obstetrical conditions, and psychosocial influences, analyzing how each of these domains interacts with maternal well-being during pregnancy. We will further discuss biological sources of stress, including epigenetic pathways. Understanding these risk factors is essential for identifying populations who may be more vulnerable to being impacted by these stressors and developing targeted interventions to support maternal mental health.

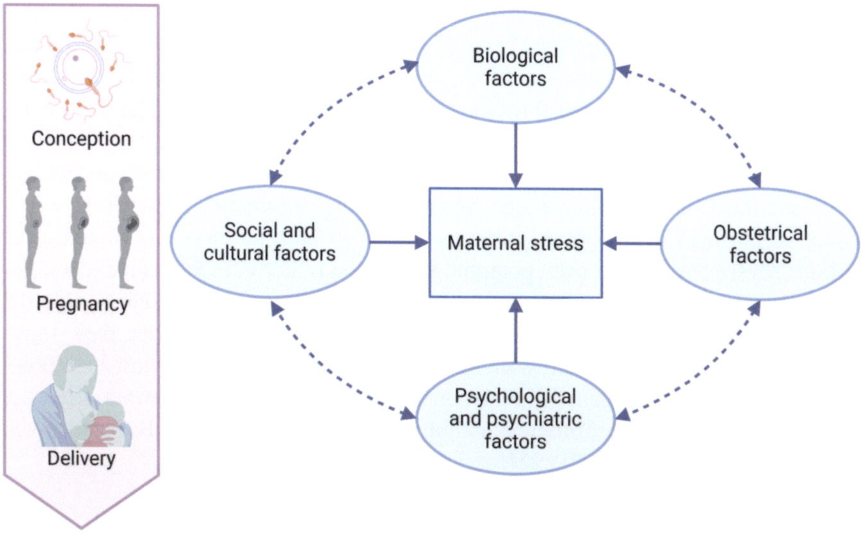

Fig. 2.1 Potential sources of maternal stress from conception to delivery. (Figure created with biorender.com)

2.2 Psychological and Psychiatric Sources of Maternal Stress

Psychological and psychiatric factors play a crucial role on maternal stress development during pregnancy. These conditions can significantly affect a mother's mental health and her ability to cope with pregnancy-related demands, potentially impacting pregnancy outcomes. Such factors cover a broad range of the mother's perception of previous, present, and future stressors as well as her overall mental and physical health during pregnancy. This section provides an overview of various psychological and psychiatric sources of maternal stress during pregnancy.

2.2.1 Life Events and Daily Stressors

Pregnancy is a period during which women may experience severe life events with a similar risk to those encountered by the general population. Such severe life events include catastrophic events (e.g., earthquakes, hurricanes, or terrorist attacks) [17] but also other life events which can impact women's well-being. Surveys indicate that approximately two-thirds of pregnant women report experiencing at least one major life event in the year preceding childbirth [18]. One of the most frequently reported life events during pregnancy is relocation (e.g., moving to a new address during pregnancy) that has been associated with elevated distress [19]. Additionally, serious illnesses demanding treatment or hospitalization of family members or death of a close person have been described as life events that contribute to substantial psychological distress in pregnant women. Further, job loss—whether affecting the pregnant individual or their partner—causing financial instability can increase psychological distress. Besides this, challenges in maintaining a balance between occupational responsibilities, family obligations, and personal needs during pregnancy might cause high levels of stress. This is particularly evident when the demands of caring for children and job-related tasks are overstraining. In addition, one-third of pregnant women report ongoing arguments with partners [20] which might lead to relationship dissatisfaction in both partners and increase the risk for severe conflicts or even potential separation or divorce. Such repeated arguments do not only contribute to negative partner satisfaction but also to conflictual family situation and increased chronic stress during pregnancy. Further, these interpersonal difficulties can manifest themselves in more extreme forms in which pregnant women feel threatened, as in the context of abuse or intimate partner violence, which often leads to psychological and physical harm and high levels of perceived stress in pregnant women [21, 22].

2.2.2 Pregnancy-Related Concerns

Pregnancy is further a critical period characterized by heightened maternal concerns about their own health and the fetal well-being. These maternal concerns may be particularly pronounced in relation to fetal development and can intensify when potential health complications are suspected. Prenatal screening, which aims to detect major developmental abnormalities, is a routine procedure; however, a significant proportion of women experience considerable psychological distress during this process [20]. Pregnancy is also a period of significant physiological changes resulting in ongoing body size changes over pregnancy and might cause weight-related concerns and body dissatisfaction (referring to negative thoughts and feelings one has toward one's body appearance), contributing to high levels of distress. However, recent data revealed that body dissatisfaction is not clearly different in pregnant and nonpregnant women [23]. Instead, whether pregnancy is individually perceived as a deviation from or a liberation from social ideals may determine if body dissatisfaction increases or even decreases during pregnancy.

2.2.3 Mental Health Concerns

Pregnancy is the early stage of a transition period to parenthood for both partners. This might cause concerns related to the future role as parent and to the potential life changes for both parents. Besides this, worries and ruminative thoughts about pregnancy-related complications, about the birth, and about potential birth complications can cause distress in pregnant women but also in their partners and might increase the risk of a vicious circle of increased worries in both partners. Such worries and ruminative thoughts during pregnancy are frequently associated with anxiety symptoms [24], which can interfere at one point with a woman's everyday life and result in clinically relevant anxiety disorders. Pooled prevalence rates for general anxiety disorders are at 3% and remain at this level over all gestational trimesters according to a systematic review [25]. Viswasam et al. [25] also found that panic disorder is more common during pregnancy than according to the expected lifetime prevalence of women outside of pregnancy. In contrast, prevalences of other anxiety disorders including specific phobia, generalized anxiety disorder, and posttraumatic stress disorder are lower than in the general population, whereas social anxiety disorder has a similar prevalence in pregnancy to women in the general population [25]. Further, prevalence rates for specific phobia are reaching 6% in pregnant women and vary between 4% and 15% over the three trimesters [25]. These anxiety disorders may emerge for the first time during pregnancy, or they may have preexisted before conception and worsen due to the challenging circumstances a woman may face during pregnancy [26]. Additionally, the onset of obsessive–compulsive disorder (OCD) during pregnancy is not uncommon, affecting 3%–4% of women, with the majority of cases emerging in the second trimester [25]. While OCD typically develops during the second trimester, women with preexisting OCD are more likely to experience a worsening of symptoms during pregnancy rather than improvements.

Depression during pregnancy is also a highly prevalent mental health problem. One of five pregnant mothers show depressive symptoms during pregnancy, and 15% fulfill the criteria of a major depression during that time [27]. Several factors contribute to the development of depression during pregnancy such as a history of depression, a lack of social support (including partner support), experiencing violence, an unplanned pregnancy, being a single parent, being unemployed, smoking including a history of smoking or current smoking during pregnancy, and a significant proportion of pregnant women also experience comorbid anxiety disorders [27, 28]. The prevalence of depression remains consistent across the three trimesters. However, higher rate of depressed pregnant woman in low- and lower-to-middle-income countries has been reported as compared to high-income countries.

In addition, there are other mental health challenges with lower prevalence rates, such as psychotic symptoms and substance use, which can impact the well-being of pregnant women and potentially lead to adverse outcomes for their offspring.

2.3 Obstetrical Sources of Maternal Stress

Numerous obstetric events have been linked to various forms of prenatal stress, with effects that, while often subtle, can hold significant clinical implications [29]. The studies reported in this section have demonstrated associations, including potential bi-directionality in the relationship between some obstetric events and maternal prenatal stress.

2.3.1 Intrauterine Growth Restriction (IUGR)

Intrauterine growth restriction (IUGR) is a significant factor contributing to perinatal complications, including increased rates of mortality, morbidity, and developmental issues in newborns. IUGR is characterized by fetal growth that is below the tenth percentile for gestational age, often resulting from restricted nutrient and oxygen supply due to uteroplacental insufficiency [30].

Although genetic factors account for roughly one-third of the variation in birth weight, environmental factors play a much larger role, contributing to approximately two-thirds of the variation. In up to 40% of IUGR cases, however, the underlying cause remains unidentified. IUGR is typically detected when there is suboptimal weight gain during the third trimester, often below the expected rate of 100–200 g/week, or through ultrasound findings indicating smaller-than-expected fetal measurements for the corresponding gestational age [31].

Research has highlighted that the development of IUGR is linked to maternal psychological stress, which may trigger the release of catecholamines, leading to reduced placental blood flow, limiting oxygen and nutrients to the fetus, and potentially causing restricted growth or preterm birth [32]. Other mechanisms may involve elevated levels of stress-related hormones like corticosteroids or opiates, which can increase maternal susceptibility to infections, exacerbate neuromuscular responses, and elevate oxytocin secretion [33]. On the other hand, some studies suggest that the management of IUGR, including hospitalization, plays a more critical role in increasing maternal stress responses, with diagnostic timing having less impact on long-term stress outcomes [34]. For example, Tsakiridis et al. [35] found that nearly one-third of women hospitalized due to IUGR pregnancies experience depressive symptoms, a finding consistent with other studies in this field. Additionally, a systematic review by Lewis et al. [36] further supports the link between maternal mental health and impaired fetal growth. Nevertheless, distinguishing the precise interaction between IUGR and depression remains challenging, and the direction of their causal relationship continues to be uncertain.

2.3.2 Maternal Diabetes

Gestational diabetes mellitus (GDM) is defined as diabetes diagnosed in second and third trimesters of pregnancy and is characterized by abnormal glucose tolerance [37]. The global prevalence of GDM has been steadily rising, emerging as a major public health concern [38]. According to the Diabetes Atlas by the International Diabetes Federation [39], GDM affects approximately one in six live births worldwide, with an estimated 20.4 million pregnancies involving women with hyperglycemia. Among these, 83.6% of adverse perinatal outcomes are attributed to GDM, while 7.9% are related to preexisting diabetes. Common complications associated with GDM include an increased risk of cesarean delivery, preeclampsia, hypertension, and the development of type 2 diabetes mellitus later in life [39].

While the precise etiology of GDM remains unclear, emerging evidence suggests that maternal psychological stress may be linked to GDM [40]. Stress, in various forms, triggers gluconeogenesis by activating the hypothalamic–pituitary–adrenal (HPA) axis, which in turn stimulates the release of glucocorticoids and corticotropin-releasing hormones. This cascade leads to hyperglycemia and potentially impaired insulin production [41]. In a study comparing women with a GDM diagnosis with healthy pregnant women, it was determined that being diagnosed with GDM caused an increase in the stress levels of pregnant women. The women with GDM reported worse health perceptions and felt less positive about their pregnancy, with higher stress levels particularly evident among those requiring insulin treatment [42]. Similarly, another study conducted between 33 and 37 weeks of gestation found that over half of the women with GDM continued to experience distress related to their diagnosis, the high-risk nature of their pregnancy, and the management of their condition, including anxiety over potential complications. Again, women who required insulin therapy experienced greater stress compared to those managed solely with diet [43].

Other research has identified elevated stress levels as a significant factor contributing to the development of GDM [44]. For example, among antenatal Indian and Hispanic populations, increased maternal stress from early to midpregnancy was associated with a 2.6-fold increase in the odds of developing GDM [41, 44]. In a prospective cohort study by Chasan-Taber [45] involving Hispanic women, a strong association was observed between high perceived stress levels and an increased likelihood of GDM. Depression was also found to be a significant risk factor, with depressed participants showing higher odds of GDM compared to those who were not depressed. In contrast, some studies have suggested that stress and anxiety levels are not significantly different in women with and without GDM diagnosis [46, 47]. Furthermore, some research indicated that stress levels in women with a GDM diagnosis tend to decrease over the course of pregnancy, aligning more closely with the stress levels of women with normal pregnancies by the end of gestation [48].

2.3.3 Fetal Anomalies

Fetal anomalies encompass a broad range of structural, functional, behavioral, and metabolic abnormalities, which can vary from minor malformations to severe, life-threatening conditions [49]. These anomalies may require intervention either before or after birth to enhance the infant's health and support survival [50]. Also known as birth defects or congenital abnormalities, fetal anomalies pose significant public health challenges, as they can lead to infant mortality and long-term disabilities [49]. While antenatal screening has significantly advanced to detect severe fetal abnormalities, the incidence of these anomalies varies across different regions [51]. Regardless of geographic location, however, fetal anomalies remain a leading cause of neonatal death, with approximately 2%–4% of pregnancies worldwide being affected by such conditions, often identified through ultrasound examination [52].

The awareness of a fetal anomaly can profoundly impact the quality of life for expectant parents, often triggering significant psychological distress [53]. The disclosure of a life-threatening congenital malformation is typically a traumatic and shocking experience for parents, who may find it emotionally overwhelming [54]. Additionally, fetal anomalies present varying prognoses and treatment plans, which can further intensify the emotional burden on families. Parents facing life-limiting fetal anomalies are at heightened risk for developing perinatal depression, traumatic stress, grief, and anxiety [55].

Research has shown that anxiety levels in expectant mothers are significantly impacted by the diagnosis of a fetal anomaly. For example, anxiety levels were found to peak in the second trimester and then temporarily decrease before rising again in the final month of pregnancy [56]. In a study by Nes et al. [57], which focused on Down syndrome and cleft lip and/or palate, women carrying fetuses with abnormalities exhibited moderate distress during pregnancy. However, the level of distress varied based on the type of anomaly; for example, anxiety levels remained stable for Down syndrome diagnoses and decreased for cleft lip and palate cases during the third trimester. Other studies have highlighted that the severity of the anomaly and diagnostic uncertainty are strongly correlated with maternal stress levels, with severe anomalies like congenital heart disease being particularly linked to heightened psychological distress [58, 59]. For instance, a study involving women carrying fetuses diagnosed with complex congenital heart disease revealed that 65% of mothers experienced significant psychological distress, compared to only 25% of those carrying healthy fetuses [60]. Similarly, a study by Rey-Bellet and Hohlfeld [61] found that while most expectant parents reacted with severe psychological shock to the diagnosis of cleft lip and/or palate, the possibility of corrective treatment offered some relief.

The psychological impact of fetal anomaly diagnoses is influenced by various factors. Greater disease severity and poorer prognoses are associated with heightened anxiety and symptoms of posttraumatic stress disorder (PTSD), particularly intrusive thoughts and avoidance behaviors [62]. Early diagnosis tends to elicit stronger emotional responses, with greater distress reported when anomalies are detected in the earlier stages of pregnancy, compared to diagnoses made later. Postnatal diagnoses, in contrast, are typically linked to lower levels of psychological distress, underscoring the importance of addressing the prolonged concern that accompanies fetal anomaly diagnoses during pregnancy [63]. Moreover, maternal psychological distress often persists into the postnatal period, with women who received fetal diagnoses being at increased risk for developing PTSD symptoms including intrusive memories, hyperarousal, and avoidance behaviors [57]. Recent research has suggested that diagnostic ambiguity is an independent predictor of elevated traumatic stress trajectories, regardless of the severity of the anomaly. Some have even posited that the uncertainty surrounding a diagnosis may be more distressing than knowing about a poor prognosis [62].

In addition to anxiety, depressive symptoms are commonly observed among women with pregnancies complicated by fetal anomalies. Hansen et al. [64] found that 31.9% of women with fetal anomalies screened positive for depressive symptoms, which is nearly double the prevalence seen across all pregnancies. Depression screening rates have varied widely across studies ranging from 21% to 72%, with the highest rates observed immediately following the diagnosis [65, 66]. Persistent depressive symptoms have also been reported among women carrying pregnancies with fetal anomalies, particularly toward the end of gestation. Furthermore, women who choose to terminate their pregnancies due to fetal anomalies exhibit higher rates of depression compared to those whose pregnancies continue, emphasizing the need for comprehensive mental health support during this challenging period [55].

2.3.4 Preterm Premature Rupture of the Membranes (PPROM)

Preterm premature rupture of membranes (PPROM) is a condition characterized by the rupture of the fetal membranes before 37 weeks of gestation. This significant obstetric complication occurs in approximately 3%–4% of all pregnancies and is responsible for 40%–50% of preterm births. PPROM results from a complex interplay of factors, including maternal reproductive tract infections, behavioral influences (e.g., smoking), obstetric complications (e.g., an incompetent cervix), and environmental stressors. Genetic predisposition has also been suggested as a contributing factor [67].

PPROM is a highly distressing event for both patients and their families, often leading to significant psychological and emotional challenges. In about 50% of cases, labor begins within 1 week of membrane rupture. Additionally, PPROM increases the risk of severe complications such as sepsis, placental abruption, and umbilical cord prolapse, all of which further compound the potential risks to maternal and fetal health [68].

Women who experience adverse obstetric events, such as PPROM, often exhibit high rates of anxiety, depression, and PTSD. Specifically, women with PPROM are at a heightened risk for antenatal anxiety and postnatal depression [69]. A retrospective study that followed women admitted for PPROM over a 6-year period found that 18.9% of women developed postpartum depression. The study further highlighted that earlier gestational age at the time of membrane rupture and neonatal morbidity or mortality were significantly associated with an increased risk of postpartum depression [70].

2.3.5 Preeclampsia

Preeclampsia is a prevalent pregnancy-related syndrome, characterized by hypertension and proteinuria after the 20th week of gestation. It is a major contributor to maternal and perinatal morbidity and mortality, affecting approximately 2%–8% of pregnancies globally [71]. For the fetus, preeclampsia can lead to complications such as intrauterine growth restriction, preterm birth, hypoxia, and fetal death. For the mother, the condition poses significant risks, including placental abruption, end-organ damage due to accelerated hypertension, stroke, and in severe cases maternal death [72]. Although the exact pathogenesis of preeclampsia remains unclear, it is believed to arise from abnormal placentation early in pregnancy, potentially influenced by immunological, genetic, and environmental factors. Maternal risk factors, including advanced age, obesity, chronic hypertension, diabetes mellitus, and preexisting renal or connective tissue diseases, are well-established contributors to the development of preeclampsia [73].

The mechanisms through which stress may be linked to the risk of preeclampsia are not yet fully understood, though several plausible pathways have been proposed. Chronic activation of the HPA axis, along with factors such as sleep disturbances, anxiety, and depressive symptoms, may contribute to the development of preeclampsia [74]. These factors can induce physiological changes, including vasoconstriction, altered immune and coagulation responses [75], and disruptions in uteroplacental blood flow [76]. Research has shown that women with preeclampsia have higher levels of cortisol-releasing hormone and exhibit signs of heightened sympathetic nervous system activity compared to women with normal pregnancies, suggesting a potential link between stress and the pathophysiology of preeclampsia [77, 78].

Importantly, the relationship between stress and preeclampsia in pregnant women remains contentious. Some studies have reported an increased risk of preeclampsia in women experiencing prenatal stress [72, 79], while others have found no significant association [80, 81]. Epidemiological studies exploring this relationship have produced inconsistent findings. On the one hand, a study using data from the complete national birth cohort in Germany, conducted by Schneider et al. [82], found that pregnant women experiencing high levels of psychosocial stress had a significantly higher risk of developing preeclampsia. Similarly, research by Yu et al. [72] demonstrated that psychosocial stress, when combined with chronic hypertension, may further elevate the risk of preeclampsia. Moreover, work-related stress and depression/anxiety have also been associated with an increased risk of preeclampsia. One prospective study indicated that women with depression, anxiety, or both had a 3.1-fold increased risk of preeclampsia compared to women without these conditions [83]. Similarly, a study by Qiu et al. [84] found that a history of maternal mood or anxiety disorders was associated with a 2.12-fold increased risk of developing preeclampsia. However, others have failed to establish a clear link between work stress, anxiety, depression, or pregnancy-related anxiety and the subsequent development of preeclampsia [81].

Multiple studies have reported that preeclampsia patients have higher rates of psychiatric disorders including depression, PTSD, and anxiety following preeclampsia diagnosis, in the immediate postpartum and over a decade later [85, 86]. However, the literature presents inconsistent findings regarding the relationship between the severity of preeclampsia and mental health outcomes [87]. While some studies suggest that more severe hypertensive pregnancy disorders, characterized by higher levels of hypertension, proteinuria, and related complications, are linked to worse outcomes in depression, anxiety, and PTSD [88, 89], others report no significant association between the severity of preeclampsia and mental health, cognitive function, or quality of life [90].

These conflicting findings highlight the complexity of the relationship between maternal stress and preeclampsia, suggesting that further research is necessary to better understand the mechanisms underlying this association. Clarifying how prenatal stress influences the development of preeclampsia and vice versa could have important implications for prevention and management strategies, particularly for women identified as being at high risk for the condition.

2.4 Biological Sources of Maternal Stress

Pregnancy is characterized by profound changes in the regulation of biological systems, including the neuroendocrine and immune systems [91, 92], which adapt to support the growth and development of the fetus. These physiological adaptations are essential for a healthy pregnancy progression but can also influence maternal health and psychological well-being, making pregnancy a particularly vulnerable period for mental health challenges [93–95]. Stress can further disrupt the delicate balance of these physiological systems. When experienced intensely or over prolonged period, stress can dysregulate stress-related biological systems, exacerbating the risk of psychological distress. During pregnancy, this dysregulation increases the likelihood of mood disturbances and carries significant implications for fetal development, emphasizing the need to understand the underlying mechanisms.

Research into the pathophysiology of perinatal stress, such as depression or anxiety symptoms, has primarily focused on hormonal imbalances, biochemical factors, influence of monoaminergic system, dysregulation of the stress response systems, and contributions of the immune system [96]. These factors not only provide insight into the biological underpinnings of maternal stress during pregnancy but also highlight potential targets for intervention to support maternal well-being. This section illustrates the key biological pathways implicated in maternal stress during pregnancy, with an emphasis on neuroendocrine, immune, biochemical, and genetic/epigenetic factors (Table 2.1). By examining these pathways, we aim to provide a comprehensive understanding of the physiological processes at play, setting the stage for further exploration of their potential implications for maternal and fetal health.

2.4.1 Neuroendocrine Pathways

The hypothalamus–pituitary–adrenal (HPA) axis and the sympathetic nervous system (SNS) are key components of the stress response system, orchestrating a coordinated biobehavioral response to challenges. These systems also support essential processes like immunity, growth, and reproduction [97]. During pregnancy, their regulation undergoes profound adaptations to support fetal development while minimizing exposure to maternal stress hormones.

Table 2.1 Summarized biological mediators and pathways to maternal antenatal stress

Biological pathways	Biological mediators	Pregnancy-related changes	Stress-related changes	Implications for maternal mental health
Neuroendocrine pathways	Cortisol Catecholamines (e.g., epinephrine and norepinephrine)	↑ Baseline cortisol ↑ Catecholamine levels ↓ Stress reactivity	↑ Cortisol ↑ Catecholamines	Dysregulations of these systems during the perinatal period might negatively affect maternal mental health
Inflammatory and monoaminergic pathways	Cytokines (e.g., TNF-α, IL-6) Acute-phase proteins (e.g., C-reactive protein) Tryptophan–kynurenine pathway metabolites	↑ Pro-inflammatory activity in early and late pregnancy ↓ Inflammation in midpregnancy	↑ Inflammation and altered cytokine profiles ↓ Tryptophan—metabolism shifted toward the kynurenine pathway, via heightened inflammation	↑ Inflammation and ↓ tryptophan concentrations might increase the risk for mental health disorders
Biochemical factors	Micronutrient status (e.g., iron, folate) Lipid metabolism (e.g., fatty acids) Vitamin D	↑ Micronutrient demands. Altered lipid metabolism	Stress impacts the body's ability to absorb and utilize essential micronutrients and alter lipid profiles ↓ Vitamin D levels	Altered micronutrient levels and lipid metabolism can contribute to mood disorders
Genetic factors	Genetic polymorphisms in key stress-related genes	–	Genetic predisposition influences individual's stress reactivity	Increased risk for perinatal mood disturbances
Epigenetic modifications	DNA methylation Histone modifications Noncoding RNAs	Pregnancy can induce epigenetic adaptations especially in the placenta	Stress induces epigenetic changes (such as increased DNA methylation), leading to altered gene expression	Epigenetic changes may increase the risk of mental health disorders

Cortisol, the hormonal end product of the HPA axis, acts in the brain by binding to glucocorticoid and mineralocorticoid receptors and exerts negative-feedback control over the activity of the HPA axis, in order to prevent detrimental consequences related to a prolonged and excessive stress response [98, 99]. Pregnancy introduces substantial changes to the HPA axis regulation, largely driven by the placental production of corticotropin-releasing hormone (CRH), which stimulates maternal cortisol secretion. Unlike the typical negative-feedback loop in nonpregnant individuals, maternal cortisol enhances placental CRH synthesis, creating a positive feed-forward loop. This results in dramatic elevations in CRH and cortisol across gestation [100, 101] that peak near delivery [102, 103]. Cortisol diurnal pattern, characterized by high levels of cortisol at waking, a steep increase 30–45 min after awakening, and a gradual decline throughout the day, is mainly preserved during pregnancy [104, 105]. In contrast, HPA axis stress reactivity is significantly dampened during pregnancy [106, 107], preventing mother and fetus from excessive exposure to stress hormones and alterations in cardiovascular parameters affecting uterine blood flow.

A dysregulation of the HPA axis plays a central role in the pathophysiology of several mental health conditions [108]. It has been proposed that the profound alterations of this system during the perinatal period might influence the risk for adverse maternal mental health [94, 109. Although more studies are needed, evidence indicates that individual dysregulation in cortisol levels, either diurnal or in response to stress, across gestation can predict less favorable maternal perinatal mental health. For example, the cortisol diurnal rhythm has been found to be altered in women reporting higher than typical depressive [110, 111] and anxiety symptoms [112, 113]. Furthermore, higher morning cortisol levels in women with a comorbid diagnosis of depressive and anxiety disorder, as compared to controls, have been found [114, 115]. Initial evidence also suggests that women with a more pronounced cortisol response to psychosocial stressors may be more vulnerable to develop depressive symptoms during and after pregnancy. Urizar and colleagues [116] found increased cortisol responses to a laboratory stressor among pregnant women at high risk for depression, while Nierop and colleagues [117] reported that women with greater cortisol stress responses in midpregnancy had significantly more depressive symptoms 2 weeks after delivery.

The SNS governs rapid "fight-or-flight" responses, releasing catecholamines such as epinephrine (E) and norepinephrine (NE) during stress. During pregnancy, SNS regulation changes to accommodate increasing cardiovascular demands [118, 119]. Furthermore, SNS stress reactivity is significantly dampened [120–122] as pregnancy advances. Although a dysregulation of the SNS has been involved in depressive or anxiety disorder in nonpregnant population [123, 124], available literature during the perinatal period is limited. Higher NE and lower dopamine levels in depressed pregnant women have been found in some studies [125–127], and a lack of dampening of SNS stress reactivity was shown in anxious women [128]. Lastly, diurnal levels of salivary α-amylase (sAA), a noninvasive marker of SNS activity [129], were found to be altered in association with maternal symptoms of psychological distress [110, 130, 131].

2.4.2 Inflammatory and Monoaminergic Pathways

During pregnancy, the maternal immune system undergoes significant changes to balance the need for pathogen defense while preventing fetal rejection [132]. Pregnancy is now understood to be a period of immunomodulation with early and late pregnancy being characterized by greater inflammation or pro-inflammatory to anti-inflammatory activity (Th1 > Th2 activity), while midpregnancy is characterized by lower inflammation (Th2 > Th1 activity) (e.g., [132, 133]). Both pro-inflammatory and anti-inflammatory cytokines show mild increases during pregnancy [134, 135], while the third trimester sees attenuated pro-inflammatory cytokine responses to immune challenges, possibly to protect the fetus from excessive maternal inflammation [91, 136].

Stress has been shown to alter immune function, resulting in elevated pro-inflammatory cytokines and stronger inflammatory responses to psychological stressors and immune challenges [137, 138]. Furthermore, inflammation plays a significant role in mental health conditions, particularly major depression [139]. Depressed individuals exhibit elevated pro-inflammatory cytokines such as IL-1β, IL-6, and TNF-α, alongside increased acute-phase reactants like C-reactive protein (CRP) [140, 141], with several evidences supporting an etiopathogenetic role of inflammation in the development of depression [142–145]. Based on this, it has been proposed that pregnancy-related alterations in the immune system during the perinatal period might play a role in the development of depression during the perinatal period (e.g., [146]). However, this is still a relatively new and unexplored area of inquiry. A number of studies reported higher levels of pro-inflammatory cytokines, such as IL-1β, IL-6, TNF-α, CRP, or IFN-gamma, in depressed pregnant women regardless of gestational timing [110, 147–149]. Furthermore, Christian et al. [150] showed that depressive symptoms predict exaggerated inflammatory responses to influenza virus vaccination during pregnancy, suggesting a sensitization of the inflammatory response related to depression during the antenatal period. An elevation in pro-inflammatory cytokines was also recently reported in anxious pregnant women [148], suggesting that inflammation might be a common pathway for several conditions that affect maternal mental health.

In the last decades, tryptophan metabolism—the pathway responsible for producing the neurotransmitter serotonin—has attracted considerable attention due to its role in the onset of depression mediated by inflammation [151]. Increasing evidence suggests that depression may depend on the activation of the kynurenine pathway which reduces circulating tryptophan levels and, consequently, its availability in the brain for serotonin synthesis [152–154]. This greater degradation of tryptophan into kynurenine results from heightened inflammation which upregulates the widely distributed enzyme indoleamine 2,3-dioxygenase (IDO) and/or the stress-related activation of the HPA axis which stimulates the hepatic enzyme tryptophan 2,3-dioxygenase (TDO) [155]. Both enzymes, although through different mechanisms, convert tryptophan into kynurenine that is then transformed into downstream metabolites [156]. Growing evidence highlights that these mechanisms might be in place also during the perinatal period and be involved in perinatal depressive symptoms [151, 157]. Several studies have shown associations between increased degradation of tryptophan into kynurenine and depressive symptoms during pregnancy or postpartum [158–161]. Notably, the link between increased inflammation and activation of the kynurenine pathway has been recently demonstrated to be involved in higher depressive symptoms in late pregnancy and with their trajectory from pregnancy to 12 months postpartum in a low-risk sample [162] as well as in severe postpartum depression with suicidal thoughts [157].

2.4.3 Biochemical Factors

Several biochemical factors, including micronutrient status, lipid metabolism, and vitamin D, are thought to contribute to antenatal stress and have been extensively studied in the last years [96]. These elements interact with maternal physiology, shaping vulnerability to stress and mood disturbances during pregnancy.

Deficiencies in micronutrients have been examined for their role in maternal mental health, although evidence is inconsistent. Lower serum zinc has been linked to higher prenatal depressive symptoms [163], while no clear association exists for magnesium, iron, folate, and vitamin B12 [164–167]. A recent meta-analytical work [168] examined the association between dairy consumption and depressive symptoms or disorders and found only inconsistent or conflicting associations depending on dairy type, gender, or population group.

Vitamin D plays a role in immune function and neurosteroid activity, with lower levels being hypothesized to increase susceptibility to depression. Studies indicate a negative association between maternal vitamin D levels during pregnancy and prenatal [149, 169, 170] as well as postnatal [171, 172] depressive symptoms. Recent meta-analytical evidence [109] suggests that vitamin D supplementation can improve depressive symptoms in adults with primary depression and baseline concentrations of 25-hydroxyvitamin D (25(OH)D) levels higher than 50 nmol/L but has no effects if baseline concentrations of 25(OH)D levels are lower than this.

Lipid metabolism has also been linked to maternal mental health during pregnancy. Higher concentrations of HDL cholesterol have been associated with lower depressive symptoms during pregnancy [174]. Long-chain polyunsaturated fatty acids (LC-PUFA), particularly docosahexaenoic acid (DHA) and arachidonic acid, play crucial roles in fetal and infant development, and observational studies have suggested a potential association with maternal psychological distress during the perinatal period, such as stress and depressive or anxiety symptoms [175]. A recent meta-analysis indicates lower levels of omega-3 PUFAs and DHA in patients with perinatal depression [176]. Furthermore, DHA supplementation during pregnancy has been shown to lower perceived stress and modulate cortisol responses to stress in African American women [177]. Lastly, lower plasma total omega-3 PUFA concentrations were associated with increased anxiety symptoms during pregnancy [178]. However, other studies have not found significant benefits of DHA supplementation in preventing prenatal depressive symptoms [179], indicating that further investigation is needed to clarify the role of LC-PUFA in maternal antenatal stress.

2.4.4 Genetic and Epigenetic Pathways

As for other psychiatric symptoms, perinatal anxiety or depressive disorders are at least partially genetically determined. The largest and most comprehensive genetic epidemiological study of perinatal depression estimates heritability of perinatal depression to vary between 44% and 54% [180], with heritability of antenatal depression being at 37% and postnatal depression at 40% and the remaining variance being explained by nonshared environment. Several genetic polymorphisms—naturally occurring variations in a specific DNA sequence that can influence gene function and expression—are thought to be implicated in increasing vulnerability for the development of depressive or anxiety symptoms across the perinatal period such as the serotonin-transporter-linked polymorphic region (5-HTTLPR) [181–183], the BDNF gene Val66Met polymorphism [184, 185], the polymorphisms in estrogen receptor alpha gene [186], genetic variants in the glucocorticoid receptor (NR3C1) and corticotropin-releasing hormone receptor 1 (CRHR1) genes [187], and the polymorphisms of tryptophan hydroxylase 2 (TPH2) gene [188, 189].

Epigenetic mechanisms provide a complementary framework to understand how maternal antenatal stress can leave lasting molecular imprints on both maternal and fetal physiologies [190]. Epigenetics refers to heritable changes in gene expression that do not involve alterations in the DNA sequence, primarily mediated by mechanisms like DNA methylation, histone modification, and micro-RNA [191]. These mechanisms are highly sensitive to environmental factors, including stress, and play a role in dysregulated stress responses and immune function in mothers during pregnancy, ultimately influencing maternal health and psychological well-being [192]. DNA methylation, the most studied epigenetic mechanisms, involves the addition of a methyl group to a cytosine base within a cytosine–phosphate–guanine (CpG) sequence [193]. This modification can alter the accessibility of the gene coding region to transcriptional machinery, potentially resulting in altered gene expression. Evidence links environmental adversity to the methylation of stress-related genes, such as NR3C1 and SCL6A4, in the general population [194, 195]. Emerging research suggests that similar patterns are observed during pregnancy. For instance, Kertes and colleagues [196] found an association between chronic stress and levels of maternal NR3C1 gene methylation in a sample of women exposed to severe war-related stressors during pregnancy. Further, changes in methylation of NR3C1 gene were reported in women who were exposed to interpersonal violence [197], to racial discrimination episodes [198], and to the Tutsi genocide during pregnancy [199]. Recently, maternal exposure to the pandemic lockdown during the second and third trimesters has been linked to increased methylation of SLC6A4 and NR3C1 genes [200]. Noteworthy, increased methylation of the NR3C1 gene in cord blood mononuclear cells was associated with maternal depression and anxiety during pregnancy [201–203], whereas Devlin and colleagues [204] reported a negative association between maternal depressive symptoms in the second trimester of pregnancy and maternal methylation levels in the SLC6A4 gene. Albeit preliminary, these findings suggest that alterations in maternal epigenome during pregnancy might accompany maternal experience of stress.

In conclusion, the intricate interplay of neuroendocrine, immune, biochemical, and genetic/epigenetic pathways forms a critical biological foundation for understanding maternal stress during pregnancy. Dysregulation within these systems, often exacerbated by stress exposure, can increase vulnerability to psychological distress and adverse pregnancy outcomes. Further research into these biological mechanisms holds significant promise for identifying novel targets for early intervention and personalized support to promote maternal well-being throughout the perinatal period.

2.5 Social and Cultural Sources of Maternal Stress

The World Health Organization [205] describes social determinants of health as the conditions in which individuals are born, live, and grow, underscoring the significant influence of the surrounding environment in shaping long-term health and well-being. Social determinants include, but are not limited to, economic factors, housing security, healthcare access, and racism. In this section, we discuss several key social and cultural determinants of health that have been studied during the perinatal period. While acknowledging the existence of other relevant factors, our focus will be on a select few to illustrate how these can impact pregnancy-related outcomes, with stress often serving as an important mechanism. Given the well-established association of these factors on health and other outcomes, in the perinatal period and across generations [206], this underscores the importance of clinically assessing for these potential sources of stress and mitigating the effects with evidence-based interventions.

2.5.1 Immigration

Immigration refers broadly to the process of crossing international borders, regardless of documentation status, the voluntary or involuntary nature, the reasons for migration, or the duration of stay. The immigrant population includes a wide range of individuals—refugees, asylum seekers, undocumented migrants, and both economic and transient immigrants—who often face unique challenges when navigating new environments [207]. These challenges may be particularly acute during pregnancy and the postpartum period, given women may encounter unfamiliar healthcare systems, language barriers, and limited access to care, causing heightened maternal stress. Such conditions have been shown to increase the risk for adverse perinatal outcomes, including depression, anxiety, preterm birth, and poor maternal–infant bonding [208].

The reasons for migration are multifactorial, often reflecting a complex interplay of structural and personal forces, including political instability, economic hardship, educational opportunity, and acute crises such as war, violence, and natural disasters [209]. Understanding the intersection of migration with perinatal health is critical to addressing the needs of immigrant families and promoting equitable maternal and child health outcomes [210]. Stress related to immigration may be related to trauma of immigration itself and stressors in transition from country of origin to host country, immigration policies of the host country, and acculturation [209] and may be experienced as highly stressful during pregnancy. The term *acculturative stress* describes the reaction to adapting to a host culture (e.g., learning a new language [211]). Immigrants and later generations can experience acculturative stress which may explain some of the adverse effects seen in perinatal individuals.

Overall, studies largely show disparities in health and mental health outcomes of immigrant and native populations, particularly in pregnant patients. However, effects of immigration on health outcomes have been heterogeneous. For example, a meta-analysis involving 11,320,674 pregnant women with an immigration background and 56,102,698 pregnant women as the native-origin population [212] showed that pregnant immigrant women had a significantly higher risk to have an emergency cesarean section, shoulder dystocia, GDM, small-for-gestational-age infant, low clinical condition of the newborn after birth (5-min Apgar less than 7), and oligohydramnios, as compared to women of native origin. However, immigrant women had a lower risk of labor induction, pregnancy-induced hypertension, preeclampsia, macrosomia, and large for gestational age. Although the relationship between immigration and adverse perinatal outcomes appears heterogeneous, immigrant women are at an increased risk of some important adverse pregnancies.

Immigration policies have been shown to affect the health of immigrant women during the perinatal period [213]. For example, a study of Mexican perinatal women living on the United States–Mexican border showed that, from 2008 to 2016, women experienced more depression symptoms when anti-immigration policies were being implemented [214]. Other studies showed that implementation of such anti-immigrant policies was related to an immediate reduction in healthcare participation in immigrants [215]. Further, a systematic review demonstrated multiple adverse effects of punitive immigration policies in the United States besides impact on healthcare utilization, including impact on women's and children's health, access to mental health services, and general mental health [216].

Acculturative stress, in particular, has been associated with adverse effects among immigrant women during the perinatal period. A cross-sectional study of immigrant women of Arabic descent in the United States demonstrated a significant association between higher levels of acculturative stress and postpartum depression [217]. Similarly, a study of pregnant women of Mexican descent in the United States demonstrated that acculturative stress and perceived stress, but not acculturation, were associated with elevated depressive symptoms in pregnancy [218]. This study suggests that acculturative stress, rather than acculturation itself, may be linked to maternal mental health. Another study, a 5-year longitudinal investigation involving Mexican-origin families with pregnant adolescent mothers, explored the relationship between acculturative stress and various family health outcomes [219]. Higher levels of cumulative family discrimination and acculturation-related stress, experienced from pregnancy through the first 2 years postpartum, were associated with increased depressive symptoms in adolescent mothers and more disrupted maternal–child interaction at ages 2 and 3. In turn, maternal depressive symptoms were associated with greater behavioral and emotional difficulties in children at 60 months. Furthermore, higher acculturative stress was associated with poor academic performance.

2.5.2 Racism

Racism has been defined as a set of practices or systems that perpetuate or worsen inequities in power, access to resources, and opportunities among different racial, ethnic, cultural, or religious groups [220]. Multiple types of racism exist, including structural, personally mediated or discrimination, and internalized [221]. Discrimination and racism are pervasive sources of maternal stress, particularly for Black, Indigenous, and people of color. As aforementioned, immigration can also be associated with discrimination and other forms of racism. Several studies have demonstrated an association between various forms of racism and adverse health outcomes, highlighting the need to address this social determinant. Proposed mechanisms for these effects include the impact of racism on stress-related biological pathways and allostatic load [222].

Epidemiological studies suggest disparities in pregnancy outcomes across various racial/ethnic groups. For example, in the United States, Black women and American Indian/Alaska Native women have, respectively, 3.3 and 2.5 times the rate of mortality, compared to non-Hispanic White women [223]. A systematic review examining the association between maternal experiences of discrimination and birth outcomes demonstrated that higher interpersonal discrimination was associated with adverse birth outcomes such as preterm birth, low birth weight, and increased stress markers during pregnancy and postpartum for both women and children [224]. Associations varied by type of discrimination experience, timing, frequency, and pervasiveness. A cross-sectional study involving Black and White, non-Latino, US-born postpartum women suggests that chronic worry about racial discrimination was associated with preterm birth among Black women before and after adjustment of covariates [225]. This indicates that worry associated with discrimination may contribute to some of the observed racial/ethnic disparities in obstetric outcomes. Qualitative studies also suggest discrimination in the healthcare settings. For example, Hoang et al. [226] conducted focus groups interviewing perinatal Black, Indigenous, and other people of color (BIPOC) about their experiences in healthcare interactions. The women described experiencing racial trauma during healthcare encounters, including witnessing and personally encountering anti-Black bias, having their pain dismissed and care withheld, and facing race-based mistreatment such as a persistent lack of bodily autonomy. Other data [227] found strong associations between lifetime and past experience of ethnically motivated interpersonal attacks and unfair treatment on mother's mental health in Māori, Pacific, and Asian women. Women who experienced unfair treatment by a health professional in their lifetime were 66% more likely to suffer from postnatal depression. This study found that maternal mental health was significantly poorer when both the mother and her partner had experienced ethnically motivated personal attacks, indicating a cumulative effect of shared racial discrimination.

2.5.3 Other Social Determinants of Health

While fewer studies exist on other social determinants of health in pregnancy and postpartum outcomes, such as housing instability, food insecurity, and poverty, available findings do suggest adverse effects. Housing instability has been consistently linked to adverse perinatal outcomes, including increased maternal stress, poor mental health, and higher risk of pregnancy complications [228]. A retrospective pregnancy cohort study showed that structural factors, such as residential redlining and segregation in housing, were associated with self-reported stress during pregnancy [229]. Beyond financial insecurity, housing instability can also lead to frequent relocations, overcrowding, and substandard living conditions, further exacerbating psychological distress particularly among vulnerable populations such as pregnant women.

Healthcare access is a critical determinant of maternal outcomes, yet systemic barriers prevent many women from receiving adequate care. Financial constraints, insurance coverage gaps, and discriminatory practices disproportionately affect BIPOC and low-income women. During the COVID-19 pandemic, structural determinants of health such as financial insecurity and lack of health insurance were associated with earlier births and heightened maternal stress [230]. In a longitudinal pregnancy cohort study during the COVID-19 pandemic, it was shown that prenatal maternal stress, related and unrelated to the pandemic, partially mediated the relationship between social determinant of health (i.e., race/ethnicity, education, financial security, health insurance, relationship status, and lifetime abuse) and lower gestational age, highlighting the compounded effects of systemic inequities.

2.6 Clinical Implications

Given the growing evidence demonstrating the significant effects of maternal stress during the preconception and perinatal period on mother–infant morbidity and mortality, it is critical to consider the clinical implications of these data. As discussed in this chapter, maternal stress originates from a multitude of interconnected stress sources, including psychological and psychiatric factors, obstetric complications, social and cultural influences, and biological vulnerabilities. These clinical considerations therefore necessitate a comprehensive approach that addresses this multifaceted nature of maternal perinatal stress and promotes the sensitization of professionals regarding the relevance of such stress conditions for the physical and mental health of pregnant women. First of all, comprehensive routine screening for maternal present stress conditions—including life event and daily stressors, social living conditions, and related discrimination—along with the identification of perinatal physical and mental health issues, is essential to obtain a holistic view of the pregnant woman's needs and ensure appropriate care. Such assessment facilitates the early identification of pregnant women at potentially higher risk for developing both obstetric and psychiatric complications. Ideally, early identification should start in the preconception period to optimize maternal physical and mental health prior to pregnancy and postpartum. However, the assessment of potential stressors and risk factors for women's health needs to be prioritized early during routine obstetric care and continue throughout the postpartum period in order to identify possible mitigating factors during different stages of pregnancy. This will also allow to connect pregnant women to relevant resources and interventions tailored to the specific sources of their stress condition. Screening for maternal mental distress and potential stressors may require the development of clinical protocols to ensure early referral to psychosocial services for perinatal care whenever needed. Additionally, providing structured support to address unmet social needs, such as connection to social services, case management, and peer support networks, may facilitate early mitigation of the effects of maternal stress during pregnancy. Although some stressors may not be modifiable, the individual response to those stressors can often be influenced through psychoeducation, stress reduction strategies, and activation of resources, which could be a core component of prenatal care and need to be considered as a public health strategy. To achieve this, it will be critical to build the capacity of healthcare providers to understand and address the effects of various stressors on perinatal morbidity and mortality.

2.7 Conclusions

Maternal stress during pregnancy is shaped by a complex interplay of psychological, obstetrical, biological, and social factors, each of which can significantly impact both maternal well-being and fetal development. Throughout this chapter, we examined how mental health conditions, pregnancy-related complications, and broader social determinants contribute to maternal stress, highlighting its pervasive and multifaceted nature. Additionally, biological mechanisms, including neuroendocrine, inflammatory, biochemical, and epigenetic pathways, further illustrate how stress influences maternal psychological well-being, with potential long-term implications for both maternal and infant physical and mental health. Despite advancements in understanding the determinants of perinatal stress, important questions remain concerning the timing and intensity of stress exposures, as well as the potential buffering effects of protective factors such as social support, resilience, and adequate access to prenatal care. While research has established clear links between maternal stress and adverse outcomes, further studies are needed to elucidate the specific mechanisms through which stress exerts its effects at different stages of pregnancy and to understand the potential accumulation effect of different maternal stress conditions.

Given the widespread impact of maternal stress, it is crucial to identify at-risk populations and implement targeted interventions that address both psychological and structural stressors. Enhancing access to mental health resources, improving healthcare equity, and fostering supportive social environments can help mitigate the negative effects of perinatal stress. Future research should also explore individualized approaches to stress reduction, incorporating biopsychosocial frameworks to better understand the interplay of risk and resilience factors. By acknowledging and addressing the diverse sources of maternal stress and fostering a distinct sensitization among professionals regarding its relevance, we can work toward improving pregnancy outcomes and promoting the long-term well-being of both mothers and their children.

References

1. DiPietro JA. Maternal stress in pregnancy: considerations for fetal development. J Adolesc Health. 2012;51(2):S3–8.
2. González-Ochoa R, Sánchez-Rodríguez EN, Chavarría A, Gutiérrez-Ospina G, Romo-González T. Evaluating stress during pregnancy: do we have the right conceptions and the correct tools to assess it? J Pregnancy. 2018;2018(1):4857065.
3. Glover V, Ahmed-Salim Y, Capron L. Maternal anxiety, depression, and stress during pregnancy: effects on the fetus and the child, and underlying mechanisms. In: Fetal development: research on brain and behavior, environmental influences, and emerging technologies. Cham: Springer International Publishing; 2016. p. 213–27.
4. Sosnowski DW, Booth C, York TP, Amstadter AB, Kliewer W. Maternal prenatal stress and infant DNA methylation: a systematic review. Dev Psychol. 2017;60:127–39.
5. Cardwell MS. Stress: pregnancy considerations. Obstet Gynecol Surv. 2013;68(2):119–29.
6. Pearlin L, Schieman S, Fazio E, Meersman S. Stress, health, and the life course: some conceptual perspectives. J Health Soc Behav. 2005;46:205–19.
7. Andersson L, Sundstrom-Poromaa I, Wulff M, Astrom M, Bixo M. Depression and anxiety during pregnancy and 6 months postpartum: a follow-up study. Acta Obstet Gynecol Scand. 2006;85(8):937–44.
8. Keenan K, Hipwell AE, Class QA, Mbayiwa K. Extending the developmental origins of disease model: impact of preconception stress exposure on offspring neurodevelopment. Dev Psychobiol. 2018;60(7):753–64.
9. Racine N, Devereaux C, Cooke JE, Eirich R, Zhu J, Madigan S. Adverse childhood experiences and maternal anxiety and depression: a meta-analysis. BMC Psychiatry. 2021;21:1–10.
10. Torche F. The effect of maternal stress on birth outcomes: exploiting a natural experiment. Demography. 2011;48:1473–91.
11. Mancuso RA, Schetter CD, Rini CM, Roesch SC, Hobel CJ. Maternal prenatal anxiety and corticotropin-releasing hormone associated with timing of delivery. Psychosom Med. 2004;66(5):762–9.
12. Wadhwa PD, Porto M, Garite TJ, Chicz-DeMet A, Sandman CA. Maternal corticotropin-releasing hormone levels in the early third trimester predict length of gestation in human pregnancy. Am J Obstet Gynecol. 1998;179(4):1079–85.
13. DeSocio JE. Epigenetics, maternal prenatal psychosocial stress, and infant mental health. Arch Psychiatr Nurs. 2018;32(6):901–6.
14. Glover V, O'Donnell KJ, O'Connor TG, Fisher J. Prenatal maternal stress, fetal programming, and mechanisms underlying later psychopathology—a global perspective. Dev Psychopathol. 2018;30(3):843–54.
15. Rodríguez-Soto NC, Buxó CJ, Morou-Bermudez E, Pérez-Edgar K, Ocasio-Quiñones IT, Surillo-González MB, Martinez KG. The impact of prenatal maternal stress due to potentially traumatic events on child temperament: a systematic review. Dev Psychobiol. 2021;63(7):e22195.

16. Veru F, Laplante DP, Luheshi G, King S. Prenatal maternal stress exposure and immune function in the offspring. Stress. 2014;17(2):133–48.
17. Dancause KN, Laplante DP, Oremus C, Fraser S, Brunet A, King S. Disaster-related prenatal maternal stress influences birth outcomes: project ice storm. Early Hum Dev. 2011;87(12):813–20.
18. Burns ER, Farr SL, Howards PP, Centers for Disease Control and Prevention (CDC). Stressful life events experienced by women in the year before their infants' births—United States, 2000–2010. MMWR Morb Mortal Wkly Rep. 2015;64(9):247–51.
19. Mukherjee S, Coxe S, Fennie K, Madhivanan P, Trepka MJ. Stressful life event experiences of pregnant women in the United States: a latent class analysis. Womens Health Issues. 2017;27(1):83–92.
20. Kingsbury M, Weeks M, MacKinnon N, Evans J, Mahedy L, Dykxhoorn J, Colman I. Stressful life events during pregnancy and offspring depression: evidence from a prospective cohort study. J Am Acad Child Adolesc Psychiatry. 2016;55(8):709–16.
21. Hill A, Pallitto C, McCleary-Sills J, Garcia-Moreno C. A systematic review and meta-analysis of intimate partner violence during pregnancy and selected birth outcomes. Int J Gynecol Obstet. 2016;133(3):269–76.
22. Shah PS, Shah J. Maternal exposure to domestic violence and pregnancy and birth outcomes: a systematic review and meta-analyses. J Women's Health. 2010;19(11):2017–31.
23. Crossland AE, Munns L, Kirk E, Preston CEJ. Comparing body image dissatisfaction between pregnant women and non-pregnant women: a systematic review and meta-analysis. BMC Pregnancy Childbirth. 2023;23(1):709.
24. Moulds ML, Bisby MA, Black MJ, Jones K, Harrison V, Hirsch CR, Newby JM. Repetitive negative thinking in the perinatal period and its relationship with anxiety and depression. J Affect Disord. 2022;311:446–62.
25. Viswasam K, Eslick GD, Starcevic V. Prevalence, onset and course of anxiety disorders during pregnancy: a systematic review and meta analysis. J Affect Disord. 2019;255:27–40.
26. Martini J, Petzoldt J, Einsle F, Beesdo-Baum K, Höfler M, Wittchen HU. Risk factors and course patterns of anxiety and depressive disorders during pregnancy and after delivery: a prospective-longitudinal study. J Affect Disord. 2015;175:385–95.
27. Yin X, Sun N, Jiang N, Xu X, Gan Y, Zhang J, et al. Prevalence and associated factors of antenatal depression: systematic reviews and meta-analyses. Clin Psychol Rev. 2021;83:101932.
28. Antoniou E, Stamoulou P, Tzanoulinou MD, Orovou E. Perinatal mental health; the role and the effect of the partner: a systematic review. Healthcare (Basel). 2021;9(11):1572. https://doi.org/10.3390/healthcare9111572.
29. Pugliese V, Bruni A, Carbone EA, Calabrò G, Cerminara G, Sampogna G, Luciano M, Steardo L Jr, Fiorillo A, Garcia CS, De Fazio P. Maternal stress, prenatal medical illnesses and obstetric complications: risk factors for schizophrenia spectrum disorder, bipolar disorder and major depressive disorder. Psychiatry Res. 2019;271:23–30.
30. Kanaka-Gantenbein C, Mastorakos G, Chrousos GP. Endocrine-related causes and consequences of intrauterine growth retardation. Ann N Y Acad Sci. 2003;997(1):150–7.
31. Vandenbosche RC. Intrauterine growth retardation. Am Fam Physician. 1998;58:1384–92.
32. Rondó PH, Ferreira RF, Nogueira F, Ribeiro MC, Lobert H, Artes R. Maternal psychological stress and distress as predictors of low birth weight, prematurity and intrauterine growth retardation. Eur J Clin Nutr. 2003;57(2):266–72.
33. Omer H. Possible psychophysiologic mechanisms in premature labor. Psychosomatics. 1986;27:580–4.
34. Geva R, Eshel R, Leitner Y, Fattal-Valevski A, Harel S. Prenatal diagnosis and management of intrauterine growth restriction: a long-term prospective study on outcome and maternal stress. Infant Mental Health Journal: Official Publication of The World Association for Infant Mental Health. 2005;26(5):481–97.
35. Tsakiridis I, Dagklis T, Zerva C, Mamopoulos A, Athanasiadis A, Papazisis G. Depression in pregnant women hospitalized due to intrauterine growth restriction: prevalence and associated factors. Midwifery. 2019;70:71–5.

36. Lewis AJ, Austin E, Galbally M. Prenatal maternal mental health and fetal growth restriction: a systematic review. J Dev Orig Health Dis. 2016;7(4):416–28.
37. American Diabetes Association. 2. Classification and diagnosis of diabetes. Diabetes Care. 2015;38(Supplement_1):S8–S16.
38. Guariguata L, Linnenkamp U, Beagley J, Whiting DR, Cho NH. Global estimates of the prevalence of hyperglycaemia in pregnancy. Diabetes Res Clin Pract. 2014;103(2):176–85.
39. Atlas D. International diabetes federation. idf diabetes atlas. Brussels: 9th edn; 2019.
40. Johns EC, Denison FC, Norman JE, Reynolds RM. Gestational diabetes mellitus: mechanisms, treatment, and complications. Trends Endocrinol Metab. 2018;29:743–54.
41. Mishra S, Shetty A, Rao CR, Nayak S, Kamath A. Effect of maternal perceived stress during pregnancy on gestational diabetes mellitus risk: a prospective case-control study. Diabetes Metab Syndr Clin Res Rev. 2020;14(5):1163–9.
42. Kim C, Vahratian A. Self-rated health and health care use among women with histories of gestational diabetes mellitus. Diabetes Care. 2010;33(1):41–2.
43. Hui AL, Sevenhuysen G, Harvey D, Salamon E. Stress and anxiety in women with gestational diabetes during dietary management. Diabetes Educ. 2014;40(5):668–77.
44. Silveira ML, Whitcomb BW, Pekow P, Braun B, Markenson G, Dole N, et al. Perceived psychosocial stress and glucose intolerance among pregnant Hispanic women. Diabetes Metab. 2014;40(6):466–75.
45. Chasan-Taber L. Lifestyle interventions to reduce risk of diabetes among high-risk pregnant and postpartum women. In: Textbook of diabetes and pregnancy. Boca Raton: CRC Press; 2018. p. 415–24.
46. Daniells S, Grenyer BF, Davis WS, Coleman KJ, Burgess JAP, Moses RG. Gestational diabetes mellitus: is a diagnosis associated with an increase in maternal anxiety and stress in the short and intermediate term? Diabetes Care. 2003;26(2):385–9.
47. Langer N, Langer O. Emotional adjustment to diagnosis and intensified treatment of gestational diabetes. Obstet Gynecol. 1994;84(3):329–34.
48. Feng Y, Feng Q, Qu H, et al. Stress adaptation is associated with insulin resistance in women with gestational diabetes mellitus. Nutr Diabetes. 2020;10:4.
49. WHO. Congenital anomalies [internet]. Geneva: WHO; 2016. https://www.who.int/news-room/fact-sheets/detail/congenital-anomalies
50. National Health Service (NHS). Fetal anomaly screening programme standards 2015–16. Lewes: Crown; 2015.
51. Irving C, Richmond S, Wren C, Longster C, Embleton ND. Changes in fetal prevalence and outcome for trisomies 13 and 18: a population-based study over 23 years. J Matern Fetal Neonatal Med. 2011;24(1):137–41.
52. Dolk H, Loane M, Garne E. The prevalence of congenital anomalies in Europe. In: de la Paz MP, Groft SC, editors. Rare diseases epidemiology [web]. Dordrecht: Springer; 2010. p. 349–64. (Advances in experimental medicine and biology; bd. 686).
53. Fonseca A, Nazaré B, Canavarro MC. Parental psychological distress and confidence after an infant's birth: the role of attachment representations in parents of infants with congenital anomalies and parents of healthy infants. J Clin Psychol Med Settings. 2013;20:143–55.
54. Fleming V, Iljuschin I, Pehlke-Milde J, Maurer F, Parpan F. Dying at life′ s beginning: experiences of parents and health professionals in Switzerland when an 'in utero' diagnosis incompatible with life is made. Midwifery. 2016;34:23–9.
55. Kaydırak MM, Balkan E, Bacak N, Kızoglu F. Perceived social support and depression, anxiety and stress in pregnant women diagnosed with foetal anomaly. J Adv Nurs. 2025;81(8):4591–9.
56. Titapant V, Chuenwattana P. Psychological effects of fetal diagnoses of non-lethal congenital anomalies on the experience of pregnant women during the remainder of their pregnancy. J Obstet Gynaecol Res. 2015;41(1):77–83.
57. Nes RB, Røysamb E, Hauge LJ, Kornstad T, Landolt MA, Irgens LM, et al. Adaptation to the birth of a child with a congenital anomaly: a prospective longitudinal study of maternal Well-being and psychological distress. Dev Psychol. 2014;50(6):1827.

58. Aite L, Zaccara A, Trucchi A, Brizzi C, Nahom A, Iacobelli B, et al. When uncertainty generates more anxiety than severity: the prenatal experience with cystic adenomatoid malformation of the lung. J Perinat Med. 2009;37(5):539–42.
59. Bekkhus M, Oftedal A, Braithwaite E, Haugen G, Kaasen A. Paternal psychological stress after detection of fetal anomaly during pregnancy. A prospective longitudinal observational study. Front Psychol. 2020;11:1848.
60. Wu Y, Kapse K, Jacobs M, Niforatos-Andescavage N, Donofrio MT, Krishnan A, et al. Association of maternal psychological distress with in utero brain development in fetuses with congenital heart disease. JAMA Pediatr. 2020; 174(3):e195316.
61. Rey-Bellet C, Hohlfeld J. Prenatal diagnosis of facial clefts: evaluation of a specialised counseling. Swiss Med Wkly. 2004;134:640–4.
62. Oftedal A, Bekkhus M, Haugen GN, Czajkowski NO, Kaasen A. The impact of diagnosed fetal anomaly, diagnostic severity and prognostic ambiguity on parental depression and traumatic stress: a prospective longitudinal cohort study. Acta Obstet Gynecol Scand. 2022;101(11):1291–9.
63. Timmer-Murillo SC, Mowrer A, Wang AZ, Jazinski-Chambers K, Piña I, Rundell MR, et al. Examining emotion regulation and inflammation as predictors of maternal mental health after fetal anomaly diagnosis. Brain Behav Immun. 2024;122:1–8.
64. Hansen K, Kukora SK, Sherman A, Feldman K. Mental health in pregnancy complicated by fetal anomaly: depression screening and referrals in a single fetal care center. J Perinatol. 2025;45(6):726–31.
65. Beauquier-Maccotta B, Chalouhi GE, Picquet AL, Carrier A, Bussières L, Golse B, Ville Y. Impact of monochorionicity and twin to twin transfusion syndrome on prenatal attachment, post traumatic stress disorder, anxiety and depressive symptoms. PLoS One. 2016;11(1):e0145649.
66. Mangin-Heimos KS, Strube M, Taylor K, Galbraith K, O'Brien E, Rogers C, et al. Trajectories of maternal and paternal psychological distress after fetal diagnosis of moderate–severe congenital heart disease. J Pediatr Psychol. 2023;48(4):305–16.
67. Menon R, Richardson LS. Preterm prelabor rupture of the membranes: a disease of the fetal membranes. In: Seminars in perinatology, vol. 41(No. 7). Philadelphia: WB Saunders; 2017. p. 409–19.
68. Thomson AJ. Care of women presenting with suspected preterm prelabour rupture of membranes from 24+ 0 weeks of gestation: Green-top Guideline No. 73. BJOG Int J Obstet Gynaecol. 2019;126(9):e152–66.
69. Zemtsov GE, Avram CM, Darling A, Dillon J, Wheeler S, Dotters-Katz SK. Incidence and risk factors for postpartum depression among women with preterm prelabor rupture of membranes. Am J Perinatol. 2022;39(08):797–802.
70. Challacombe FL, Suchomelova Z, Zampieri C, Hall M, Curran C, Shennan A, Story L. Preterm premature rupture of the membranes (PPROM): a study of patient experiences and support needs. J Reprod Infant Psychol. 2025;43(4):926–43.
71. Zhang S, Ding Z, Liu H, Chen Z, Wu J, Zhang Y, Yu Y. Association between mental stress and gestational hypertension/preeclampsia: a meta-analysis. Obstet Gynecol Surv. 2013;68(12):825–34.
72. Yu Y, Zhang S, Wang G, Hong X, Mallow EB, Walker SO, et al. The combined association of psychosocial stress and chronic hypertension with preeclampsia. Am J Obstet Gynecol. 2013;209(5):438-e1–438.e12.
73. Sibai B, Dekker G, Kupferminc M. Pre-eclampsia. Lancet. 2005;365(9461):785–99.
74. László KD, Liu XQ, Svensson T, Wikström AK, Li J, Olsen J, et al. Psychosocial stress related to the loss of a close relative the year before or during pregnancy and risk of preeclampsia. Hypertension. 2013;62(1):183–9.
75. Coussons-Read ME, Lobel M, Carey JC, Kreither MO, D'Anna K, Argys L, et al. The occurrence of preterm delivery is linked to pregnancy-specific distress and elevated inflammatory markers across gestation. Brain Behav Immun. 2012;26(4):650–9.

76. von Känel R, Mills PJ, Fainman C, Dimsdale JE. Effects of psychological stress and psychiatric disorders on blood coagulation and fibrinolysis: a biobehavioral pathway to coronary artery disease? Biopsychosoc Sci Med. 2001;63(4):531–44.
77. Greenwood JP, Stoker JB, Walker JJ, Mary DA. Sympathetic nerve discharge in normal pregnancy and pregnancy-induced hypertension. J Hypertens. 1998;16(5):617–24.
78. Rang S, Wolf H, Montfrans GA, Karemaker JM. Serial assessment of cardiovascular control shows early signs of developing pre-eclampsia. J Hypertens. 2004;22(2):369–76.
79. Shamsi U, Hatcher J, Shamsi A, Zuberi N, Qadri Z, Saleem S. A multicentre matched case control study of risk factors for preeclampsia in healthy women in Pakistan. BMC Womens Health. 2010;10:1–7.
80. Andersson L, Sundstrom-Poromaa I, Wulff M, et al. Implications of antenatal depression and anxiety for obstetric outcome. Obstet Gynecol. 2004;104:467Y476.
81. Vollebregt KC, Van Der Wal MF, Wolf H, Vrijkotte TG, Boer K, Bonsel GJ. Is psychosocial stress in first ongoing pregnancies associated with pre-eclampsia and gestational hypertension? BJOG Int J Obstet Gynaecol. 2008;115(5):607–15.
82. Schneider S, Freerksen N, Maul H, et al. Risk groups and maternal-neonatal complications of preeclampsia: current results from the national German perinatal quality registry. J Perinat Med. 2011;39:257Y265.
83. Kurki T, Hiilesmaa V, Raitasalo R, Mattila H, Ylikorkala O. Depression and anxiety in early pregnancy and risk for preeclampsia. Obstet Gynecol. 2000;95(4):487–90.
84. Qiu C, Williams MA, Calderon-Margalit R, Cripe SM, Sorensen TK. Preeclampsia risk in relation to maternal mood and anxiety disorders diagnosed before or during early pregnancy. Am J Hypertens. 2009;22(4):397–402.
85. Gaugler-Senden IP, Duivenvoorden HJ, Filius A, De Groot CJ, Steegers EA, Passchier J. Maternal psychosocial outcome after early onset preeclampsia and preterm birth. J Matern Fetal Neonatal Med. 2012;25(3):272–6.
86. Postma IR, Bouma A, De Groot JC, Aukes AM, Aarnoudse JG, Zeeman GG. Cerebral white matter lesions, subjective cognitive failures, and objective neurocognitive functioning: a follow-up study in women after hypertensive disorders of pregnancy. J Clin Exp Neuropsychol. 2016;38(5):585–98.
87. Caropreso L, de Azevedo Cardoso T, Eltayebani M, Frey BN. Preeclampsia as a risk factor for postpartum depression and psychosis: a systematic review and meta-analysis. Arch Womens Ment Health. 2020;23:493–505.
88. Cetin O, Guzel Ozdemir P, Kurdoglu Z, Sahin HG. Investigation of maternal psychopathological symptoms, dream anxiety and insomnia in preeclampsia. J Matern Fetal Neonatal Med. 2017;30(20):2510–5.
89. Porcel J, Feigal C, Poye L, Postma IR, Zeeman GG, Olowoyeye A, et al. Hypertensive disorders of pregnancy and risk of screening positive for posttraumatic stress disorder: a cross-sectional study. Pregnancy Hypertens. 2013;3(4):254–60.
90. Abedian Z, Soltani N, Mokhber N, Esmaily H. Depression and anxiety in pregnancy and postpartum in women with mild and severe preeclampsia. Iran J Nurs Midwifery Res. 2015;20(4):454–9.
91. Christian LM. Psychoneuroimmunology in pregnancy: immune pathways linking stress with maternal health, adverse birth outcomes and fetal development. Neurosci Biobehav Rev. 2012;36(1):350–61. https://doi.org/10.1016/j.pestbp.2011.02.012.
92. Sherer ML, Posillico CK, Schwarz JM. An examination of changes in maternal neuroimmune function during pregnancy and the postpartum period. Brain Behav Immun. 2017;66:201–9. https://doi.org/10.1016/j.bbi.2017.06.016.
93. Gold PW, Chrousos GP. Organization of the stress system and its dysregulation in melancholic and atypical depression: high vs low CRH/NE states. Mol Psychiatry. 2002;7(3):254.
94. Kammerer M, Taylor A, Glover V. The HPA axis and perinatal depression: a hypothesis. Arch Womens Ment Health. 2006;9(4):187–96. https://doi.org/10.1007/s00737-006-0131-2.
95. Osborne LM, Monk C. Perinatal depression—the fourth inflammatory morbidity of pregnancy?: theory and literature review. Psychoneuroendocrinology. 2013;38(10):1929–52. https://doi.org/10.1016/j.psyneuen.2013.03.019.

96. Serati M, Redaelli M, Buoli M, Altamura AC. Perinatal major depression biomarkers: a systematic review. J Affect Disord. 2016;193:391–404. https://doi.org/10.1016/j.jad.2016.01.027.
97. de Kloet E, Ron O, M. S., & Joëls, M. Stress and cognition: are corticosteroids good or bad guys? Trends Neurosci. 1999;22(10):422–6.
98. de Kloet E, Ronald. Brain corticosteroid receptor balance and homeostatic control. Front Neuroendocrinol. 1991;12:95–164.
99. Joëls M, Baram TZ. The neuro-symphony of stress. Nat Rev Neurosci. 2009;10(6):459.
100. Mastorakos G, Ilias I. Maternal and fetal hypothalamic-pituitary-adrenal axes during pregnancy and postpartum. Ann N Y Acad Sci. 2003;997:136–49. https://doi.org/10.1196/annals.1290.016.
101. O'Keane V, Lightman S, Marsh M, Pawlby S, Papadopoulos AS, Taylor A, Moore R, Patrick K. Increased pituitary-adrenal activation and shortened gestation in a sample of depressed pregnant women: a pilot study. J Affect Disord. 2011;130(1–2):300–5. https://doi.org/10.1016/j.jad.2010.10.004.
102. Chandna AR, Kuhlmann N, Bryce CA, Greba Q, Campanucci VA, Howland JG. Chronic maternal hyperglycemia induced during mid-pregnancy in rats increases RAGE expression, augments hippocampal excitability, and alters behavior of the offspring. Neuroscience. 2015;303:241–60. https://doi.org/10.1016/j.neuroscience.2015.06.063.
103. Lindsay JR, Nieman LK. The hypothalamic-pituitary-adrenal axis in pregnancy: challenges in disease detection and treatment. Endocr Rev. 2005;26(6):775–99.
104. Hellgren C, Åkerud H, Skalkidou A, Sundström-Poromaa I. Cortisol awakening response in late pregnancy in women with previous or ongoing depression. Psychoneuroendocrinology. 2013;38(12):3150–4. https://doi.org/10.1016/j.psyneuen.2013.08.007.
105. Kivlighan KT, DiPietro JA, Costigan KA, Laudenslager ML. Diurnal rhythm of cortisol during late pregnancy: associations with maternal psychological well-being and fetal growth. Psychoneuroendocrinology. 2008;33(9):1225–35. https://doi.org/10.1016/j.psyneuen.2008.06.008.
106. De Weerth C, Buitelaar JK. Physiological stress reactivity in human pregnancy—a review. Neurosci Biobehav Rev. 2005;29(2):295–312. https://doi.org/10.1016/j.neubiorev.2004.10.005.
107. Kammerer M, Adams D, von Castelberg Bv B, Glover V. Pregnant women become insensitive to cold stress. BMC Pregnancy Childbirth. 2002;2(1):8. https://doi.org/10.1186/1471-2393-2-8.
108. Baumeister D, Lightman SL, Pariante CM. The interface of stress and the HPA axis in behavioural phenotypes of mental illness. In: Behavioral neurobiology of stress-related disorders. Berlin: Springer; 2014. p. 13–24.
109. Glynn LM, Davis EP, Sandman CA. New insights into the role of perinatal HPA-axis dysregulation in postpartum depression. Neuropeptides. 2013;47(6):363–70. https://doi.org/10.1016/j.npep.2013.10.007.
110. Nazzari S, Fearon P, Rice F, Ciceri F, Molteni M, Frigerio A. The biological underpinnings of perinatal depressive symptoms: a multi-systems approach. J Affect Disord. 2020a;274(May):1004–12. https://doi.org/10.1016/j.jad.2020.05.023.
111. O'Connor TG, Tang W, Gilchrist MA, Moynihan JA, Pressman EK, Blackmore ER. Diurnal cortisol patterns and psychiatric symptoms in pregnancy: short-term longitudinal study. Biol Psychol. 2014;96(1):35–41. https://doi.org/10.1016/j.biopsycho.2013.11.002.
112. Van Den Heuvel MI, Van Assen MALM, Glover V, Claes S, Van Den Bergh BRH. Associations between maternal psychological distress and salivary cortisol during pregnancy : a mixed-models approach. Psychoneuroendocrinology. 2018;96(May):52–60. https://doi.org/10.1016/j.psyneuen.2018.06.005.
113. Kane HS, Dunkel Schetter C, Glynn LM, Hobel CJ, Sandman CA. Pregnancy anxiety and prenatal cortisol trajectories. Biol Psychol. 2014;100(1):13–9. https://doi.org/10.1016/j.biopsycho.2014.04.003.
114. Evans LM, Myers MM, Monk C. Pregnant women's cortisol is elevated with anxiety and depression — but only when comorbid. Arch Womens Ment Health. 2008;11(3):239–48. https://doi.org/10.1007/s00737-008-0019-4.Pregnant.

115. Monk C, Fifer WP, Myers MM, Bagiella E, Duong JK, Chen IS, Leotti L, Altincatal A. Effects of maternal breathing rate, psychiatric status, and cortisol on fetal heart rate. Dev Psychobiol. 2011;53(3):221–33. https://doi.org/10.1002/dev.20513.
116. Urizar GG Jr, Yim IS, Kofman YB, Tilka N, Miller K, Freche R, Johnson A. Ethnic differences in stress-induced cortisol responses: increased risk for depression during pregnancy. Biol Psychol. 2019;147:107630.
117. Nierop A, Bratsikas A, Klinkenberg A, Nater UM, Zimmermann R, Ehlert U. Prolonged salivary cortisol recovery in second-trimester pregnant women and attenuated salivary α-amylase responses to psychosocial stress in human pregnancy. J Clin Endocrinol Metab. 2006a;91(4):1329–35. https://doi.org/10.1210/jc.2005-1816.
118. DiPietro JA, Costigan KA, Gurewitsch ED. Maternal psychophysiological change during the second half of gestation. Biol Psychol. 2005;69(1 SPEC. ISS):23–38. https://doi.org/10.1016/j.biopsycho.2004.11.003.
119. Silversides CK, Colman JM. Physiological changes in pregnancy. Heart Dis Pregnancy. 2007;2:6–17.
120. Entringer S, Buss C, Shirtcliff EA, Cammack AL, Yim IS, Chicz-DeMet A, Sandman CA, Wadhwa PD. Attenuation of maternal psychophysiological stress responses and the maternal cortisol awakening response over the course of human pregnancy. Stress. 2010;13(3):258–68.
121. Klinkenberg AV, Nater UM, Nierop A, Bratsikas A, Zimmermann R, Ehlert U. Heart rate variability changes in pregnant and non-pregnant women during standardized psychosocial stress 1. Acta Obstet Gynecol Scand. 2009;88(1):77–82.
122. Nierop A, Bratsikas A, Zimmermann R, Ehlert U. Are stress-induced cortisol changes during pregnancy associated with postpartum depressive symptoms? Psychosom Med. 2006b;68(6):931–7. https://doi.org/10.1097/01.psy.0000244385.93141.3b.
123. Moret C, Briley M. The importance of norepinephrine in depression. Neuropsychiatr Dis Treat. 2011;7(SUPPL):9–13. https://doi.org/10.2147/NDT.S19619.
124. Schumann A, Andrack C, Bär KJ. Differences of sympathetic and parasympathetic modulation in major depression. Prog Neuro-Psychopharmacol Biol Psychiatry. 2017;79(July):324–31. https://doi.org/10.1016/j.pnpbp.2017.07.009.
125. Diego MA, Jones NA, Field T, Hernandez-Reif M, Schanberg S, Kuhn C, Gonzalez-Garcia A. Maternal psychological distress, prenatal cortisol, and fetal weight. Psychosom Med. 2006;68(5):747–53. https://doi.org/10.1097/01.psy.0000238212.21598.7b.
126. Field T, Diego M, Hernandez-Reif M. Prenatal depression effects on the fetus and newborn. Infant Behav Dev. 2004;29(3):445–55. https://doi.org/10.1016/j.infbeh.2006.03.003.
127. Lundy BL, Jones NA, Field T, Nearing G, Davalos M, Pietro P, Schanberg S, Kuhn C. Prepartum depression effects on neonates. Infant Behav Dev. 1999;22(1):121–37. https://doi.org/10.1016/S0163-6383(99)80009-5.
128. Braeken MAKA, Jones A, Otte RA, Widjaja D, Van Huffel S, Monsieur GJYJ, van Oirschot CM, Van den Bergh BRH. Anxious women do not show the expected decrease in cardiovascular stress responsiveness as pregnancy advances. Biol Psychol. 2015;111:83–9. https://doi.org/10.1016/j.biopsycho.2015.08.007.
129. Nater UM, Rohleder N. Salivary alpha-amylase as a non-invasive biomarker for the sympathetic nervous system: current state of research. Psychoneuroendocrinology. 2009;34(4):486–96. https://doi.org/10.1016/j.psyneuen.2009.01.014.
130. Braithwaite EC, Ramchandani PG, Lane TA, Murphy SE. Symptoms of prenatal depression are associated with raised salivary alpha-amylase levels. Psychoneuroendocrinology. 2015;60:163–72. https://doi.org/10.1016/j.psyneuen.2015.06.013.
131. Giesbrecht GF, Campbell T, Letourneau N, Kaplan BJ, Field CJ, Dewey D, Bell RC, Bernier FP, Cantell M, Casey LM, Eliasziw M, Farmer A, Gagnon L, Giesbrecht GF, Goonewardene L, Johnston DW, Kooistra L, Letourneau N, Manca DP, et al. Sexually dimorphic adaptations in basal maternal stress physiology during pregnancy and implications for fetal development. Psychoneuroendocrinology. 2015;56:168–78. https://doi.org/10.1016/j.psyneuen.2015.03.013.

132. La Rocca C, Carbone F, Longobardi S, Matarese G. The immunology of pregnancy: regulatory T cells control maternal immune tolerance toward the fetus. Immunol Lett. 2014;162(1):41–8.
133. Sykes L, MacIntyre DA, Yap XJ, Teoh TG, Bennett PR. The Th1:Th2 dichotomy of pregnancy and preterm labour. Mediat Inflamm. 2012;2012:967629. https://doi.org/10.1155/2012/967629.
134. Christian LM, Porter K. Longitudinal changes in serum proinflammatory markers across pregnancy and postpartum: effects of maternal body mass index. Am J Manag Care. 2014;20(11):887–93. https://doi.org/10.1016/j.pestbp.2011.02.012.
135. Curry AE, Vogel I, Skogstrand K, Drews C, Schendel DE, Flanders WD, Hougaard DM, Thorsen P. Maternal plasma cytokines in early- and mid-gestation of normal human pregnancy and their association with maternal factors. J Reprod Immunol. 2008;77(2):152–60. https://doi.org/10.1016/j.jri.2007.06.051.
136. Gillespie S, Porter K, Christian L. Adaptation of the inflammatory immune response across pregnancy and postpartum in Black and White women. J Reprod Immunol. 2016;114:27–31. https://doi.org/10.1016/j.jri.2016.02.001.
137. Dunn AJ, Swiergiel AH. Effects of interleukin-1 and endotoxin in the forced swim and tail suspension tests in mice. Pharmacol Biochem Behav. 2005;81(3):688–93.
138. Yang EV, Glaser R. Stress-induced immunomodulation and the implications for health. Int Immunopharmacol. 2002;2(2–3):315–24. https://doi.org/10.1016/S1567-5769(01)00182-5.
139. Miller AH, Raison CL. The role of inflammation in depression: from evolutionary imperative to modern treatment target. Nat Rev Immunol. 2016;16(1):22–34. https://doi.org/10.1038/nri.2015.5.
140. Dowlati Y, Herrmann N, Swardfager W, Liu H, Sham L, Reim EK, Lanctôt KL. A meta-analysis of cytokines in major depression. Biol Psychiatry. 2010;67(5):446–57. https://doi.org/10.1016/j.biopsych.2009.09.033.
141. Valkanova V, Ebmeier KP, Allan CL. CRP, IL-6 and depression: a systematic review and meta-analysis of longitudinal studies. J Affect Disord. 2013;150(3):736–44. https://doi.org/10.1016/j.jad.2013.06.004.
142. Au B, Smith KJ, Gariépy G, Schmitz N. The longitudinal associations between C-reactive protein and depressive symptoms: evidence from the English longitudinal study of ageing (ELSA). Int J Geriatr Psychiatry. 2015;30(9):976–84.
143. Bonaccorso S, Marino V, Puzella A, Pasquini M, Biondi M, Artini M, Almerighi C, Verkerk R, Meltzer H, Maes M. Increased depressive ratings in patients with hepatitis C receiving interferon-α-based immunotherapy are related to interferon-α-induced changes in the serotonergic system. J Clin Psychopharmacol. 2002;22(1):86–90.
144. Capuron L, Gumnick JF, Musselman DL, Lawson DH, Reemsnyder A, Nemeroff CB, Miller AH. Neurobehavioral effects of interferon-α in cancer patients: phenomenology and paroxetine responsiveness of symptom dimensions. Neuropsychopharmacology. 2002;26(5):643.
145. Gimeno D, Kivimäki M, Brunner EJ, Elovainio M, De Vogli R, Steptoe A, Kumari M, Lowe GDO, Rumley A, Marmot MG. Associations of C-reactive protein and interleukin-6 with cognitive symptoms of depression: 12-year follow-up of the Whitehall II study. Psychol Med. 2009;39(3):413–23.
146. Corwin EJ, Pajer K. The psychoneuroimmunology of postpartum depression. J Women's Health. 2008;17(9):1529–34. https://doi.org/10.1089/jwh.2007.0725.
147. Christian LM, Franco A, Glaser R, Iams JD. Depressive symptoms are associated with elevated serum proinflammatory cytokines among pregnant women. Brain Behav Immun. 2009;23(6):750–4. https://doi.org/10.1016/j.bbi.2009.02.012.
148. Osborne LM, Yenokyan G, Fei K, Kraus T, Moran T, Monk C, Sperling R. Innate immune activation and depressive and anxious symptoms across the peripartum: an exploratory study. Psychoneuroendocrinology. 2019;99(August 2018):80–6. https://doi.org/10.1016/j.psyneuen.2018.08.038.

149. Cassidy-Bushrow AE, Peters RM, Johnson DA, Templin TN. Association of depressive symptoms with inflammatory biomarkers among pregnant African-American women. J Reprod Immunol. 2012b;94(2):202–9. https://doi.org/10.1016/j.jri.2012.01.007.
150. Christian LM, Franco A, Iams JD, Sheridan J, Glaser R. Depressive symptoms predict exaggerated inflammatory responses to an in vivo immune challenge among pregnant women. Brain Behav Immun. 2010;24(1):49–53. https://doi.org/10.1016/j.bbi.2009.05.055.
151. Maes M, Leonard BE, Myint AM, Kubera M, Verkerk R. The new "5-HT" hypothesis of depression: cell-mediated immune activation induces indoleamine 2,3-dioxygenase, which leads to lower plasma tryptophan and an increased synthesis of detrimental tryptophan catabolites (TRYCATs), both of which contribute to the onset of depression. Prog Neuro-Psychopharmacol Biol Psychiatry. 2011;35(3):702–21. https://doi.org/10.1016/j.pnpbp.2010.12.017.
152. Manchia M, Carpiniello B, Valtorta F, Comai S. Serotonin dysfunction, aggressive behavior, and mental illness: exploring the link using a dimensional approach. ACS Chem Neurosci. 2017;8(5):961–72. https://doi.org/10.1021/acschemneuro.6b00427.
153. Myint AM, Kim YK. Cytokine-serotonin interaction through IDO: a neurodegeneration hypothesis of depression. Med Hypotheses. 2003;61(5–6):519–25. https://doi.org/10.1016/S0306-9877(03)00207-X.
154. Savitz J. The kynurenine pathway: a finger in every pie. Mol Psychiatry. 2019;25(1):131–47. https://doi.org/10.1038/s41380-019-0414-4.
155. Comai S, Costa CVL, Ragazzi E, Bertazzo A, Allegri G. The effect of age on the enzyme activities of tryptophan metabolism along the kynurenine pathway in rats. Clin Chim Acta. 2005;360(1–2):67–80.
156. Comai S, Bertazzo A, Brughera M, Crotti S. Tryptophan in health and disease. Adv Clin Chem. 2020;95:165–218.
157. Achtyes E, Keaton S, Smart L, Burmeister A, Heilman P, Krzyzanowski S, Nagalla M, Guillemin G, Escobar Galvis M, Lim C, Muzik M, Postolache T, Leach R, Brundin L. Inflammation and kynurenine pathway dysregulation in post-partum women with severe and suicidal depression. Brain Behav Immun. 2020;83:239–47. https://doi.org/10.1016/j.bbi.2019.10.017.
158. Kohl C, Walch T, Huber R, Kemmler G, Neurauter G, Fuchs D, Sölder E, Schröcksnadel H, Sperner-Unterweger B. Measurement of tryptophan, kynurenine and neopterin in women with and without postpartum blues. J Affect Disord. 2005;86(2–3):135–42. https://doi.org/10.1016/j.jad.2004.12.013.
159. M'Baïlara K, Henry C, Lestage J, Launay JM, Parrot F, Swendsen J, Sutter AL, Roux D, Dallay D, Demotes-Mainard J. Decreased brain tryptophan availability as a partial determinant of post-partum blues. Psychoneuroendocrinology. 2006;31(3):407–13. https://doi.org/10.1016/j.psyneuen.2005.10.001.
160. Scrandis DA, Langenberg P, Tonelli LH, Sheikh TM, Manogura AC, Alberico LA, Hermanstyne T, Fuchs D, Mighty H, Hasday JD, Boteva K, Postolache TT. Prepartum depressive symptoms correlate positively with C-reactive protein levels and negatively with tryptophan levels: a preliminary report. Int J Child Health Hum Dev. 2008;1(2):167–74.
161. Teshigawara T, Mouri A, Kubo H, Nakamura Y, Shiino T, Okada T, Morikawa M, Nabeshima T, Ozaki N, Yamamoto Y, Saito K. Changes in tryptophan metabolism during pregnancy and postpartum periods: potential involvement in postpartum depressive symptoms. J Affect Disord. 2019;255(April):168–76. https://doi.org/10.1016/j.jad.2019.05.028.
162. Nazzari S, Molteni M, Valtorta F, Comai S, Frigerio A. Prenatal IL-6 levels and activation of the tryptophan to kynurenine pathway are associated with depressive but not anxiety symptoms across the perinatal and the post-partum period in a low-risk sample. Brain Behav Immun. 2020b;89(March):175–83. https://doi.org/10.1016/j.bbi.2020.06.015.
163. Wójcik J, Dudek D, Schlegel-Zawadzka M, Grabowska M, Marcinek A, Florek E, Piekoszewski W, Nowak RJ, Opoka W, Nowak G. Antepartum/postpartum depressive symptoms and serum zinc and magnesium levels. Pharmacol Rep. 2006;58(4):571.

164. Armony-Sivan R, Shao J, Li M, Zhao G, Zhao Z, Xu G, Zhou M, Zhan J, Bian Y, Ji C. No relationship between maternal iron status and postpartum depression in two samples in China. J Pregnancy. 2012;2012(1):521431.
165. Bodnar LM, Wisner KL, Luther JF, Powers RW, Evans RW, Gallaher MJ, Newby PK. An exploratory factor analysis of nutritional biomarkers associated with major depression in pregnancy. Public Health Nutr. 2012;15(6):1078–86.
166. Chong MFF, Wong JXY, Colega M, Chen L-W, van Dam RM, Tan CS, Lim AL, Cai S, Broekman BFP, Lee YS. Relationships of maternal folate and vitamin B12 status during pregnancy with perinatal depression: the GUSTO study. J Psychiatr Res. 2014;55:110–6.
167. Lewis SJ, Araya R, Leary S, Smith GD, Ness A. Folic acid supplementation during pregnancy may protect against depression 21 months after pregnancy, an effect modified by MTHFR C677T genotype. Eur J Clin Nutr. 2012;66(1):97–103.
168. Hockey M, McGuinness AJ, Marx W, Rocks T, Jacka FN, Ruusunen A. Is dairy consumption associated with depressive symptoms or disorders in adults? A systematic review of observational studies. Crit Rev Food Sci Nutr. 2020;60(21):3653–68.
169. Brandenbarg J, Vrijkotte TGM, Goedhart G, van Eijsden M. Maternal early-pregnancy vitamin D status is associated with maternal depressive symptoms in the Amsterdam born children and their development cohort. Biopsychosoc Sci Med. 2012;74(7):751–7.
170. Miyake Y, Tanaka K, Okubo H, Sasaki S, Arakawa M. Dietary vitamin D intake and prevalence of depressive symptoms during pregnancy in Japan. Nutrition. 2015;31(1):160–5.
171. Gur EB, Gokduman A, Turan GA, Tatar S, Hepyilmaz I, Zengin EB, Eskicioglu F, Guclu S. Mid-pregnancy vitamin D levels and postpartum depression. Eur J Obstet Gynecol Reprod Biol. 2014;179:110–6.
172. Robinson M, Whitehouse AJO, Newnham JP, Gorman S, Jacoby P, Holt BJ, Serralha M, Tearne JE, Holt PG, Hart PH. Low maternal serum vitamin D during pregnancy and the risk for postpartum depression symptoms. Arch Womens Ment Health. 2014;17:213–9.
173. Wang R, Xu F, Xia X, Xiong A, Dai D, Ling Y, et al. The effect of vitamin D supplementation on primary depression: a meta-analysis. J Affect Disord. 2024;344:653–61.
174. Teofilo MMA, Farias DR, Pinto TDJP, Vilela AAF, dos Santos Vaz J, Nardi AE, Kac G. HDL-cholesterol concentrations are inversely associated with Edinburgh postnatal depression scale scores during pregnancy: results from a Brazilian cohort study. J Psychiatr Res. 2014;58:181–8.
175. Shiraishi M, Matsuzaki M, Yatsuki Y, Murayama R, Severinsson E, Haruna M. Associations of dietary intake and plasma concentrations of eicosapentaenoic and docosahexaenoic acid with prenatal depressive symptoms in Japan. Nurs Health Sci. 2015;17(2):257–62.
176. Lin PY, Chang CH, Chong MFF, Chen H, Su KP. Polyunsaturated fatty acids in perinatal depression: a systematic review and meta-analysis. Biol Psychiatry. 2017;82(8):560–9.
177. Keenan K, Hipwell AE, Bortner J, Hoffmann A, McAloon R. Association between fatty acid supplementation and prenatal stress in African Americans: a randomized controlled trial. Obstet Gynecol. 2014;124(6):1080–7.
178. Chong MFF, Ong Y-L, Calder PC, Colega M, Wong JXY, Tan CS, Lim AL, Fisk HL, Cai S, Pang WW. Long-chain polyunsaturated fatty acid status during pregnancy and maternal mental health in pregnancy and the postpartum period: results from the GUSTO study. J Clin Psychiatry. 2015;76(7):10546.
179. Mozurkewich EL, Clinton CM, Chilimigras JL, Hamilton SE, Allbaugh LJ, Berman DR, Marcus SM, Romero VC, Treadwell MC, Keeton KL. The mothers, Omega-3, and mental health study: a double-blind, randomized controlled trial. Am J Obstet Gynecol. 2013;208(4):313–e1.
180. Viktorin A, Meltzer-Brody S, Kuja-Halkola R, Sullivan PF, Landén M, Lichtenstein P, Magnusson PKE. Heritability of perinatal depression and genetic overlap with nonperinatal depression. Am J Psychiatry. 2016;173(2):158–65. https://doi.org/10.1176/appi.ajp.2015.15010085.

181. Binder EB, Newport DJ, Zach EB, Smith AK, Deveau TC, Altshuler LL, Cohen LS, Stowe ZN, Cubells JF. A serotonin transporter gene polymorphism predicts peripartum depressive symptoms in an at-risk psychiatric cohort. J Psychiatr Res. 2010;44(10):640–6.
182. Tavares Pinheiro R, da Cunha M, Coelho F, Azevedo da Silva R, Amaral Tavares Pinheiro K, Pierre Oses J, de Avila Quevedo L, Dias de Mattos Souza L, Jansen K, Maria Zimmermann Peruzatto J, Gus Manfro G. Association of a serotonin transporter gene polymorphism (5-HTTLPR) and stressful life events with postpartum depressive symptoms: a population-based study. J Psychosom Obstet Gynecol. 2013;34(1):29–33.
183. Zhang X, Wang L, Huang F, Li J, Xiong L, Xue H, Zhang Y. Evaluation of the promoter region polymorphism (5-HTTLPR) in the serotonin transporter gene in females with postpartum depression. Exp Ther Med. 2015;9(1):245–9.
184. Comasco E, Sylvén SM, Papadopoulos FC, Oreland L, Sundström-Poromaa I, Skalkidou A. Postpartum depressive symptoms and the BDNF Val66Met functional polymorphism: effect of season of delivery. Arch Womens Ment Health. 2011;14(6):453–63.
185. Figueira P, Malloy-Diniz L, Campos SB, Miranda DM, Romano-Silva MA, De Marco L, Neves FS, Correa H. An association study between the Val66Met polymorphism of the BDNF gene and postpartum depression. Arch Womens Ment Health. 2010;13:285–9.
186. Pinsonneault JK, Sullivan D, Sadee W, Soares CN, Hampson E, Steiner M. Association study of the estrogen receptor gene ESR1 with postpartum depression—a pilot study. Arch Womens Ment Health. 2013;16(6):499–509. https://doi.org/10.1007/s00737-013-0373-8.
187. Engineer N, Darwin L, Nishigandh D, Ngianga-Bakwin K, Smith SC, Grammatopoulos DK. Association of glucocorticoid and type 1 corticotropin-releasing hormone receptors gene variants and risk for depression during pregnancy and post-partum. J Psychiatr Res. 2013;47(9):1166–73.
188. Fasching PA, Faschingbauer F, Goecke TW, Engel A, Häberle L, Seifert A, Voigt F, Amann M, Rebhan D, Burger P, Kornhuber J, Ekici AB, Beckmann MW, Binder EB. Genetic variants in the tryptophan hydroxylase 2 gene (TPH2) and depression during and after pregnancy. J Psychiatr Res. 2012;46(9):1109–17. https://doi.org/10.1016/j.jpsychires.2012.05.011.
189. Lin Y-MJ, Ko H-C, Chang F-M, Yeh T-L, Sun HS. Population-specific functional variant of the TPH2 gene 2755C> a polymorphism contributes risk association to major depression and anxiety in Chinese peripartum women. Arch Womens Ment Health. 2009;12:401–8.
190. Kundakovic M, Jaric I. The epigenetic link between prenatal adverse environments and neurodevelopmental disorders. Genes. 2017;8(3):104. https://doi.org/10.3390/genes8030104.
191. Meaney MJ, Szyf M, Seckl JR. Epigenetic mechanisms of perinatal programming of hypothalamic-pituitary-adrenal function and health. Trends Mol Med. 2007;13(7):269–77. https://doi.org/10.1016/j.molmed.2007.05.003.
192. Cao-Lei L, de Rooij SR, King S, Matthews SG, Metz GAS, Roseboom TJ, Szyf M. Prenatal stress and epigenetics. Neurosci Biobehav Rev. 2020;117(November 2016):198–210. https://doi.org/10.1016/j.neubiorev.2017.05.016.
193. Meaney MJ. Epigenetics and the biological definition of gene x environment interactions. Child Dev. 2010;81(1):41–79. https://doi.org/10.1111/j.1467-8624.2009.01381.x.
194. McGowan PO, Matthews SG. Prenatal stress, glucocorticoids, and developmental programming of the stress response. Endocrinology. 2018;159(1):69–82. https://doi.org/10.1210/en.2017-00896.
195. Turecki G, Meaney MJ. Effects of the social environment and stress on glucocorticoid receptor gene methylation: a systematic review. Biol Psychiatry. 2016;79(2):87–96. https://doi.org/10.1016/j.biopsych.2014.11.022.
196. Kertes DA, Kamin HS, Hughes DA, Rodney NC, Bhatt S, Mulligan CJ. Prenatal maternal stress predicts methylation of genes regulating the hypothalamic-pituitary-adrenocortical system in mothers and newborns in the Democratic Republic of Congo. Child Dev. 2016;87(1):61–72. https://doi.org/10.1111/cdev.12487.
197. Schechter DS, Moser DA, Paoloni-Giacobino A, Stenz L, Gex-Fabry M, Aue T, Adouan W, Cordero MI, Suardi F, Manini A, Sancho Rossignol A, Merminod G, Ansermet F, Dayer AG, Rusconi Serpa S. Methylation of NR3C1 is related to maternal PTSD, parenting stress

and maternal medial prefrontal cortical activity in response to child separation among mothers with histories of violence exposure. Front Psychol. 2015;6(May):1–12. https://doi.org/10.3389/fpsyg.2015.00690.
198. Santos HP Jr, Bhattacharya A, Martin EM, Addo K, Psioda M, Smeester L, Joseph RM, Hooper SR, Frazier JA, Kuban KC, O'Shea T, Fry RC, Investigators, for the E. Epigenome-wide DNA methylation in placentas from preterm infants: association with maternal socioeconomic status. Epigenetics. 2019;14(8):751–65. https://doi.org/10.1080/15592294.2019.1614743.
199. Perroud N, Rutembesa E, Paoloni-Giacobino A, Mutabaruka J, Mutesa L, Stenz L, Malafosse A, Karege F. The Tutsi genocide and transgenerational transmission of maternal stress: epigenetics and biology of the HPA axis. World J Biol Psychiatry. 2014;15(4):334–45. https://doi.org/10.3109/15622975.2013.866693.
200. Nazzari S, Grumi S, Mambretti F, Villa M, Giorda R, Provenzi L, Borgatti R, Biasucci G, Decembrino L, Giacchero R, Magnani ML, Nacinovich R, Prefumo F, Spinillo A, Veggiotti P. Maternal and infant NR3C1 and SLC6A4 epigenetic signatures of the COVID-19 pandemic lockdown: when timing matters. Transl Psychiatry. 2022;12(1):386. https://doi.org/10.1038/s41398-022-02160-0.
201. Dereix AE, Ledyard R, Redhunt AM, Bloomquist TR, Brennan KJ, Baccarelli AA, Hacker MR, Burris HH. Maternal anxiety and depression in pregnancy and DNA methylation of the NR3C1 glucocorticoid receptor gene. Epigenomics. 2021;13(21):1701–9. https://doi.org/10.2217/epi-2020-0022.
202. Hompes T, Izzi B, Gellens E, Morreels M, Fieuws S, Pexsters A, Schops G, Dom M, Van Bree R, Freson K, Verhaeghe J, Spitz B, Demyttenaere K, Glover V, Van den Bergh B, Allegaert K, Claes S. Investigating the influence of maternal cortisol and emotional state during pregnancy on the DNA methylation status of the glucocorticoid receptor gene (NR3C1) promoter region in cord blood. J Psychiatr Res. 2013;47(7):880–91. https://doi.org/10.1016/j.jpsychires.2013.03.009.
203. Oberlander TF, Weinberg J, Papsdorf M, Grunau R, Misri S, Devlin AM. Prenatal exposure to maternal depression, neonatal methylation of human glucocorticoid receptor gene (NR3C1) and infant cortisol stress responses. Epigenetics. 2008;3(2):97–106. https://doi.org/10.4161/epi.3.2.6034.
204. Devlin AM, Brain U, Austin J, Oberlander TF. Prenatal exposure to maternal depressed mood and the MTHFR C677T variant affect SLC6A4 methylation in infants at birth. PLoS One. 2010;5(8):2–9. https://doi.org/10.1371/journal.pone.0012201.
205. World Health Organization. Social determinants of health. 2025. https://www.who.int/health-topics/social-determinants-of-health#tab=tab_2. Accessed on 15 Mar 2025.
206. Fortuna LR, Tobón AL, Anglero YL, Postlethwaite A, Porche MV, Rothe EM. Focusing on racial, historical and intergenerational trauma, and resilience: a paradigm to better serving children and families. Child Adolesc Psychiatr Clin N Am. 2022;31(2):237–50.
207. Smelser NJ. Review of the international Encyclopedia of the social sciences. Soc Forces. 1970;48:534–7.
208. Toledo-Corral CM, Gao L, Chavez T, Grubbs B, Habre R, Dunton GF, et al. Role of race, ethnicity, and immigration in perceived stress and depressive symptomatology trends during pregnancy. J Immigr Minor Health. 2022;24(3):561–9.
209. Wickramage K, Vearey J, Zwi AB, Robinson C, Knipper M. Migration and health: a global public health research priority. BMC Public Health. 2018;18:1–9.
210. Almeida LM, Caldas JP, Ayres-de-Campos D, Dias S. Assessing maternal healthcare inequities among migrants: a qualitative study. Cad Saude Publica. 2014;30:333–40.
211. Berry JW. Acculturation and adaptation in a new society. Int Migr. 1992;30:69.
212. Behboudi-Gandevani S, Bidhendi-Yarandi R, Panahi MH, Mardani A, Paal P, Prinds C, Vaismoradi M. Adverse pregnancy outcomes and international immigration status: a systematic review and meta-analysis. Ann Glob Health. 2022;88(1):44. https://doi.org/10.5334/aogh.3591. PMID: 35854922; PMCID: PMC9248985.

213. Londoño Tobón A, Berry OO, Gorelik S, Ryou HS, Byatt N, Cardoza K, et al. A call to address the political determinants of perinatal mental health. Health Aff Forefront. 2024. https://doi.org/10.1377/forefront.20240822.518945.
214. Salerno Valdez E, Sabo S, Butler M, Camplain R, Simpson R, Castro Y. Perinatal depression symptom prevalence on the U.S.–Mexico border. J Rural Ment Health. 2019;43(1):38–44.
215. Rhodes SD, Mann L, Simán FM, Song E, Alonzo J, Downs M, et al. The impact of local immigration enforcement policies on the health of immigrant Hispanics/Latinos in the United States. Am J Public Health. 2015;105(2):329–37.
216. Vernice NA, Pereira NM, Wang A, Demetres M, Adams LV. The adverse health effects of punitive immigrant policies in the United States: a systematic review. PLoS One. 2020;15(12):e0244054.
217. Alhasanat-Khalil D, Fry-McComish J, Dayton C, Benkert R, Yarandi H, Giurgescu C. Acculturative stress and lack of social support predict postpartum depression among US immigrant women of Arabic descent. Arch Psychiatr Nurs. 2018;32(4):530–5.
218. D'Anna-Hernandez KL, Aleman B, Flores AM. Acculturative stress negatively impacts maternal depressive symptoms in Mexican-American women during pregnancy. J Affect Disord. 2015;176:35–42.
219. Zeiders KH, Umaña-Taylor AJ, Jahromi LB, Updegraff KA, White RM. Discrimination and acculturation stress: a longitudinal study of children's well-being from prenatal development to 5 years of age. J Dev Behav Pediatr. 2016;37(7):557–64.
220. Paradies Y, Truong M, Priest N. A systematic review of the extent and measurement of healthcare provider racism. J Gen Intern Med. 2014;29:364–87.
221. Paradies Y, Ben J, Denson N, Elias A, Priest N, Pieterse A, et al. Racism as a determinant of health: a systematic review and meta-analysis. PLoS One. 2015;10(9):e0138511.
222. Williams DR, Lawrence JA, Davis BA. Racism and health: evidence and needed research. Annu Rev Public Health. 2019;40(1):105–25.
223. Petersen EE. Vital signs: pregnancy-related deaths, United States, 2011–2015, and strategies for prevention, 13 states, 2013–2017. MMWR Morb Mortal Wkly Rep. 2019;68:423–9.
224. Larrabee Sonderlund A, Schoenthaler A, Thilsing T. The association between maternal experiences of interpersonal discrimination and adverse birth outcomes: a systematic review of the evidence. Int J Environ Res Public Health. 2021;18(4):1465.
225. Braveman P, Heck K, Egerter S, Dominguez TP, Rinki C, Marchi KS, Curtis M. Worry about racial discrimination: a missing piece of the puzzle of Black-White disparities in preterm birth? PLoS One. 2017;12(10):e0186151.
226. Hoang TMH, Lee BA, Hsieh WJ, Lukacena KM, Tabb KM. Experiences of racial trauma among perinatal women of color in seeking healthcare services. Gen Hosp Psychiatry. 2023;84:60–6.
227. Bécares L, Atatoa-Carr P. The association between maternal and partner experienced racial discrimination and prenatal perceived stress, prenatal and postnatal depression: findings from the growing up in New Zealand cohort study. Int J Equity Health. 2016;15:1–12.
228. DiTosto JD, Holder K, Soyemi E, Beestrum M, Yee LM. Housing instability and adverse perinatal outcomes: a systematic review. Am J Obstet Gynecol MFM. 2021;3(6):100477.
229. Mendez DD, Hogan VK, Culhane JF. Stress during pregnancy: the role of institutional racism. Stress Health. 2013;29(4):266–74.
230. Preis H, Wang W, Zhu W, Mahaffey B, Lobel M. Social determinants of health, prenatal maternal stress, and earlier birth during the COVID-19 pandemic. Soc Personal Psychol Compass. 2023;17(7):e12751.

3 The Overlooked Burden: Maternal Stress in the Postpartum Period

Sandra Nakić Radoš, Maja Žutić, and Lucija Kolić

Abstract

The postpartum period represents a time of significant physical, psychological, and social changes where mothers face numerous specific stressors and demands. They may experience substantial postpartum stress—a specific form of stress triggered by postpartum stressors (events, situations, or daily challenges which cause discomfort) occurring within the first postpartum year. Most significant stressors during this period can be categorised into parenting roles, tasks, resources, and relationships, which more specifically refer to infant care, physical changes and overload, lack of sleep, lifestyle changes, returning to work, isolated motherhood, changes in body and sexuality, and breastfeeding.

Global prevalence rates ranging from 8% to 68% point to postpartum stress being a widespread health issue. Additionally, prolonged exposure to stress can lead to many adverse effects, such as health problems in mothers and infants and a strained mother-infant relationship. Postpartum stress is complex as it is shaped by various biological (e.g. neuroendocrine, genetic and epigenetic, obstetric, maternal health), psychological (e.g. pregnancy plans, maternal personal characteristics), and social (e.g. sociodemographic, infant characteristics, social support) factors. Unfortunately, for years, it was widely unrecognised or investigated only as a risk factor for other peripartum difficulties; however, addressing and mitigating postpartum stress is crucial for improving outcomes for both mothers and children.

S. Nakić Radoš (✉) · M. Žutić
University Department of Psychology, Catholic University of Croatia, Zagreb, Croatia
e-mail: snrados@unicath.hr; maja.zutic@unicath.hr

L. Kolić
Kindergarten "Maslačak", Zadar, Croatia

R. A. Caparros-Gonzalez (ed.), *Maternal Stress during Pregnancy and Postpartum*, https://doi.org/10.1007/978-3-032-09245-8_3

This chapter puts postpartum stress into focus by examining postpartum-specific stressors, clinical presentation, prevalence and course, biopsychosocial risk factors, consequences, and assessment methods, followed by a biopsychosocial framework of postpartum stress that can guide researchers and clinicians in alleviating the personal and global burden of postpartum stress.

Keywords

Postpartum stress · Maternal stress · Stressors · Risk factors · Biopsychosocial model

3.1 Introduction

Michelle Duggar, the well-known mother featured in the TV show *19 Kids and Counting*, once wrote about a moment when, at 1 A.M., she found herself crying while folding the family's laundry. In her blog post, she shared: "I felt so inadequate! Diapers, dishes, laundry, meals, cleanup, school lessons, baths, hugs, kisses, correction… My list seemed to go on and on" [1]. While Michelle's situation is undoubtedly unique, it vividly illustrates the sense of overwhelm many mothers experience while caring for their families.

The first few months after childbirth represent a period of significant change. Immediately following delivery, women often experience pain and fatigue due to the birthing process itself, as well as additional discomforts such as sore nipples and milk leakage [2]. Alongside these physical changes, mothers invest substantial energy into building a bond with their newborn and establishing routines for feeding and sleeping. Simultaneously, if the newborn has older siblings, they may feel displaced, expressing anger or jealousy towards the new family member. During this period, the newborn asserts its needs with great urgency, requiring frequent feeding, diaper changes, and soothing to sleep [3]. Many mothers emphasise a striking difference between the idealised image of motherhood presented by society prior to childbirth and the reality of the postpartum period [4]. Therefore, the concept of the "fourth trimester" is well founded, as women face a number of specific stressors and demands, making early parenthood a critical period for their well-being.

Given that postpartum stress is only beginning to be explored as a distinct phenomenon, independent of other psychological conditions, much more research is needed to understand its prevalence, risk factors, and potential interventions. With the development of more complex research methods and designs, there has been a growing need for a more integrative model that can comprehensively capture both physical and mental health. With this paradigm shift, in 1977, Georg Engel conceptualised a biopsychosocial model of disease and health, which posits that biological, psychological, and social factors are interconnected and jointly contribute to illness and health. Although this comprehensive model emerged a long time ago, studies of postpartum stress rarely integrated Engel's theoretical framework into their research designs. For example, a recent narrative review of biopsychosocial models of peripartum depression—a construct far better investigated than peripartum stress—identified only five such models [5].

Stress is more often investigated as a predictor of peripartum depression or anxiety [6, 7] and very rarely as a primary construct of interest. Moreover, one study showed that 10% of postpartum women had symptoms of anxiety and stress without depression [8]. Some studies have drawn attention to the existence of a certain clinical and scientific preference for postpartum depression, compared to anxiety and stress, and encourage simultaneously focusing on all three constructs, with equal emphasis on each [8, 9].

This chapter puts postpartum stress into focus by examining postpartum-specific stressors, clinical presentation, prevalence and course, biopsychosocial risk factors and correlates of postpartum stress, consequences, and assessment methods. We then provide a biopsychosocial framework of postpartum stress and some research and clinical implications that we hope will encourage future research into focusing on postpartum stress as the primary construct of interest.

3.2 Postpartum-Specific Stress

Stress is often conceptualised through a well-known theoretical framework by Lazarus and Folkman [10], according to which stress occurs when the demands of the situation prevail over the person's resources to cope with them. This transactional explanation of stress highlights the cognitive processes through which individuals assign meaning to their environment. Stress typically involves a stressor and the response to it, with stressors categorised as either physical or psychological. Physical stressors may include injuries, significant physical fatigue, and exhaustion. Psychological stressors, on the other hand, can include tasks with tight deadlines, interpersonal conflicts, isolation, or unexpected events [11].

Postpartum stress is defined as an unpleasant emotional state triggered by postpartum stressors occurring up to one year postpartum [12, 13]. A key concept emphasised in this definition is the identification of postpartum stressors—events, situations, or challenges that mothers perceive as sources of psychological, emotional, or physical discomfort during the postpartum period [14]. These stressors are often not major life events but rather daily challenges that mothers face [4].

There are more than a dozen different postpartum stressors identified in the literature [13]. The most significant stressors during this period refer to infant care, significant physical changes and overload, lack of sleep, lifestyle changes, returning to work and leaving the child in someone else's care, isolated motherhood, and changes in body and sexuality [14–16]. These stressors can be categorised into parenting roles, tasks, resources, and relationships [14]. Importantly, research also highlights breastfeeding as one of the most significant postpartum stressors [4]. On the other hand, Horowitz and Damato [14] found that parenting tasks, while being sources of stress, are also sources of satisfaction—such as feelings of pride in motherhood, enjoyment in caring for a child, and the general act of providing care for the child.

3.3 Clinical Considerations

In most cases, if the postpartum emotional or behavioural changes (Criterion A) are associated with significant impairment in functioning or personal suffering (Criterion B) and could not be attributed to other mental disorders (Criterion C) or bereavement (Criterion D), these can be classified as adjustment disorder, according to DSM-5 [17]. The adjustment disorder refers to a reaction within 3 months after the stressors occur. It can be triggered by different stressors, which can be continuously present and can follow a developmental phase, such as becoming a parent. Also, it can present with dominant depressed mood, anxiety, and/or disturbance of conduct [17]. The symptoms usually resolve within 6 months, but if the stressors are continuously present, such as in parenting transition, the symptoms can be persistent. In research on postpartum stress, a clinical interview is rarely applied, so we lack a clear distinction between stress levels (usually measured by self-report scales, as described in Sect. 3.7 on the assessment), adjustment disorder, and other postpartum mental disorders. Still, one study showed that of the women who screened positive for depression symptoms, 6% were classified as having postpartum depression and 24% as having adjustment disorder using the clinical interview [18]. It seems that severe postpartum stress, presented as adjustment disorder, is quite prevalent, but still underdiagnosed.

Stress in the postpartum should be differentiated from other mental health problems that can occur in the postpartum. First of all, it should be separated from acute stress disorder (ASD) and posttraumatic stress disorder (PTSD). Following a traumatic experience, ASD is a short-term sequel which resolves within 1 month, while PTSD is a long-term mental health disorder accompanied by different sets of symptoms. One in three women perceive childbirth as a traumatic experience, with around 4% meeting diagnostic criteria for childbirth-related PTSD (CB-PTSD) and about 12% exhibiting clinically significant PTSD symptoms, according to meta-analyses [19, 20]. PTSD is characterised by intrusions or re-experiencing the traumatic event, avoidance of all reminders associated with the trauma, negative changes in cognition and mood, and elevated arousal and reactivity [17].

Although the highly intensive and abrupt experience of stress is implicated in the development of ASD and PTSD by its clinical features, these can be distinguished. Firstly, in childbirth-related PTSD, there is usually a clear single event that provokes a negative sequel in cognition and emotions, such as negative birth experience, preterm birth, obstetrical interventions, etc. [21]. On the other hand, in postpartum stress, several stressors provoke unpleasant emotions, and these are not necessarily attributed to a specific event. Instead, the uncontrollability and unpredictability of daily events are what provoke stressful experiences, per the transactional model of stress [10]. Many things are unpredictable in the early postpartum stage, including the course of postpartum recovery, baby sleep intervals, and the next feeding time, to mention some of them. Secondly, the intensity of the symptoms in childbirth-related PTSD is, on a clinical level, so high that it affects the daily and social functioning of a woman and demands treatment [22]. In contrast, in postpartum stress, daily functioning can be preserved, although social support is essential to help mothers cope with daily tasks and to deal with the lack of time [23]. Nevertheless, despite conceptual and clinical differences between postpartum stress and PTSD following childbirth, a meta-analysis showed the association between the two [24].

3.4 Prevalence and Course of Postpartum Stress

Overall, studies show that 10–30% of postpartum women experience some form of mental health difficulty, including stress [8, 25, 26]. In studies using instruments designed to measure general stress, it was found that in South Korea 8% of mothers experience severe stress, while the average reports indicate moderate stress levels [27]. In Ireland, as many as 20% of mothers experience moderate to severe stress [28], with similar results in Canada, where 19% of mothers experience moderate to severe stress [29]. In the United States, mothers report high levels of stress, with 50–68% experiencing at least moderate stress [6, 30]. In Croatia, most mothers report moderate levels of postpartum stress, with 17% reporting high stress levels [31]. Similarly, mothers in the Czech Republic report moderate stress levels [32], with comparable results observed in Spain [33]. Conversely, in China, most mothers report low levels of stress [34].

Stress is not only a key factor implicated in various health issues, but limited research on the trajectories or duration of maternal postpartum stress suggests that stress levels can remain elevated over extended time. Specifically, maternal psychological distress—such as stress, anxiety, and depression—tends to persist from the third trimester of pregnancy to 6 months postpartum [35], with some studies showing that postpartum stress actually reaches its peak around 3 months [27] or even 6 months postpartum [28]. Overload, as the most predominant postpartum stressor, was at the highest level at 9–12 months postpartum, compared to 5–8 months or 13 months and more [15].

Another study even found that maternal distress gradually increased in primiparous women from pregnancy to 2 years postpartum [36]. However, prolonged exposure to stress can lead to many adverse effects with an increasing number of studies linking postpartum stress to health problems in mothers and infants [37]. Given these risks, addressing and mitigating postpartum stress is crucial for improving outcomes for both mothers and children.

3.5 Risk Factors and Correlates of Postpartum Stress

3.5.1 Bio-obstetric Factors

3.5.1.1 Neuroendocrine System

The hypothalamic-pituitary-adrenal (HPA) axis plays a key role in stress response [38]. Homeostasis is maintained by regulating the circulating levels of glucocorticoid hormones, with cortisol serving as the primary downstream glucocorticoid

[38]. Corticotropin-releasing hormone (CRH) is the main regulator of the HPA axis which stimulates the release of adrenocorticotropic hormone (ACTH), subsequently involved in the release of glucocorticoids, including cortisol [39, 40]. The postpartum period is marked by placental CRH withdrawal, resulting in transient suppression of hypothalamic CRH release and HPA axis dysregulation [41], which some suggest to be involved in postpartum mood disorders.

Empirical findings on the relationship between stress and neuroendocrine factors are sparse and ambiguous. One study found that at 25 weeks of pregnancy, placental CRH (but not cortisol or ACTH) was a strong predictor of depression symptoms 8 weeks postpartum [41]. Another study found that the natural decrease in cumulative hair cortisol concentration from the third trimester to 12 weeks postpartum was significant in the non-depressed and adjustment disorder groups, but not in the postpartum depression group [42], suggesting different trajectories of cortisol regulation. One study found that at 6 months postpartum, depressive symptoms were related to a smaller increase in the cortisol awakening response, a steeper cortisol decline across the day, and higher average cortisol levels, while women with elevated anxiety had lower overall cortisol output, and, interestingly, stress showed no association with any cortisol measure [43]. This finding suggests that postpartum stress is less associated with changes in cortisol levels compared to more severe forms of psychological distress, like depression or anxiety; however, further replication is needed.

3.5.1.2 Genetic and Epigenetic Factors

Due to a lack of studies, no genetic, epigenetic, or other biological risk factors for postpartum stress are conclusively elucidated. Present research primarily focuses on postpartum depression, disabling definitive conclusions about the specific biological risk factors of postpartum stress. Some studies confirmed the diathesis-stress hypothesis where peripartum women had a heightened risk for postpartum depression when gene x stress interactions were included in models [44]. Such studies showed that stress could adversely impact maternal mental health, with this association depending on certain genetic predispositions (most commonly studied is polymorphism in the promoter of the serotonin transporter gene (5-HTTLPR)) [45–47].

Epigenetic mechanisms such as DNA methylation (DNAm) are even more understudied, although they received more attention in recent years as they have been associated with stress responses and increased susceptibility to depression in the general population [48]. One epigenome-wide meta-analysis found associations between maternal prenatal stress and differential DNAm of infants at several sites [49]. Moreover, stressor-specific areas of conflict with family/friends, abuse (physical, sexual, and emotional), and loss of a close person were associated with differential infant methylation, thus identifying genes linked to adverse foetal outcomes and supporting the role of DNAm in the relationship between maternal stress and child health [49].

3.5.1.3 Obstetric Factors

Most studies suggest that first-time mothers are at a higher risk of experiencing elevated levels of postpartum stress [13, 50–52]. This association can be attributed to the fact that first-time mothers typically have lower self-confidence during the initial postpartum weeks as they are still learning to interpret their baby's cues, which contributes to heightened stress levels. In contrast, multiparous mothers benefit from prior experience in newborn care and generally have a clearer understanding of what to expect. Nonetheless, as mothers gradually become more attuned to their baby's needs, their self-confidence tends to increase, leading to a reduction in perceived stress levels [53]. In this context, parental mastery has been identified as a protective factor against the development of severe stress [30]. On the other hand, Krieg [54] found that multiparous mothers experience higher stress levels despite their competence in basic childcare tasks, as they face the additional challenge of managing the care of multiple children simultaneously. Additionally, mothers who had three or more births experience more stress related to physical changes due to pregnancy and birth than primiparas [32]. These findings suggest that distinct stressors lead to elevated stress in first-time and experienced mothers.

Processing the childbirth experience is considered the first formal task of motherhood, which subsequently influences parental behaviour in the early weeks postpartum [55]. Beyond its significant impact on mental health, a negative childbirth experience can lead to decreased self-esteem and self-efficacy in mothers [56], contributing to higher stress levels, particularly during the period of acquiring parental skills [53]. Several studies have found no association between the mode of delivery and stress levels [27, 30, 32, 33], while others suggest that mothers who have undergone caesarean sections report higher levels of stress [28, 31, 35]. Additionally, lower birth satisfaction is associated with higher levels of postpartum stress [31, 51, 56].

3.5.1.4 Maternal Physical Health

Physical health conditions, such as postpartum pain or complications during or after childbirth, may exacerbate maternal mental health challenges, with research primarily focusing on its relationship to elevated anxiety and depression [57, 58]. Studies identified a wide range of physical symptoms that may impact mothers' health status and quality of life in the two years postpartum, including physical exhaustion, sleeping problems, sexual concerns, constipation, and breast problems [59]. Therefore, as postpartum pain and health issues bring upon additional difficulties and discomfort, its relationship with worse mental health might be mediated by elevated stress levels.

Some also found that mothers with a higher body mass index (BMI) reported more severe stress [37]. This may be because higher BMI is generally associated with lower engagement in health-promoting behaviour, which, in turn, is linked to more adverse outcomes during the postpartum period [60]. Similarly, one intervention that has proven effective in reducing stress among new mothers is participating in physical activities for 130 min per week during the nine months following childbirth. This approach resulted in greater stress reduction compared to interventions focused on wellness and self-care activities [61].

3.5.1.5 Sleep

Sleep disturbances are a great source of distress during early parenthood. Studies found that mothers who experienced shorter, later, and more variable sleep had higher levels of stress [62]. Others found that greater variability in parental sleep up to a year postpartum was associated with household chaos (the absence of organisation in the home) [63]. A study investigating maternal mental health found that the lack of sleep and the inability to establish a child's sleep rhythm are at the core of postpartum mental health difficulties [64]. Also, interventions focused on the promotion of healthy sleep and physical exercise were key factors in reducing symptoms of depression and stress after childbirth [61].

3.5.1.6 Breastfeeding

Breastfeeding is often cited as one of the most significant stressors in the postpartum period, especially for the first-time mothers [13, 50], with pain experienced during breastfeeding identified as the most negative aspect [4]. Also, mothers who suffered from dysphoric milk ejection reflex (D-MER), which is characterised as a surge of unpleasant emotions occurring just before or during the first minutes of milk let-down, had significantly higher stress, depression, and anxiety levels, compared to women without D-MER [65].

Moreover, the notion that breastfeeding is a key element of maternal identity still persists [66], and mothers place great importance on breastfeeding success, perceiving it as an indicator of being a "good mother" [4]. Societal pressure and breastfeeding idealisation can trigger guilt and inadequacy in mothers who are unable to exclusively breastfeed [4, 67]. Therefore, it is not surprising that research shows supplementing breastfeeding with infant formula is a stressor [31, 52, 67–69]. Some authors also note that this relationship can be bidirectional, where higher levels of stress from other sources can affect a woman's milk supply and lactation, leading to breastfeeding issues or the decision to introduce infant formula [68].

3.5.2 Psychological Factors

3.5.2.1 Pregnancy Plans

Several studies exploring the connection between planning of a pregnancy and stress have yielded mixed results. Some authors found that women with unplanned pregnancies exhibited higher levels of postpartum stress [31, 70, 71], while others identified a link with postpartum depression but not with stress [35]. Nevertheless, this area still lacks sufficient research, particularly concerning moderators that potentially contribute to the relationship between pregnancy planning and postpartum psychological difficulties, such as social support [31, 71].

3.5.2.2 Maternal Personal Characteristics

It is considered that some types of people are more susceptible to stress or adverse mental health, due to personal characteristics like neuroticism, coping strategies, resilience, and other. According to Charney and Manji [72], stressful life events are not experienced randomly, rather some individuals tend to put themselves in situations that are highly likely to produce a stressful life event. For example, one study highlighted that emotional stability was the most important predictor of subjective well-being (stress, anxiety, and depression symptoms) during pregnancy and the first year postpartum [73]. Interestingly, in this study, besides emotional stability, a higher relationship satisfaction predicted lower stress but only among mothers and nonpregnant women.

In another study, among the five primary used coping strategies, two correlated with stressors; coping by taking time for respite or recovery was negatively correlated with changes in body and sexuality, and coping by managing emotions and thoughts was positively correlated with parenting demands [15]. A study on three resilience resources, mastery, self-esteem, and perceived social support, revealed that mastery and self-esteem moderated (and attenuated) the positive association between prenatal life stressors and early postpartum depressive symptoms [74]. Moreover, a multiple mediation analysis in another study found that resilience, postpartum stress, and sleep problems fully mediated the effects of social support on postpartum anxiety symptoms [64]. One randomised controlled trial found that an intervention programme about mindfulness-based childbirth and parenting significantly reduced postpartum self-perceived stress and depression [75]. Therefore, factors such as coping strategies, mindfulness, and resilience may have an impact on reducing the effects of stress and mental health outcomes, which warrants further investigation.

3.5.3 Social and Contextual Factors

3.5.3.1 Sociodemographic Factors

Delaying parenthood until the late 20s or early 30s, when both partners feel more secure in their adult roles, is known to facilitate the transition to parenthood [3]. Numerous studies have identified a relationship between maternal age and postpartum stress levels. However, some suggest that older mothers report higher stress levels [16, 32], while others find that younger mothers experience greater stress [28, 31]. A study on Spanish mothers did not find a significant association between maternal age and stress levels but noted that younger mothers were more preoccupied with bodily changes that occur during and after pregnancy [33]. Further research is needed to determine potential moderators of this relationship, as younger maternal age at first birth has also been linked to poorer mental health outcomes later in life [76].

A potential moderator of the relationship between sociodemographic factors and postpartum stress is the mother's socioeconomic status. Clout and Brown [35] suggest that the absence of a correlation between age and postpartum stress in their study might be due to their sample predominantly comprising participants from higher socioeconomic backgrounds. Indeed, studies that included participants from diverse socioeconomic statuses have shown that lower socioeconomic status is associated with higher stress levels and may even serve as a risk factor for severe stress in mothers [27, 28, 30, 77].

Similarly, the mother's level of education also appears to be associated with postpartum stress. Some authors have found that lower educational attainment is associated with higher postpartum stress [28, 78], while others report that more highly educated mothers experience higher stress levels [16, 52]. An interesting finding was observed in Croatia, where, although education level was not linked to overall postpartum stress levels, mothers with lower education were more preoccupied with stressors related to childcare and bodily changes [31].

Specific peripartum populations such as migrant women, refugees, adolescent mothers, and other marginalised groups may be a particularly high-risk group as they face unique stressors such as poverty, employment difficulties, trauma, lack of support, and discrimination, which exacerbate mental health challenges (e.g. [79, 80]).

3.5.3.2 Infant Characteristics

Not only do maternal health issues contribute to the rise of stress levels but the infant's health issues, as well. Three in four parents of premature newborns in the neonatal intensive care unit (NICU) reported experiencing high stress primarily regarding the sight and sounds of the unit, the infants' appearance, and the parent-infant relationship [81]. A recent meta-analysis showed that mothers of newborns from NICU reported a higher pooled prevalence of stress, anxiety, and depression than fathers [82].

A common issue in infancy is infant colic, with parents describing feelings of suffering alongside their child and the child's crying overshadowing all other aspects of their lives. This not only impacts their mental health but also affects the relationship, with parents reporting feelings of loneliness and helplessness [83]. It is no surprise that this experience is often described as a nightmare, not just for the child but also for the mother [84], with mothers particularly feeling unable to rely on their partner for support amidst the chaos [83]. This relationship appears to be bidirectional, where not only does infant colic contribute to increased stress but better maternal mental health also helps reduce the occurrence of infant colic in the child [85]. Furthermore, difficult infant temperament was associated with higher levels of not only maternal depression and anxiety [86] but postpartum stress, as well [87].

3.5.3.3 Social Support

The arrival of a child often results in couples having less time for each other, but this does not necessarily lead to issues in their relationships [3]. In fact, strong and supportive partnerships tend to remain stable after childbirth, while relationships characterised by high conflict before birth generally continue to be strained during the postpartum period [88]. Research has shown that first-time mothers in satisfying romantic relationships experience lower levels of postpartum stress. This protective effect extends beyond first-time mothers, benefiting those adjusting to life with multiple children as well [6, 27, 28, 30, 31, 37, 89].

Partner support plays a crucial role, with women who feel strongly supported by their partners reporting reduced stress levels both during pregnancy and after childbirth [90]. Conversely, single mothers often report lower levels of perceived social support, reduced social inclusion, and less frequent contact with family and friends [91] as the absence of a partner may limit opportunities for social interactions and reduce access to supportive relationships [92]. This highlights the importance of social support from family and friends for maternal well-being [6, 27, 31].

3.5.3.4 Structural Factors

In the initial days postpartum, hospital staff are a key source of social support for mothers. However, research indicates that women are often dissatisfied with the emotional support provided by healthcare professionals and expect a more open and informative approach from midwives. Additionally, many mothers express a desire for continued midwife visits after leaving the hospital, as challenges such as breastfeeding issues, sleep disturbances, and developmental concerns often emerge later as the child grows [4]. Midwife-led interventions aimed at reducing postpartum stress and enhancing mothers' confidence in childcare have shown positive effects, even among mothers lacking other forms of social support. This further emphasises the critical role of healthcare professionals in supporting new mothers [93].

Next, maternity leave policies are one of the structural factors that may impact maternal well-being, as they are a core element of health and economic protection of women across the peripartum period [94]. They offer women a period to adapt to their new role, provide care for the newborn, and help prevent or mitigate stress arising from early parenthood [95]. A recent systematic review identified that paid and longer maternity leave was associated with a reduction of postpartum depression symptoms in high-income countries [95] but not specifically examined in the association with postpartum stress.

3.6 Consequences of Postpartum Stress

3.6.1 Mother

3.6.1.1 Mental Health Problems

Maternal postpartum stress has been implicated in many adverse outcomes, both for the mother and the baby. Substantial evidence corroborates that stress has a central role in peripartum mental health difficulties. Namely, experience of stress is particularly important as it is one of the strongest predictors of both peripartum depression and anxiety [96–98]. A recent umbrella review demonstrated that among the main psychological correlates of peripartum depression were factors associated with stress, namely, stressful life events and childcare stress [99]. If left untreated, peripartum depression can subsequently have a number of short- and long-term negative effects on women and children [100].

A more recently coined term, called parental burnout, has received scientific attention in the last decades. Parental burnout stems from a prolonged and chronic stress experienced in parenting [101]. It is a serious condition characterised by intense exhaustion related to parenting, emotional distancing from children, and a lack of fulfilment in parenting [102]. Global worldwide prevalence of parental burnout is around 5–8% [103]. Among mothers with children up to 5 years, 3.5% had elevated burnout, with sociodemographic characteristics (higher parity, urban residence), personality traits (low emotional stability, low agreeableness, high perfectionism), and low parenting self-efficiency as risk factors [104]. At particularly high risk of parental burnout may be parents of chronically ill children (e.g. diabetes, inflammatory bowel diseases) [105], who may face specific chronic stressors (e.g. financial difficulties, uncertainty surrounding child's health, etc.).

3.6.1.2 Maternal Health Outcomes

Chronic stress is believed to affect health outcomes through a number of ways, including systemic inflammation brought on by immune system dysregulation (e.g. elevated C-reactive protein and inflammatory cytokines). In one study, chronic financial stress at one month postpartum predicted higher CRP levels at six and twelve months postpartum, even after adjusting for multiple confounders [106]. Another study found that in postpartum and only in African Americans, poor sleep and stress predicted greater stimulated proinflammatory cytokine production [107]. Also, in this study, parenting stress was both a mediator and a predictor linking sleep and enhanced inflammatory responding, demonstrating the bidirectionality of these constructs at postpartum. However, another study found no significant relationships between immune, endocrine, and stress factors among mothers up to months postpartum [108].

Stress may impact the brain in several ways. One review pointed to three categories of stressful experiences related to maternal brain outcomes: first is stress from the mother's childhood that may have a long-term impact on her brain, second are psychosocial and environmental stressors during the perinatal period, and third are specific stressors related to childbirth or parenting [109]. One neuroimaging study among first-time mothers showed that higher perceived stress was associated with heightened right dorsolateral prefrontal cortex (DLPFC) activity while engaging in cognitive reappraisal task (to decrease the intensity of their negative emotions) versus naturally responding to a negative stimuli which was further associated with elevated parenting stress [110]. Such findings indicate that stress and everyday reappraisal use is reflected in maternal neural regulation of emotion.

3.6.2 Mother-Infant Relationship

One of the main concerns a woman has after childbirth, apart from her own health and postpartum recovery, is the care for the newborn. Showing love and affection to the baby is a major part of the mother-infant bonding process that starts to develop from pregnancy to postpartum period but increases in quality and intensity after childbirth [111]. Mother-infant bonding refers to the strong and enduring emotional, cognitive, behavioural, and neurobiological tie that a mother develops towards the baby [112]. The mother-infant bonding process is largely affected by maternal mental health, including symptoms of postpartum depression [113], anxiety [86, 114], and posttraumatic stress disorder [113]. Studies examining stress in relation to mother-infant bonding has been scarce, as noted by an earlier review on bonding correlates [115]. Still, more recent studies show that higher levels of stress were associated with poor mother-infant bonding [116–118], which has been confirmed in a recent systematic review [119].

3.6.3 Infant

Many hypothesise that exposure to adversities during the peripartum period can have long-term effects through epigenetic mechanisms on infant health and development. One study revealed that maternal postpartum stress is associated with a higher risk of developmental delays in toddlers, and no such associations were found for prenatal stress, perinatal complications, or postpartum depression, suggesting that maternal postpartum stress could serve as an important target for psychosocial interventions [120]. On the other hand, another study found that symptoms of depression, anxiety, and stress predicted mental health outcomes among adult offspring only when experienced antenatally and not in postpartum [9], which could suggest an intrauterine biological mechanism important for the observed relationships. The authors suggest that possible alterations of the HPA axis among women with elevated depression, anxiety, and stress levels might have permanently influenced a dysregulation in foetal HPA axis, which was implicated in later adverse health outcomes. In addition, the aforementioned study found a weaker association between women who experienced high perceived stress at all time points both antenatally and postnatally, with offspring behavioural problems and depressive symptoms, which may imply that internalising issues in adulthood are more specifically related to maternal peripartum stress, rather than other conditions [9]. As previously mentioned, recent studies investigated epigenetic changes in the offspring of mothers who suffered from peripartum mental health difficulties. Studies found that antenatal and postnatal stress and depression were related with epigenomic changes in the foetus and the first year of infant's life [49, 121].

3.6.4 Family and Society

Although maternal mortality during childbirth remains the most significant challenge in perinatal care, the World Health Organization (WHO) recognises maternal mental health difficulties as one of the most critical public health issues, with efforts to address them only recently beginning [122]. Margiotta et al. [123] calculated that untreated mental health issues in mothers cost the state of Texas as much as $2.2 billion in a single year, placing a significant burden on public health and society as a whole. In the United Kingdom, it is reported that changes in medical practices for treating maternal mental health issues could save £52 million for the NHS [124]. Several interventions aimed at promoting competent childcare and improving family conditions have shown promising results. For example, *the Nurse-Family Partnership*, implemented in the United States, Australia, Canada, the Netherlands, and the United Kingdom, has led to better intelligence test scores and academic success among children of participating mothers. These mothers also experienced longer intervals between births, increased contact with the child's father, more stable close relationships, and a greater sense of control over their lives. Furthermore, this intervention has resulted in a fivefold reduction in state expenses in caring for at-risk families [3].

3.7 Assessment Methods

3.7.1 Biological Measures

Stress during pregnancy and postpartum can be measured both subjectively and objectively. However, measuring it is challenging due to individual variations and the multifaceted nature of stressful experiences [125]. As stress activates the sympathetic nervous system, resulting in various physiological responses [126], many studies attempted to objectively measure stress through measuring certain hormones (e.g. cortisol from different sample types [e.g. blood, saliva, hair, urine]), inflammatory markers (e.g. CRP and proinflammatory cytokines like IL-6 and IL-1β), heart rate variability, sleep patterns, genetic polymorphisms (e.g. *5-HTTLPR* polymorphism), epigenetic changes (e.g. DNA methylation), and other biomarkers. Importantly, genetic and epigenetic profiling may not serve as direct markers of stress but can reveal susceptibility to stress and individual variability in stress responses and outcomes. Although not typically used to measure stress, neuroimaging may provide insight into functional or structural brain alterations related to stress. Functional neuroimaging (fMRI) approach may depict the relationship between stress and neural activity and uncover the mechanisms behind emotion processing in the postpartum [110, 127].

With recent modern advances and innovations, a new era in stress monitoring has emerged [128], where different devices and tools can easily be used in measuring physiological and behavioural indicators of stress. For example, wearable devices, such as smartwatches, seem to be a feasible and accessible method to measure heart rate variability [126] which reflects autonomic nervous system functioning and the body's coping with stress. These can also be used to measure sleep patterns, physical activity, and other behavioural factors. Wearable devices enable real-time and continuous tracking of persons' stress responses, providing an objective and easy way to assess indicators of stress over a longer period of time. Such monitoring, paired with machine-learning algorithms, may provide a personalised assessment of risk, alongside fostering early detection and better stress management.

A useful framework for understanding how stress affects maternal health is the allostatic load theory, where allostatic load refers to the cumulative dysregulations of various physiological systems as a response to chronic stress [129–131]. Allostatic load index (ALI) can be calculated by combining multiple measures, including biomarkers and anthropometric indicators including body mass index, waist-hip ratio, resting systolic and diastolic blood pressure, heart rate, CRP, glycosylated haemoglobin, cholesterol (total and high-density lipoprotein), and salivary cortisol diurnal slope [129, 131]. Findings show that ALI is a good measure of chronic stress during the peripartum period, but it is important to account for several relevant factors, such as gestational age [129].

3.7.2 Psychological Measures

Psychological measures of the stress during postpartum are self-report scales which can be differentiated between measures of general stress administered in the postpartum period and postpartum-specific measures. According to a scoping review [132], out of 15 instruments, four general measures are used to assess stress in the postpartum period, such as Perceived Stress Scale [133] and Depression Anxiety Stress Scale (DASS)—the stress subscale [134].

On the other hand, 11 parental measures of stress were identified, focused mainly on mothers, and for a period up to 12 months postpartum, with focus on the first 6 months in majority. However, the psychometric properties of these instruments have been insufficiently studied, and only seven of the 15 identified instruments were psychometrically validated [132]. A promising new postpartum-specific stress self-report tool has been developed and validated recently, Maternal Postpartum Stress Scale [13], which can be used in the whole first year postpartum. The MPSS demonstrated good psychometric properties, with high reliability and consistent factor structure across different countries [33, 34, 135].

3.8 Postpartum Stress Within a Biopsychosocial Framework

It is known that a paradigm or theoretical lenses through which clinicians view a disease, determine its treatment [136]. Therefore, to improve the understanding of the complexity of postpartum stress, an overview of stress through a biopsychosocial perspective is necessary. In sum, the most prominent biopsychosocial correlates and consequences of postpartum stress are presented in Fig. 3.1.

3.9 Research and Clinical Implications

3.9.1 Research Implications

As postpartum stress has received little specific research attention, there are many topics that future studies should address:

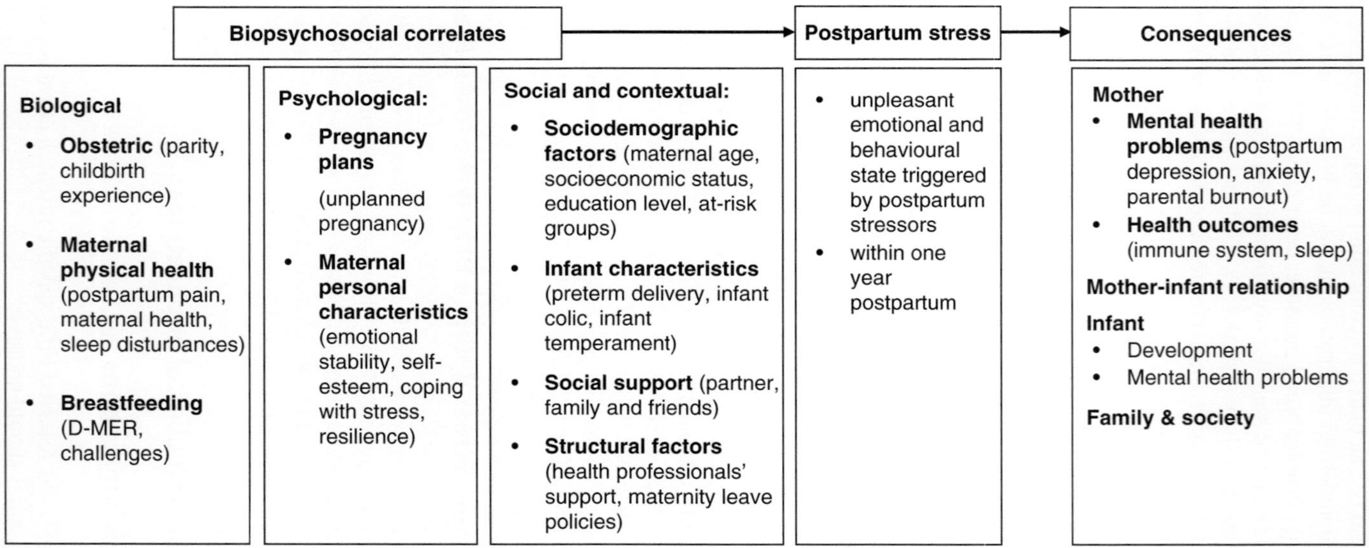

Fig. 3.1 Correlates and consequences of postpartum stress from a biopsychosocial perspective

1. *Stress as a primary construct*: Most research focuses on stress as a predictor of peripartum depression or anxiety, but there is a need to study stress as a focal construct, not just as a risk factor of other mental health issues. Simultaneously investigating depression, anxiety, and stress, with equal emphasis on all three constructs, should be considered in future studies.
2. *Developing biopsychosocial models of peripartum stress*: Considering that present research rarely integrates all aspects of postpartum stress, there is a strong need to incorporate biological and psychosocial dimensions of stress both during pregnancy and postpartum and their interrelationships through a biopsychosocial theoretical framework.
3. *Investigating protective factors of postpartum stress*: As many studies focused on risk factors of peripartum mental health difficulties, a paradigm shift towards exploring protective factors and their buffering effects may benefit the understanding of different outcomes of peripartum stress.
4. *Improvement of research designs and measurements*: Due to many methodological diversities among studies that disable mutual comparison, the standardisation of postpartum stress assessment is needed, with incorporating more modern measures of stress monitoring (e.g., wearable devices). Fostering longitudinal study designs and differentiating between certain types of stressors, sensitive time periods for heightened vulnerability to stressors, and differences between the duration of stress may aid in better understanding peripartum stress. Larger and more representative postpartum populations, including both mothers and fathers, are needed. Marginalised groups (adolescents, immigrants, etc.) may be of interest to future research due to exposure to specific psychological stress.
5. *Prevention and intervention programme effectiveness*: There is a lack of prevention and intervention programmes specifically focused on postpartum stress compared to other postpartum mental health difficulties. Development of such programmes and investigating their feasibility and cost-effectiveness is essential.

3.9.2 Clinical Implications

Considering the vast impact of postpartum stress on the entire family system, there are several steps that may be taken to improve the outcomes and alleviate the personal and global burden of postpartum stress:

1. *Implementation of prevention programmes*: As stress is a factor that can be mitigated through improving coping strategies, strengthening resilience, and prompting relying on social support, cost-effective prevention programmes should be implemented. Utilising modern technology, i.e. mobile applications, may offer a practical and feasible way of mental health monitoring and psychoeducation on stress management.
2. *Pregnancy courses enrichment*: Many pregnant women attend pregnancy courses, which are a great opportunity for mental health education on stress management and techniques for well-being and better coping with parenting

stress (e.g., mindfulness, breathing techniques), which may alleviate challenges in the postpartum period.

3. *Strengthening partner dyad*: Good partner support is proven to be essential for peripartum mental health. Therefore, including partners in education on parenting, recognising mental health difficulties in themselves and their partner, encouraging them in active caregiving, and improving communication skills, sexuality, and other topics may be beneficial for better adaptation to parenthood.
4. *Routine screening for postpartum stress*: Assessing stress as part of postpartum mental health issues seems crucial for identifying women who are struggling but do not meet criteria for other mental health disorders. Screening for elevated stress during the entire peripartum period should be routinely implemented.
5. *Availability of psychological support*: Mothers with high levels of general or postpartum-specific stress should be referred to professionals (preferably specialised experts in peripartum mental health), and this help should be easily accessible and timely. Peripartum women should be priority groups for psychological support.

3.10 Conclusion

Recognising that the postpartum period is accompanied by specific challenges, changes, and demands, and that it is fundamentally different from other periods of life, is essential. Despite ongoing research, stress, especially in the postpartum period, still seems elusive to comprehensive conceptualisation. Postpartum stress, as an emotional and behavioural reaction to specific stressors within the first postpartum year, is still underresearched, unrecognised, and untreated, even though multitude of evidence confirms stress as one of the central factors implicated in poor mental health. Still, there is much to learn and uncover about the complex mechanisms through which postpartum stress is shaped, expressed, and transmitted to the offspring. It remains to distinguish between general and postpartum specific stress, as well as how it interacts with different biological and psychosocial elements. Finally, we have to move further and work towards implementing effective programmes to prevent postpartum stress and alleviate its adverse effects for mothers, infants, and their families.

References

1. Duggar M. Where God guides, he provides! A note to Mothers. The Duggar Family [Internet]. 2016 Apr 21 [cited Feb 10 2025]. Available from: https://www.duggarfamily.com/2016/04/where-god-guides-he-provides-a-note-to-mothers/.
2. Hung CH. Correlates of first-time mothers' postpartum stress. Kaohsiung J Med Sci. 2006;22(10):500–7. https://doi.org/10.1016/s1607-551x(09)70344-4.
3. Berk LE. Development through the lifespan. 7th ed. Pearson; 2018.

4. Razurel C, Bruchon-Schweitzer M, Dupanloup A, Irion O, Epiney M. Stressful events, social support and coping strategies of primiparous women during the postpartum period: a qualitative study. Midwifery. 2011;27(2):237–42. https://doi.org/10.1016/j.midw.2009.06.005.
5. Žutić M. Biopsychosocial models of Peripartum depression: a narrative review. Clínica y Salud. 2023;34(2):91–9. https://doi.org/10.5093/clysa2023a16.
6. Rabinowitz EP, Kutash LA, Richeson AL, Sayer MA, Samii MR, Delahanty DL. Depression, anxiety, and stress in pregnancy and postpartum: a longitudinal study during the COVID-19 pandemic. Midwifery. 2023;121:103655. https://doi.org/10.1016/j.midw.2023.103655.
7. Schalla MA, Stengel A. The role of stress in perinatal depression and anxiety - a systematic review. Front Neuroendocrinol. 2024;72:101117. https://doi.org/10.1016/j.yfrne.2023.101117.
8. Miller RL, Pallant JF, Negri LM. Anxiety and stress in the postpartum: is there more to postnatal distress than depression? BMC Psychiatry. 2006;6:12. https://doi.org/10.1186/1471-244X-6-12.
9. Betts KS, Williams GM, Najman JM, Alati R. The relationship between maternal depressive, anxious, and stress symptoms during pregnancy and adult offspring behavioral and emotional problems. Depress Anxiety. 2015;32(2):82–90. https://doi.org/10.1002/da.22272.
10. Lazarus R, Folkman S. Stress, appraisal, and coping. New York: Springer; 1984.
11. McEwen BS. Central role of the brain in stress and adaptation: allostasis, biological embedding, and cumulative change. In: Fink G, editor. Stress: concepts, cognition, emotion, and behavior. Elsevier; 2016. p. 40–52.
12. Hung CH. The construct of postpartum stress: a concept analysis. J Nurs. 2001;48:69–76.
13. Nakić Radoš S, Brekalo M, Matijaš M. Measuring stress after childbirth: development and validation of maternal postpartum stress scale. J Reprod Infant Psychol. 2023;41(1):65–77. https://doi.org/10.1080/02646838.2021.1940897.
14. Horowitz JA, Damato EG. Mothers' perceptions of postpartum stress and satisfaction. J Obstet Gynecol Neonatal Nurs. 1999;28(6):595–605. https://doi.org/10.1111/j.1552-6909.1999.tb02168.x.
15. Walker LO, Murry N. Maternal stressors and coping strategies during the extended postpartum period: a retrospective analysis with contemporary implications. Womens Health Rep. 2022;3(1):104–14. https://doi.org/10.1089/whr.2021.0134.
16. Wang Y, Wang Y, Huang W, Deng J, Gu J. Association of maternal postpartum depression, anxiety, and stress symptoms: a network analysis. BMC Psychiatry. 2024;24(1):940. https://doi.org/10.1186/s12888-024-06412-9.
17. American Psychiatric Association. Diagnostic and statistical manual of mental disorders. 5th ed. Text revision. Arlington: American Psychiatric Publishing; 2022.
18. Ferrari B, Mesiano L, Benacchio L, Ciulli B, Donolato A, Riolo R. Prevalence and risk factors of postpartum depression and adjustment disorder during puerperium–a retrospective research. J Reprod Infant Psychol. 2021;39(5):486–98. https://doi.org/10.1080/02646838.2020.1786035.
19. Dikmen Yildiz P, Ayers S, Phillips L. Longitudinal trajectories of post-traumatic stress disorder (PTSD) after birth and associated risk factors. J Affect Disord. 2018;229:377–85. https://doi.org/10.1016/j.jad.2017.12.074.
20. Heyne CS, Kazmierczak M, Souday R, Horesh D, Lambregtse-van den Berg M, Weigl T, et al. Prevalence and risk factors of birth-related posttraumatic stress among parents: a comparative systematic review and meta-analysis. Clin Psychol Rev. 2022;94:102157. https://doi.org/10.1016/j.cpr.2022.102157.
21. Horsch A, Garthus-Niegel S, Ayers S, Chandra P, Hartmann K, Vaisbuch E, et al. Childbirth-related posttraumatic stress disorder: definition, risk factors, pathophysiology, diagnosis, prevention, and treatment. Am J Obstet Gynecol. 2024;230(3):S1116–27. https://doi.org/10.1016/j.ajog.2023.09.089.
22. Ayers S, Wright DB, Thornton A. Development of a measure of postpartum PTSD: the city birth trauma scale. Front Psychiatry. 2018;9:409. https://doi.org/10.3389/fpsyt.2018.00409.

23. Albanese AM, Geller PA, Steinkamp JM, Barkin JL. In their own words: a qualitative investigation of the factors influencing maternal postpartum functioning in the United States. Int J Environ Res Public Health. 2020;17(17):6021. https://doi.org/10.3390/ijerph17176021.
24. Ayers S, Bond R, Bertullies S, Wijma K. The aetiology of post-traumatic stress following childbirth: a meta-analysis and theoretical framework. Psychol Med. 2016;46(6):1121–34. https://doi.org/10.1017/S0033291715002706.
25. Glavin K, Leahy-Warren P. Postnatal depression is a public health nursing issue: perspectives from Norway and Ireland. Nurs Res Pract. 2013;2013:1–7. https://doi.org/10.1155/2013/813409.
26. Obrochta CA, Chambers C, Bandoli G. Psychological distress in pregnancy and postpartum. Women Birth. 2020;33(6):583–91. https://doi.org/10.1016/j.wombi.2020.01.009.
27. Lee M-S, Lee JJ, Park S, Kim S, Lee H. Is social support associated with postpartum depression, anxiety and perceived stress among Korean women within the first year postpartum? J Psychosom Obstet Gynaecol. 2023;44(1):2231629. https://doi.org/10.1080/0167482X.2023.2231629.
28. Hannon S, Gartland D, Higgins A, Brown SJ, Carroll M, Begley C, Daly D. Maternal mental health in the first year postpartum in a large Irish population cohort: the MAMMI study. Arch Womens Ment Health. 2022;25(3):641–53. https://doi.org/10.1007/s00737-022-01231-x.
29. Van Lieshout RJ, Savoy CD, Boyle MH, Georgiades K, Jack SM, Niccols A, Whitty H, Lipman EL. The mental health of young Canadian mothers. J Adolesc Health. 2020;66(4):464–9. https://doi.org/10.1016/j.jadohealth.2019.10.024.
30. Mollard E, Kupzyk K, Moore T. Postpartum stress and protective factors in women who gave birth in the United States during the COVID-19 pandemic. Womens Health. 2021;17. https://doi.org/10.1177/17455065211042190.
31. Kolić L, Nakić Radoš S. Prevalence and correlates of general and specific stress in postpartum mothers. UniCath J Biomed Bioeth. 2024;1(2):3–12. Available from: https://unij2b.unicath.hr/wp-content/uploads/2024/12/1.-Prevalence-and-Associated-Factors.pdf.
32. Dušová B, Chromá J, Greplová K, Poláková H. Maternal stress: not just a mental illness, but also a health hazard [Internet]. 2024. https://doi.org/10.21203/rs.3.rs-4411646/v1.
33. Martínez Vázquez S, Ruíz Perete A, de la Torre-Luque A, Nakić Radoš S, Brekalo M, Amezcua-Prieto C, Caparros-Gonzalez RA. Assessment of postpartum stress using the maternal postpartum stress scale (MPSS) in Spanish women. Healthcare. 2024;12:1032. https://doi.org/10.3390/healthcare12101032.
34. Wang Y, Gao Q, Liu J, Zhang F, Xu X. Translation and validation of the Chinese version of the maternal postpartum stress scale. BMC Pregnancy Childbirth. 2023;23(1):685. https://doi.org/10.1186/s12884-023-05990-y.
35. Clout D, Brown R. Sociodemographic, pregnancy, obstetric, and postnatal predictors of postpartum stress, anxiety, and depression in new mothers. J Affect Disord. 2015;188:60–7. https://doi.org/10.1016/j.jad.2015.08.054.
36. DiPietro JA, Costigan KA, Sipsma HL. Continuity in self-report measures of maternal anxiety, stress, and depressive symptoms from pregnancy through two years postpartum. J Psychosom Obstet Gynaecol. 2008;29(2):115–24. https://doi.org/10.1080/01674820701701546.
37. Wang Y, Gu J, Gao Y, Lu Y, Zhang F, Xu X. Postpartum stress in the first 6 months after delivery: a longitudinal study in Nantong, China. BMJ Open. 2023;13(10):e073796. https://doi.org/10.1136/bmjopen-2023-073796.
38. Hantsoo L, Jagodnik KM, Novick AM, Baweja R, di Scalea TL, Ozerdem A, et al. The role of the hypothalamic-pituitary-adrenal axis in depression across the female reproductive lifecycle: current knowledge and future directions. Front Endocrinol. 2023;14:1295261. https://doi.org/10.3389/fendo.2023.1295261.
39. Ketchesin KD, Stinnett GS, Seasholtz AF. Corticotropin-releasing hormone-binding protein and stress: from invertebrates to humans. Stress. 2017;20(5):449–64. https://doi.org/10.1080/10253890.2017.1322575.

40. Vuppaladhadiam L, Ehsan C, Akkati M, Bhargava A. Corticotropin-releasing factor family: a stress hormone-receptor system's emerging role in mediating sex-specific signaling. Cells. 2020;9(4):839. https://doi.org/10.3390/cells9040839.
41. Yim IS, Glynn LM, Dunkel-Schetter C, Hobel CJ, Chicz-DeMet A, Sandman CA. Risk of postpartum depressive symptoms with elevated corticotropin-releasing hormone in human pregnancy. Arch Gen Psychiatry. 2009;66(2):162–9. https://doi.org/10.1001/archgenpsychiatry.2008.533.
42. Stickel S, Eickhoff SB, Habel U, Stickeler E, Goecke TW, Lang J, Chechko N. Endocrine stress response in pregnancy and 12 weeks postpartum - exploring risk factors for postpartum depression. Psychoneuroendocrinology. 2021;125:105122. https://doi.org/10.1016/j.psyneuen.2020.105122.
43. Weiss SJ, Xu L. Postpartum symptoms of anxiety, depression and stress: differential relationships to women's cortisol profiles. Arch Womens Ment Health. 2024;27(3):435–45. https://doi.org/10.1007/s00737-024-01421-9.
44. Figueiredo FP, Parada AP, de Araujo LF, Silva WA Jr, Del-Ben CM. The influence of genetic factors on peripartum depression: a systematic review. J Affect Disord. 2015;172:265–73. https://doi.org/10.1016/j.jad.2014.10.016.
45. Mehta D, Quast C, Fasching PA, Seifert A, Voigt F, Beckmann MW, et al. The 5-HTTLPR polymorphism modulates the influence on environmental stressors on peripartum depression symptoms. J Affect Disord. 2012;136(3):1192–7. https://doi.org/10.1016/j.jad.2011.11.042.
46. Pinheiro RT, Coelho FM, Silva RA, Pinheiro KA, Oses JP, LdeÁ Q, Souza LD, Jansen K, Zimmermann Peruzatto JM, Manfro GG, Giovenardi M, Almeida S, Lucion AB. Association of a serotonin transporter gene polymorphism (5-HTTLPR) and stressful life events with postpartum depressive symptoms: a population-based study. Journal of psychosomatic obstetrics and gynaecology. 2013;34(1):29–33. https://doi.org/10.3109/0167482X.2012.759555.
47. Žutić M. Biopsihosocijalne odrednice peripartalne depresivnosti [Biopsychosocial determinants of peripartum depressiveness] [Doctoral dissertation]. University of Zagreb, Faculty of Humanities and Social Sciences; 2024. Available from: https://urn.nsk.hr/urn:nbn:hr:131:208596.
48. Sales AJ, Guimarães FS, Joca SRL. DNA methylation in stress and depression: from biomarker to therapeutics. Acta Neuropsychiatr. 2021;33(5):217–41. https://doi.org/10.1017/neu.2021.18.
49. Kotsakis Ruehlmann A, Sammallahti S, Cortés Hidalgo AP, Bakulski KM, Binder EB, Campbell ML, et al. Epigenome-wide meta-analysis of prenatal maternal stressful life events and newborn DNA methylation. Mol Psychiatry. 2023;28(12):5090–100. https://doi.org/10.1038/s41380-023-02010-5.
50. Salari P, Nazari S, Mazlom SR, Ghanbari Hashem Abadi BA. Comparing postpartum stressors and social support level in primiparous and multiparous women. J Midwifery Reprod Health. 2014;2:71–6. https://doi.org/10.22038/jmrh.2013.2000.
51. Hung CH. Predictors of postpartum women's health status. J Nurs Scholarsh. 2004;36(4):345–51. https://doi.org/10.1111/j.1547-5069.2004.04062.x.
52. Hung CH, Lin CJ, Stocker J, Yu CY. Predictors of postpartum stress. J Clin Nurs. 2011;20(5–6):666–74. https://doi.org/10.1111/j.1365-2702.2010.03555.x.
53. Kristensen IH, Simonsen M, Trillingsgaard T, Pontoppidan M, Kronborg H. First-time mothers' confidence, mood, and stress in the first months postpartum: a cohort study. Sex Reprod Healthc. 2018;17:43–9. https://doi.org/10.1016/j.srhc.2018.06.003.
54. Krieg DB. Does motherhood get easier the second time around? Examining parenting stress and marital quality among mothers having their first or second child. Parenting. 2007;7(2):149–75. https://doi.org/10.1080/15295190701306912.
55. Mercer RT. Becoming a mother: research on maternal identity from Rubin to the present. New York: Springer Publishing Company; 1995.
56. Hinic K. Understanding and promoting birth satisfaction in new mothers. MCN Am J Matern Child Nurs. 2017;42(4):210–5. https://doi.org/10.1097/nmc.0000000000000345.

57. Makeen M, Farrell LM, LaSorda KR, et al. Associations between postpartum pain, mood, and maternal–infant attachment and parenting outcomes. Sci Rep. 2022;12:17814. https://doi.org/10.1038/s41598-022-21793-1.
58. Schaffir J, Kunkler A, Lynch CD, Benedict J, Soma L, Doering A. Association between postpartum physical symptoms and mood. J Psychosom Res. 2018;107:33–7. https://doi.org/10.1016/j.jpsychores.2018.02.003.
59. Cheng CY, Li Q. Integrative review of research on general health status and prevalence of common physical health conditions of women after childbirth. Womens Health Issues. 2008;18(4):267–80. https://doi.org/10.1016/j.whi.2008.02.004.
60. Strahm AM, Mitchell AM, Pan X, Christian LM. Repetitive negative thinking during pregnancy and postpartum: associations with mental health, inflammation, and breastfeeding. J Affect Disord. 2022;319:497–506. https://doi.org/10.1016/j.jad.2022.09.067.
61. Lewis BA, Schuver K, Dunsiger S, Samson L, Frayeh AL, Terrell CA, et al. Randomized trial examining the effect of exercise and wellness interventions on preventing postpartum depression and perceived stress. BMC Pregnancy Childbirth. 2021;21(1):42. https://doi.org/10.1186/s12884-021-04257-8.
62. McQuillan ME, Bates JE, Staples AD, Deater-Deckard K. Maternal stress, sleep, and parenting. J Fam Psychol. 2019;33(3):349–59. https://doi.org/10.1037/fam0000516.
63. Whitesell CJ, Crosby B, Anders TF, Teti DM. Household chaos and family sleep during infants' first year. J Fam Psychol. 2018;32(5):622–31. https://doi.org/10.1037/fam0000422.
64. Wang Y, Gu J, Zhang F, Xu X. The multiple mediation model of social support and postpartum anxiety symptomatology: the role of resilience, postpartum stress, and sleep problems. BMC Psychiatry. 2024;24(1):630. https://doi.org/10.1186/s12888-024-06087-2.
65. Žutić M, Matijaš M, Nakić Radoš S. Dysphoric Milk ejection reflex: measurement, prevalence, clinical features, maternal mental health, and mother-infant bonding. Breastfeed Med. 2024. Advance online publication. https://doi.org/10.1089/bfm.2024.0172.
66. Grattan RE, London SM, Bueno GE. Perceived pressure to breastfeed negatively impacts postpartum mental health outcomes over time. Front Public Health. 2024;12:1357965. https://doi.org/10.3389/fpubh.2024.1357965.
67. Gila-Díaz A, Carrillo GH, López de Pablo ÁL, Arribas SM, Ramiro-Cortijo D. Association between maternal postpartum depression, stress, optimism, and breastfeeding pattern in the first six months. Int J Environ Res Public Health. 2020;17(19):7153. https://doi.org/10.3390/ijerph17197153.
68. Mezzacappa ES, Guethlein W, Vaz N, Bagiella E. A preliminary study of breast-feeding and maternal symptomatology. Ann Behav Med. 2000;22(1):71–9. https://doi.org/10.1007/bf02895170.
69. Mizuhata K, Taniguchi H, Hikita N, Shimada M, Morokuma S. Effects of breastfeeding on stress measured by saliva cortisol level and perceived stress. Asian/Pacific Island Nursing Journal. 2020;5(3):128–38. https://doi.org/10.31372/20200503.1100.
70. Chou FH, Avant KC, Kuo SH, Fetzer SJ. Relationships between nausea and vomiting, perceived stress, social support, pregnancy planning, and psychosocial adaptation in a sample of mothers: a questionnaire survey. Int J Nurs Stud. 2008;45(8):1185–91. https://doi.org/10.1016/j.ijnurstu.2007.08.004.
71. Gariepy AM, Lundsberg LS, Miller D, Stanwood NL, Yonkers KA. Are pregnancy planning and pregnancy timing associated with maternal psychiatric illness, psychological distress and support during pregnancy? J Affect Disord. 2017;205:87–94. https://doi.org/10.1016/j.jad.2016.06.058.
72. Charney DS, Manji HK. Life stress, genes and depression: multiple pathways lead to increased risk and new opportunities for intervention. Sci Signal. 2004;225:re5. https://doi.org/10.1126/stke.2252004re5.
73. Reić Ercegovac I, Penezić Z. Zadovoljstvo životom, depresivnost i stres kod žena tijekom trudnoće i prve godine postpartalno – uloga osobina ličnosti, zadovoljstva brakom i socijalne podrške [Life satisfaction, depression and stress in women during pregnancy and first year

postpartum – the role of personality traits, marital satisfaction and social support]. Klinička psihologija. 2011;1–2:5–22.
74. Julian M, Somers JA, Dunkel Schetter C, Guardino CM. Resilience resources, life stressors, and postpartum depressive symptoms in a community sample of low and middle-income Black, Latina, and White mothers. Stress Health. 2024;40(1):e3275. https://doi.org/10.1002/smi.3275.
75. Pan Y, Li F, Liang H, Shen X, Bing Z, Cheng L, et al. Effectiveness of mindfulness-based stress reduction on mental health and psychological quality of life among university students: a grade-assessed systematic review. Evid Based Complement Alternat Med. 2024;2024:1–30. https://doi.org/10.1155/2024/8872685.
76. Henretta JC, Grundy EM, Okell LC, Wadsworth ME. Early motherhood and mental health in midlife: a study of British and American cohorts. Aging Ment Health. 2008;12(5):605–14. https://doi.org/10.1080/13607860802343308.
77. Saur AM, dos Santos MA. Risk factors associated with stress symptoms during pregnancy and postpartum: integrative literature review. Women Health. 2021;61(7):651–67. https://doi.org/10.1080/03630242.2021.1954132.
78. Kubo A, Ferrara A, Brown SD, Ehrlich SF, Tsai AL, Quesenberry CP, et al. Perceived psychosocial stress and gestational weight gain among women with gestational diabetes. PLoS One. 2017;12(3):e0174290. https://doi.org/10.1371/journal.pone.0174290.
79. Lara-Cinisomo S, Girdler SS, Grewen K, Meltzer-Brody S. A biopsychosocial conceptual framework of postpartum depression risk in immigrant and U.S.-born Latina mothers in the United States. Womens Health Issues. 2016;26(3):336–43. https://doi.org/10.1016/j.whi.2016.02.006.
80. Lockwood Estrin G, Ryan EG, Trevillion K, Demilew J, Bick D, Pickles A, Howard LM. Young pregnant women and risk for mental disorders: findings from an early pregnancy cohort. BJPsych Open. 2019;5(2):e21. https://doi.org/10.1192/bjo.2019.6.
81. Hendy A, El-Sayed S, Bakry S, Mohammed SM, Mohamed H, Abdelkawy A, et al. The stress levels of premature infants' parents and related factors in NICU. SAGE Open Nurs. 2024;10:23779608241231172. https://doi.org/10.1177/23779608241231172.
82. Shetty AP, Halemani K, Issac A, Thimmappa L, Dhiraaj S, K R, Mishra P, Upadhyaya VD. Prevalence of anxiety, depression, and stress among parents of neonates admitted to neonatal intensive care unit: a systematic review and meta-analysis. Clin Exp Pediatr. 2024;67(2):104–15. https://doi.org/10.3345/cep.2023.00486.
83. Landgren K, Hallström I. Parents' experience of living with a baby with infantile colic: a phenomenological hermeneutic study. Scand J Caring Sci. 2010;25(2):317–24. https://doi.org/10.1111/j.1471-6712.2010.00829.x.
84. Türkmen H, Akın B, Aksoy YE, Erdoğan A. Maternal attachment and mental health status in mothers who have babies with infantile colic. Midwifery. 2022;110:103339. https://doi.org/10.1016/j.midw.2022.103339.
85. Garnacho-Garnacho VE, Rodríguez-López ES, Oliva-Pascual-Vaca A, Goenaga-Echave L, Otero-Campos Á. Maternal psychological well-being as a protector in infantile colic. Nutrients. 2024;16:42342. https://doi.org/10.3390/nu16142342.
86. Tolja R, Nakić Radoš S, Anđelinović M. The role of maternal mental health, infant temperament, and couple's relationship quality for mother-infant bonding. J Reprod Infant Psychol. 2020;38(4):395–407. https://doi.org/10.1080/02646838.2020.1733503.
87. Vukšić N, Žutić M, Nakić RS. Razlike u percipiranom temperamentu dojenčeta, povezivanju s dojenčetom i mentalnom zdravlju između majki koje doje i ne doje [Differences in perceived infant temperament, bonding, and mental health between breastfeeding and non-breastfeeding mothers]. Psihologijske teme. 2022;31(2):359–81. https://doi.org/10.31820/pt.31.2.8.
88. Houts RM, Barnett-Walker KC, Paley B, Cox MJ. Patterns of couple interaction during the transition to parenthood. Pers Relat. 2008;15(1):103–22. https://doi.org/10.1111/j.1475-6811.2007.00187.x.

89. Tissera H, Auger E, Séguin L, Kramer MS, Lydon JE. Happy prenatal relationships, healthy postpartum mothers: a prospective study of relationship satisfaction, postpartum stress, and health. Psychol Health. 2020;36(4):461–77. https://doi.org/10.1080/08870446.2020.1766040.
90. Stapleton LR, Schetter CD, Westling E, Rini C, Glynn LM, Hobel CJ, Sandman CA. Perceived partner support in pregnancy predicts lower maternal and infant distress. J Fam Psychol. 2012;26(3):453–63. https://doi.org/10.1037/a0028332.
91. Cairney J, Boyle M, Offord DR, Racine Y. Stress, social support and depression in single and married mothers. Soc Psychiatry Psychiatr Epidemiol. 2003;38(8):442–9. https://doi.org/10.1007/s00127-003-0661-0.
92. Marks NF, McLanahan SS. Gender, family structure, and social support among parents. J Marriage Fam. 1993;55(2):481–93. https://doi.org/10.2307/352817.
93. Navidian A, Safarzadeh Sarasiyabi A, Koochakzai M. The effect of home-based supportive-educational counseling on Primigravidas' postpartum stress. Int J Womens Health Reprod Sci. 2016;5(2):112–8. https://doi.org/10.15296/ijwhr.2017.21.
94. Addati L, Cassirer N, Gilchrist K. Maternity and paternity at work: law and practice across the world. International Labor Office; 2014. Available from: https://www.ilo.org/sites/default/files/wcmsp5/groups/public/@dgreports/@dcomm/@publ/documents/publication/wcms_242615.pdf.
95. Hidalgo-Padilla L, Toyama M, Zafra-Tanaka JH, Vives A, Diez-Canseco F. Association between maternity leave policies and postpartum depression: a systematic review. Arch Womens Ment Health. 2023;26(5):571–80. https://doi.org/10.1007/s00737-023-01350-z.
96. Beck C. Predictors of postpartum depression: an update. Nurs Res. 2001;50(5):275–85. https://doi.org/10.1097/00006199-200109000-00004.
97. Dennis CL, Falah-Hassani K, Brown HK, Vigod SN. Identifying women at risk for postpartum anxiety: a prospective population-based study. Acta Psychiatr Scand. 2016;134(6):485–93. https://doi.org/10.1111/acps.12648.
98. Hutchens BF, Kearney J. Risk factors for postpartum depression: an umbrella review. J Midwifery Womens Health. 2020;65(1):96–108. https://doi.org/10.1111/jmwh.13067.
99. Al-Abri K, Edge D, Armitage CJ. Prevalence and correlates of perinatal depression. Soc Psychiatry Psychiatr Epidemiol. 2023;58(11):1581–90. https://doi.org/10.1007/s00127-022-02386-9.
100. Slomian J, Honvo G, Emonts P, Reginster JY, Bruyère O. Consequences of maternal postpartum depression: a systematic review of maternal and infant outcomes. Womens Health. 2019;15:1745506519844044. https://doi.org/10.1177/1745506519844044.
101. Mikolajczak M, Raes M-E, Avalosse H, Roskam I. Exhausted parents: sociodemographic, child-related, parent-related, parenting and family-functioning correlates of parental burnout. J Child Fam Stud. 2018;27(2):602–14. https://doi.org/10.1007/s10826-017-0892-4.
102. Mikolajczak M, Roskam I. Parental burnout: moving the focus from children to parents. New Dir Child Adolesc Dev. 2020;174:7–13. https://doi.org/10.1002/cad.20376.
103. Roskam I, Aguiar J, Akgun E, Arikan G, Artavia M, Avalosse H, Aunola K, Bader M, Bahati C, Barham EJ, Besson E, Beyers W, Boujut E, Brianda ME, Brytek-Matera A, Carbonneau N, César F, Chen BB, Dorard G, Dos Santos Elias LC, et al. Parental burnout around the globe: a 42-country study. Affect Sci. 2021;2(1):58–79. https://doi.org/10.1007/s42761-020-00028-4.
104. Plantaš A, Nakić Radoš S. Some psychosocial predictors of parental burnout in mothers of children below five years old. Društvena istraživanja [Internet]. 2024;33(4):503–25. [Accessed 2025 Feb 10]. https://doi.org/10.5559/di.33.4.02.
105. Lindström C, Aman J, Norberg AL. Increased prevalence of burnout symptoms in parents of chronically ill children. Acta Paediatr. 2010;99(3):427–32. https://doi.org/10.1111/j.1651-2227.2009.01586.x.
106. Guardino CM, Dunkel Schetter C, Hobel CJ, Gaines Lanzi R, Schafer P, Thorp JM, et al. Chronic stress and C-reactive protein in mothers during the first postpartum year. Psychosom Med. 2017;79(4):450–60. https://doi.org/10.1097/PSY.0000000000000424.

107. Christian LM, Kowalsky JM, Mitchell AM, Porter K. Associations of postpartum sleep, stress, and depressive symptoms with LPS-stimulated cytokine production among African American and White women. J Neuroimmunol. 2018;316:98–106. https://doi.org/10.1016/j.jneuroim.2017.12.020.
108. Groer ME, Jevitt C, Ji M. Immune changes and dysphoric moods across the postpartum. Am J Reprod Immunol. 2015;73(3):193–208. https://doi.org/10.1111/aji.12322.
109. Kim P. How stress can influence brain adaptations to motherhood. Front Neuroendocrinol. 2021;60:100875. https://doi.org/10.1016/j.yfrne.2020.100875.
110. Grande LA, Olsavsky AK, Erhart A, Dufford AJ, Tribble R, Phan KL, Kim P. Postpartum stress and neural regulation of emotion among first-time mothers. Cogn Affect Behav Neurosci. 2021;21(5):1066–82. https://doi.org/10.3758/s13415-021-00914-9.
111. Rossen L, Hutchinson D, Wilson J, Burns L, Allsop S, Elliott EJ, et al. Maternal bonding through pregnancy and postnatal: findings from an Australian longitudinal study. Am J Perinatol. 2017;34(8):808–17. https://doi.org/10.1055/s-0037-1599052.
112. Nakić Radoš S, Hairston I, Handelzalts JE. The concept analysis of parent-infant bonding during pregnancy and infancy: a systematic review and meta-synthesis. J Reprod Infant Psychol. 2024;42(2):142–65. https://doi.org/10.1080/02646838.2022.
113. Nakić Radoš S, Matijaš M, Anđelinović M, Čartolovni A, Ayers S. The role of posttraumatic stress and depression symptoms in mother-infant bonding. J Affect Disord. 2020;268:134–40. https://doi.org/10.1016/j.jad.2020.03.006.
114. Nicol-Harper R, Harvey AG, Stein A. Interactions between mothers and infants: impact of maternal anxiety. Infant Behav Dev. 2007;30:161–7. https://doi.org/10.1016/j.infbeh.2006.08.005.
115. Tichelman E, Westerneng M, Witteveen AB, Van Baar AL, Van Der Horst HE, De Jonge A, et al. Correlates of prenatal and postnatal mother-to-infant bonding quality: a systematic review. PLoS One. 2019;14(9):e0222998. https://doi.org/10.1371/journal.pone.0222998.
116. Nakić Radoš S. Parental sensitivity and responsiveness as mediators between postpartum mental health and bonding in mothers and fathers. Front Psychiatry. 2021;12:723418. https://doi.org/10.3389/fpsyt.2021.723418.
117. Nordahl D, Rognmo K, Bohne A, Landsem IP, Moe V, Wang CEA, et al. Adult attachment style and maternal-infant bonding: the indirect path of parenting stress. BMC Psychol. 2020;8:1–11. https://doi.org/10.1186/s40359-020-00424-2.
118. Power C, Weise V, Mack JT, Karl M, Garthus-Niegel S. Does parental mental health mediate the association between parents' perceived stress and parent-infant bonding during the early COVID-19 pandemic? Early Hum Dev. 2024;189:105931. https://doi.org/10.1016/j.earlhumdev.2023.105931.
119. O'Dea GA, Youssef GJ, Hagg LJ, Francis LM, Spry EA, Rossen L, et al. Associations between maternal psychological distress and mother-infant bonding: a systematic review and meta-analysis. Arch Womens Ment Health. 2023;26(4):441–52. https://doi.org/10.1007/s00737-023-01332-1.
120. Schmeer KK, Guardino C, Irwin JL, Ramey S, Shalowitz M, Dunkel SC. Maternal postpartum stress and toddler developmental delays: results from a multisite study of racially diverse families. Dev Psychobiol. 2020;62(1):62–76. https://doi.org/10.1002/dev.21871.
121. Abrishamcar S, Zhuang BC, Thomas M, Gladish N, MacIsaac JL, Jones MJ, et al. Association between maternal perinatal stress and depression and infant DNA methylation in the first year of life. Transl Psychiatry. 2024;14(1):445. https://doi.org/10.1038/s41398-024-03148-8.
122. World Health Organization. Maternal mental health. Available from: https://www.who.int/teams/mental-health-and-substance-use/promotion-prevention/maternal-mental-health.
123. Margiotta C, Gao J, O'Neil S, Vohra D, Zivin K. The economic impact of untreated maternal mental health conditions in Texas. BMC Pregnancy Childbirth. 2022;22(1):50. https://doi.org/10.1186/s12884-022-05001-6.
124. Bauer A, Tinelli M, Knapp M. The economic case for increasing access to treatment for women with common mental health problems during the perinatal period. London: Care

Policy and Evaluation Centre; 2022. Available from: https://www.lse.ac.uk/cpec/assets/documents/CPEC-Perinatal-Economics-2022.pdf.
125. Štěpáníková I, Baker E, Oates G, Bienertova-Vasku J, Klánová J. Assessing stress in pregnancy and postpartum: comparing measures. Matern Child Health J. 2020;24(10):1193–201. https://doi.org/10.1007/s10995-020-02978-4.
126. Niela-Vilen H, Ekholm E, Sarhaddi F, Azimi I, Rahmani AM, Liljeberg P, et al. Comparing prenatal and postpartum stress among women with previous adverse pregnancy outcomes and normal obstetric histories: a longitudinal cohort study. Sex Reprod Healthc. 2023;35:100820. https://doi.org/10.1016/j.srhc.2023.100820.
127. Gingnell M, Toffoletto S, Wikström J, Engman J, Bannbers E, Comasco E, Sundström-Poromaa I. Emotional anticipation after delivery – a longitudinal neuroimaging study of the postpartum period. Sci Rep. 2017;7:114. https://doi.org/10.1038/s41598-017-00146-3.
128. Kafková J, Kuchár P, Pirník R, Skuba M, Tichý T, Brož J. A new era in stress monitoring: a review of embedded devices and tools for detecting stress in the workplace. Electronics. 2024;13(19):3899. https://doi.org/10.3390/electronics13193899.
129. Li Y, Dalton VK, Lee SJ, Rosemberg MS, Seng JS. Exploring the validity of allostatic load in pregnant women. Midwifery. 2020;82:102621. https://doi.org/10.1016/j.midw.2019.102621.
130. Li Y, Rosemberg MS, Seng JS. Allostatic load: a theoretical model for understanding the relationship between maternal posttraumatic stress disorder and adverse birth outcomes. Midwifery. 2018;62:205–13. https://doi.org/10.1016/j.midw.2018.04.002.
131. Ross KM, Kane HS, Guardino C, Schetter CD. Parental attachment anxiety: associations with allostatic load in mothers of 1-year-olds. J Soc Personal Relat. 2020;37(3):717–37. https://doi.org/10.1177/0265407519876717.
132. Øygarden AMU, Berg RC, Abudayya A, Glavin K, Strøm BS. Measurement instruments for parental stress in the postpartum period: a scoping review. PLoS One. 2022;17(3):e0265616. https://doi.org/10.1371/journal.pone.0265616.
133. Cohen S, Kamarck T, Mermelstein R. A global measure of perceived stress. J Health Soc Behav. 1983;24(4):385–96. https://doi.org/10.2307/2136404.
134. Lovibond PF, Lovibond SH. The structure of negative emotional states: comparison of the Depression Anxiety Stress Scales (DASS) with the Beck Depression and Anxiety Inventories. Behav Res Ther. 1995;33(3):335–43. https://doi.org/10.1016/0005-7967(94)00075-U.
135. Lochmannová A, Martin CR, Nakić Radoš S. Translation and validation of the czech version of the maternal postpartum stress scale. Int J Childbirth. 2025. https://doi.org/10.1891/IJC-2025-0004.
136. Beck CT. Theoretical perspectives of postpartum depression and their treatment implications. MCN Am J Matern Child Nurs. 2002;27(5):282–7. https://doi.org/10.1097/00005721-200209000-00008.

Intimate Partner Violence During Pregnancy and the Postpartum: An Increasing Problem Worldwide

4

Lorena Mesa-Melgarejo and Rafael A. Caparros-Gonzalez

Abstract

Intimate partner violence during pregnancy (IPV-P) is a significant yet often underrecognized public health issue with serious implications for maternal, fetal, and neonatal health. Despite global commitments to eradicate gender-based violence, IPV remains the most widespread human rights violation worldwide, disproportionately affecting women in vulnerable conditions and resource-limited settings. This chapter presents the findings of a scoping review conducted to examine the global prevalence, associated risk factors, health and social consequences, and policy and clinical challenges related to IPV-P. The aim is to contribute to the growing body of evidence that supports the need for systematic detection and intervention strategies within health systems. A systematic search was carried out across bibliographic databases without restrictions on study design or publication type. Studies published in English, Spanish, or Portuguese between 2003 and 2025 were included, yielding 75 studies from 68 countries. The analysis incorporated cross-sectional studies, systematic reviews, and cohort studies. Data were extracted on IPV prevalence, contributing factors, and reported impacts. The results show the prevalence rates of IPV-P ranged from 4% to 65%, with higher rates reported in sub-Saharan Africa, Southeast Asia, and Latin America. Emotional and psychological abuse were the most frequently reported forms of IPV during pregnancy, though physical and sexual violence were also significant. Risk

L. Mesa-Melgarejo (✉)
Institute for Health Technology Assessment (IETS), Bogotá, Colombia
e-mail: lorena.mesa@iets.org.co

R. A. Caparros-Gonzalez
Faculty of Health Sciences, Department of Nursing, University of Granada, Granada, Spain

Instituto de Investigacion Biosanitaria Ibs.GRANADA, Granada, Spain

R. A. Caparros-Gonzalez (ed.), *Maternal Stress during Pregnancy and Postpartum*, https://doi.org/10.1007/978-3-032-09245-8_4

factors were classified using an ecological model, highlighting individual (e.g., low education, early pregnancy, mental health conditions), relational (e.g., partner unemployment, substance use, lack of social support), community (e.g., normalization of violence, limited healthcare access), and structural (e.g., gender inequality, economic instability) determinants. The consequences of IPV-P were substantial and included preterm birth, low birth weight, neonatal intensive care admission, and postpartum depression. Women with disabilities, adolescents, and displaced or refugee populations were at greater risk. The findings underscore the urgency of integrating routine IPV screening into prenatal care, developing standardized surveillance systems, and ensuring that health professionals are trained in early detection and appropriate response. Furthermore, the chapter advocates for the application of an intersectional lens in public health policies to recognize and respond to the complex vulnerabilities experienced by pregnant women.

Keywords

Exposure to violence · Abuse · Pregnancy harms · Maternal welfare · Pregnancy complications

4.1 Introduction

The elimination of all forms of gender-based violence is one of the key targets of the Sustainable Development Goals (SDGs) for 2030 and a priority for achieving global equity. However, gender-based violence remains the most widespread violation of human rights [52]. According to a global study conducted by the World Health Organization (WHO) in 2021 across 159 countries, intimate partner violence (IPV) is the most prevalent form of violence against women worldwide. The study reported that 24%—that is, one in four women aged 15 to 49—experience IPV in their lifetime and 13% had experienced at least one episode of physical or sexual violence by a partner in the previous 12 months [68].

These figures are significantly higher in low-income countries and in regions such as Oceania, Southern Asia, and sub-Saharan Africa, where prevalence rates range between 33% and 51%. By contrast, "the lowest rates are found in Europe (16–23%), Central Asia (18%), Eastern Asia (20%), and South-Eastern Asia (21%)" [68] (see Fig. 4.1).

IPV encompasses a broad spectrum of behaviors and actions, including physical violence, sexual violence, coercion, economic abuse, stalking, and psychological harm inflicted by a present or former intimate partner [56]. The health consequences of IPV vary in type and severity and may result in both short- and long-term harm [4]. Nonetheless, the literature consistently acknowledges that all acts of violence leave enduring effects—not only on the victims but also on the perpetrators and the communities in which they live [56].

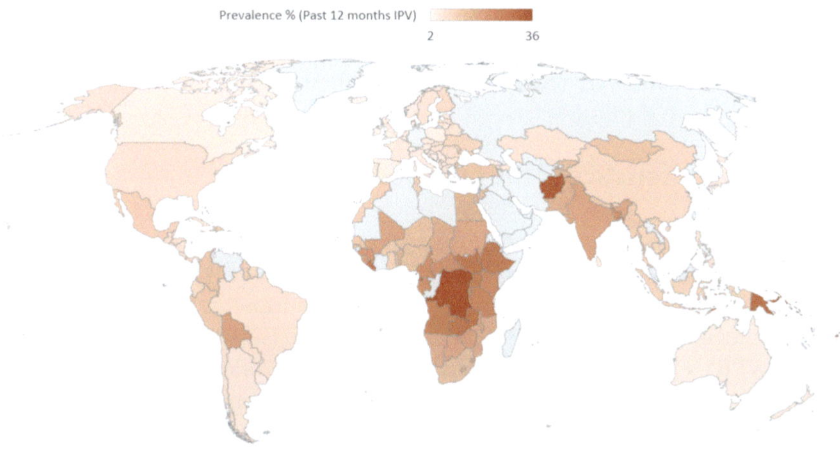

Fig. 4.1 Prevalence of IPV in women 15–49 age group, by country (2018). (Source: Prepared by the authors based on WHO [68])

In line with this, several studies suggest that the effects of IPV during pregnancy (perinatal IPV, or IPV-P) may be especially harmful, with consequences that extend to the fetus, newborn, and early childhood development [5, 34, 35, 66, 69]. While some research has suggested that IPV prevalence may decrease during pregnancy, evidence indicates that this decline is not sustained over time and may even rise during the first postpartum year [19].

Over the past decade, IPV-P has garnered increasing visibility and attention due to its relevance and the urgent need for integrated interventions. Prenatal screening for IPV is a crucial strategy to mitigate the negative impact of violence on pregnant women and their children and also to identify risk factors that can inform appropriate responses within the health system. This requires acknowledging both the scope of IPV and the specific patterns and impacts associated with the perinatal period.

In this context, the present chapter presents the findings of a scoping review on the prevalence, risk factors, and health and social consequences of perinatal partner violence, as well as the challenges this phenomenon poses for clinicians and policymakers.

4.2 Methodological Considerations

This chapter is based on a scoping review [54], which included a systematic search of the literature across bibliographic databases, followed by a selection and synthesis process of relevant publications. Since this is a scoping review with a systematic and comprehensive approach, no restrictions were placed on study design or publication type. A formal quality appraisal of the included studies was not conducted. Studies published in English, Spanish, and Portuguese, and available in full-text format, were considered eligible. The search yielded a total of 7141 references, of which 351 were selected based on title screening. After applying the inclusion criteria, 75 publications were retained for final synthesis.

4.2.1 Characteristics of the Included Studies

The studies included span the period from 2003 to 2025 and cover data from 68 different countries. Two studies reported findings according to WHO regions: African region (AFR), region of the Americas (AMR), Southeast Asian region (SEAR), European region (EUR), Eastern Mediterranean region (EMR), and Western Pacific region (WPR). One study presented findings based on World Bank income classification (low-, lower-middle-, upper-middle-, and high-income countries). The largest number of studies was conducted in sub-Saharan African countries, followed by those from Asia and Europe.

The year 2024 accounted for the highest number of publications, with a total of 18 studies. The figure depicting the number of studies per year shows a growing trend in publications addressing IPV-P, particularly during the last decade and even more so in the post-COVID-19 pandemic years (Fig. 4.2). In terms of study design, cross-sectional studies represented 65% of the sample, followed by systematic reviews and cohort studies.

4.2.2 Methodological Challenges

The included studies employed a wide variety of instruments and methodological approaches to estimate IPV-P prevalence. Variations were identified in the types of violence assessed, the measurement timepoints (e.g., lifetime, prepregnancy, during pregnancy, postpartum), and the definitions of IPV, all of which limit comparability

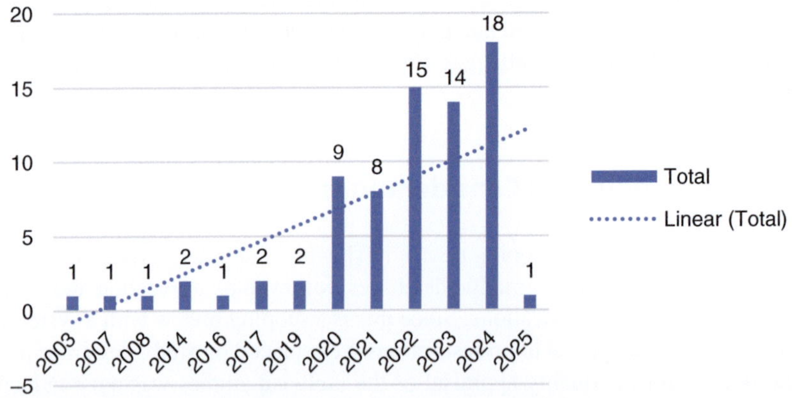

Fig. 4.2 Number of studies by year. (Source: Prepared by the authors)

across contexts and countries. Most studies were cross-sectional, which constrains the ability to establish causal relationships between IPV and maternal or neonatal outcomes. Nonetheless, the findings represent a rich source of hypotheses and potential lines of inquiry for further research.

It is noteworthy that vulnerable populations—including adolescents, refugees, women with disabilities, and migrants—were considered in several of the included studies. This contributes to closing the knowledge gaps surrounding IPV-P among these populations. However, the majority of studies were conducted in urban areas with access to healthcare services, which may lead to underestimation of IPV prevalence in rural or remote settings—a factor identified as critical in the general population of women [68].

According to the authors of the included studies, the main challenges in IPV-P research lie in ethical, methodological, and social dimensions. These include the normalization of violence, fear of stigma or retaliation from partners, and economic dependence, all of which act as barriers to disclosure for pregnant women. Such barriers likely contribute to systematic underreporting of IPV, thereby obscuring the true magnitude of the problem.

4.3 Global Prevalence of Partner Violence During Pregnancy and the Postpartum Period

Intimate partner violence against pregnant women is a widespread and persistent global phenomenon, as evidenced by the findings of this review, which synthesizes data from diverse cultural, economic, and geographic contexts. Despite methodological variations across studies, a concerning pattern of exposure to various forms of violence, physical, sexual, and emotional, during pregnancy is consistently identified, with significant implications for maternal, fetal, and neonatal health.

The reported prevalence rates in the included studies are alarming. In some contexts, more than 50% of pregnant or postpartum women reported having experienced IPV. For instance, rates as high as 61.5% in Papua New Guinea [3], 64.1% in Malaysia [48], and 52.2% in Brazil [15] have been documented. Table 4.1 summarizes the prevalence rates reported across the included studies in this scoping review.

From a global perspective, the meta-analysis by Chen et al. [19] estimates that 12.8% of pregnant women have experienced IPV during pregnancy. This is lower than the reported lifetime or prepregnancy prevalence (21.2%) but increases again in the postpartum period (14.7%), especially beyond the first 12 months after childbirth. The study also highlights substantial regional and income-based disparities, with higher prevalence rates observed in low- and middle-income countries, particularly in Southeast Asia and the Eastern Mediterranean region. These findings were further supported by Wong et al. [66] and Mella et al. [43], who reported prevalence estimates of 28.4% for emotional IPV, 13.8% for physical IPV, and 8% for sexual IPV, with significantly higher rates in countries with greater gender inequality and sociocultural norms that justify violence against women.

Table 4.1 IPV-P prevalence reported by studies included

Item	Authors	Year	Country	Study objective	Reported IPV-P prevalence (pregnancy)
1	Abrha et al.	2024	Ethiopia	To determine the prevalence of IPV during pregnancy and its correlates using PMA data	16.7% (12.5% sexual, 7% physical)
2	Abujilban et al.	2021	Jordan	To compare the prevalence of IPV before and during pregnancy and identify predictors of physical violence	Control 93.1%, psychological 66%, physical 31.2%, and sexual 8.9%
3	Adebowale et al.	2020	Nigeria	To determine the prevalence of IPV and its association with psychiatric morbidity and alcohol use by the partner	24.8% IPV in last 12 months (mostly emotional)
4	Agyemang-Duah et al.	2024	Papua New Guinea	To analyze the relationship between IPV and pregnancy termination using national survey data	61.5% of women reported IPV; 6.3% had terminated at least one pregnancy
5	Al Shidhani et al.	2020	Oman	To identify the prevalence of domestic violence (emotional and physical) during lifetime, year before pregnancy, and during pregnancy and its effects on perinatal outcomes	16.8% lifetime; 2.7% year before; 1.6% during pregnancy (Oman sample)
6	Albini et al.	2023	USA	To characterize injuries and identify risk factors of IPV in pregnant women attending emergency departments	Hospital data: 556 IPV-P cases between 2010 and 2014
7	Alhusen et al.	2024	USA	To compare the prevalence of perinatal IPV in women with and without disabilities	Women with disabilities: 2.6 times higher odds of IPV before and during pregnancy
8	Alhusen et al.	2019	USA	To review the effects of IPV on maternal and neonatal health during pregnancy	3–9%, up to 50% in high-risk groups
9	Al-Marhabi et al.	2023	Saudi Arabia	To evaluate maternal and fetal outcomes among pregnant women exposed to violence	42.9% of women reported some form of violence during pregnancy

(continued)

Table 4.1 (continued)

Item	Authors	Year	Country	Study objective	Reported IPV-P prevalence (pregnancy)
10	Ambachew Kebede et al.	2022	Ethiopia	To evaluate the magnitude of IPV during pregnancy and its association with social support and decision-making power	48.6% in postpartum women in Gondar
11	Aslam et al.	2024	Pakistan	To explore factors associated with domestic violence among pregnant women and its impact on maternal and perinatal health	Total 31.4% (psychological 16.4%, sexual 9.5%, physical 1.8%)
12	Atilla et al.	2023	Turkey	To determine the prevalence of IPV during the COVID-19 pandemic and associated factors in pregnant women	44.1% during the pandemic
13	Atsbaha et al.	2022	Ethiopia	To estimate the prevalence of IPV among pregnant women attending health services and its determinants	36.3%
14	Barreto et al.	2016	Brazil	To identify the prevalence and sociodemographic factors associated with physical violence during pregnancy	Not exact percentage reported, but considered high
15	Barzola et al.	2020	Peru	To determine the prevalence and associated factors of domestic violence in a specialized hospital	Total 29.4%; psychological 27.8%, physical 8.3%, and sexual 3.3%
16	Belay et al.	2019	Ethiopia	To measure the prevalence of IPV and depression in pregnant women and their association	21%
17	Boru Biffto et al.	2022	Ethiopia	To estimate the combined prevalence of IPV and its factors through systematic review and meta-analysis	Global pregnancy IPV: 37% (physical 24%, sexual 21%, psychological 27%)
18	Boyacioğlu et al.	2021	Turkey	To systematically review the prevalence and risk factors of IPV in pregnancy in Turkey	Between 0.9% and 57.1% depending on study

(continued)

Table 4.1 (continued)

Item	Authors	Year	Country	Study objective	Reported IPV-P prevalence (pregnancy)
19	Chen et al.	2024	Multinational	Meta-analysis on prevalence of IPV before, during, and after pregnancy	Before, 21.2%; during, 12.8%; and after, 14.7% (24% >1 year postpartum)
20	Chen et al.	2022	Hong Kong	To examine longitudinal changes in IPV exposure from before pregnancy to 3 years postpartum	IPV before pregnancy 22.9%, during 13.5%, 4 weeks postpartum 14.7%, and at 3 years 11.8%
21	D'Angelo et al.	2023	USA	To determine the prevalence of physical, emotional, and sexual violence during pregnancy and its distribution by demographic characteristics and risk factors using PRAMS data from six US states	5.7% experienced some form of violence during pregnancy (emotional 5.4%, physical 1.5%, sexual 0.9%)
22	Domingos Biagio et al.	2024	Brazil	To investigate the relationship between violence, mental health, and nutritional status in pregnant women	52.2% any violence; psychological 19.5%
23	Eikemo et al.	2024	Sweden	To describe the prevalence of IPV in pregnant women, compare exposure before and during pregnancy, and examine screening frequency and women's willingness to disclose violence in healthcare settings	6.2% reported IPV before pregnancy; 2.1% during pregnancy (some only during)
24	Eikemo et al.	2023	Sweden	To estimate the prevalence of IPV during pregnancy and its association with sociodemographic and health characteristics	2.1% total; psychological 1.8%, physical 0.6%, and sexual 0.1%

(continued)

Table 4.1 (continued)

Item	Authors	Year	Country	Study objective	Reported IPV-P prevalence (pregnancy)
25	Fan et al.	2024	China	To review the literature on IPV against pregnant women in contemporary China	2.5–31.3% depending on study; psychological violence most common
26	Fernandez et al.	2024	Spain and Denmark	To estimate the prevalence and associated factors of IPV in pregnant women through digital screening	Spain 13.7%, Denmark 6.9%
27	Ferrari et al.	2008	Brazil	To identify factors associated with domestic violence in pregnant women using the public health system	Psychological 19.1%, physical/sexual 6.5%
28	Galbally et al.	2024	Australia	To examine the relationship between childhood trauma, stressful events, depression, and perinatal IPV	Not numerically specific, but compared women with and without perinatal depression
29	Gebreslasie et al.	2024	Ethiopia	To analyze the relationship between IPV during pregnancy and neonatal asphyxia in Tigray	7.3% IPV during pregnancy; 12.7% of neonates with asphyxia
30	Ghoneim et al.	2021	Egypt	To evaluate the relationship between IPV and depression during pregnancy in Egyptian women	Not generally estimated (case-control: 158 with IPV vs. 158 without)
31	Hou et al.	2020	China	To study the effect of IPV on the trajectory of perinatal depression in a Chinese cohort	Psychological 9.2%, physical 4.5%, and sexual 2.3% (last 12 months)
32	Huldani et al.	2022	Multinational	To estimate the combined prevalence of IPV against pregnant women during the COVID-19 pandemic	IPV during COVID-19: 22% (95% CI: 4–40%) globally; psychological 24%, physical 14%, and sexual 6%

(continued)

Table 4.1 (continued)

Item	Authors	Year	Country	Study objective	Reported IPV-P prevalence (pregnancy)
33	Iyengar et al.	2020	India	To evaluate psychiatric comorbidity associated with IPV in pregnant women	35% IPV history (42.8% psychological, 57.1% physical/sexual)
34	Izaguirre et al.	2014	Spain	To explore narratives of maternal experience of women victims of IPV during pregnancy	Qualitative, no exact percentage
35	Jarihulu et al.	2021	Bangladesh	To study patterns of violence before, during, and after pregnancy	Physical: before 52.8%, during 35.2%, and postpartum 32.2%; psychological: 67.4%, 65%, and 60.8%
36	Laughon et al.	2025	USA	To compare IPV screening in the perinatal period by disability status in a population-based sample	4–9% overall; two to four times higher among people with disabilities
37	Lin et al.	2023	Taiwan	To explore the association between domestic violence and adverse obstetric outcomes	No specific prevalence reported; previous studies: 1.2–7.3% pregnant women with domestic violence
38	Lin et al.	2022	Taiwan	To evaluate the relationship between domestic violence and low birth weight in term newborns	4.9% low birth weight in women with violence vs. 3.3% without
39	Lockington et al.	2023	Australia	To evaluate maternal and perinatal outcomes in women exposed to IPV in a tertiary hospital	7.2% (2017–2021)
40	Luhumyo et al.	2020	Kenya	To estimate the prevalence and determinants of IPV during pregnancy in Eldoret	34.1% total; physical/sexual 22.8%, psychological 27.4%

(continued)

Table 4.1 (continued)

Item	Authors	Year	Country	Study objective	Reported IPV-P prevalence (pregnancy)
41	Manongi et al.	2020	Tanzania	To evaluate the association between IPV and depressive symptoms in pregnant women	38.8% experienced some type of IPV; 11.5% depression
42	Maruyama et al.	2023	Japan	To explore the prevalence and risk factors of IPV in urban pregnant women	13.4%
43	McGing et al.	2024	USA	To describe characteristics of pregnant patients with suspected IPV in hospital records	0.02% with hospital diagnosis of intentional IPV
44	Mekuriaw et al.	2022	Ethiopia	To estimate the magnitude and associated factors of IPV during pregnancy in Ethiopia	28.7% (emotional violence 24.1%)
45	Melby et al.	2022	Norway	To investigate the association between antenatal depression and IPV in culturally diverse women	14% depression; 15.4% reported IPV
46	Melkam et al.	2024	Sub-Saharan Africa	To estimate the prevalence and associated factors of IPV in pregnant women using DHS data	41.94%
47	Mella et al.	2021	Chile	To determine the prevalence and risk factors of IPV in pregnant and postpartum women in Santiago	5.7% pregnancy, 5.9% postpartum
48	Mishkin et al.	2022	Iraq	To study the prevalence and associated factors of IPV in displaced pregnant women	13%
49	Monterrosa et al.	2017	Colombia	To characterize pregnant adolescents and determine the prevalence of types of violence	7.1% partner violence; physical 6.7%, psychological 3.7%, and sexual 2.2%
50	Muldoon et al.	2021	Canada	To determine the prevalence and risk factors of perinatal IPV during the COVID-19 pandemic	24.07% perinatal IPV; 17.13% coercive control; 4.17% both

(continued)

Table 4.1 (continued)

Item	Authors	Year	Country	Study objective	Reported IPV-P prevalence (pregnancy)
51	Narayanan et al.	2024	Malaysia	To study determinants of antenatal depression and its association with IPV in pregnant women	Total IPV: 64.1% (emotional 30%, physical 2.4%, sexual 3.5%)
52	Nassir et al.	2003	Developing countries	To review evidence on prevalence, risk factors, and impacts of violence in pregnancy in developing countries	4–29% during pregnancy
53	Nepal et al.	2022	South Asia	To systematically review the prevalence of IPV in pregnancy in South Asia	23.4% (physical 13.6%, sexual 8.5%, emotional 20.2%)
54	Nigusie et al.	2023	Ethiopia	To estimate the proportion and associated factors of sexual IPV in pregnant women	19.8% sexual violence during pregnancy
55	Nyemgahm et al. [51]	2024	Sub-Saharan Africa	To review evidence on IPV in pregnancy among adolescents	8.3–41% (depending on study)
56	Opoku et al.	2023	Sub-Saharan Africa	To evaluate prevalence and associated factors of physical IPV during pregnancy in 26 African countries	6% (range: 2.1–14%)
57	Oseso et al.	2023	Kenya	To analyze whether a history of IPV predicts violence during pregnancy and postpartum	12.2% incident IPV during pregnancy or postpartum
58	Pastor-Moreno et al.	2020	Various	Meta-analysis of prevalence of IPV during pregnancy and its relationship with socioeconomic context	Global IPV: 9.2% (physical 5.0%, sexual 1.4%, emotional 4.7%)
59	Rahnavardi et al.	2023	Iran	To study protective and risk factors of domestic violence in pregnant adolescents	Physical 13.3%, emotional 23.5%, sexual 9.0%
60	Risco-Sanchez et al.	2022	Brazil	To evaluate prevalence and associated factors of domestic violence/IPV in pregnant and postpartum women in a public hospital	23% any violence; physical during pregnancy 2.3%, last year 5.3%; IPV pregnancy/postpartum 6.7%

(continued)

Table 4.1 (continued)

Item	Authors	Year	Country	Study objective	Reported IPV-P prevalence (pregnancy)
61	Savvoudi et al.	2024	Multinational	To review prevalence, associated factors, and consequences of DV/IPV during pregnancy in the pandemic	Higher than before the pandemic (no global figure)
62	Silva and Leite	2020	Brazil	To estimate IPV prevalence in pregnancy and associate it with sociodemographic and clinical characteristics	Psychological 16.1%, physical 7.6%, and sexual 2.7%
63	Silva et al.	2022	Brazil	To analyze characteristics of the partner associated with violence during pregnancy	Not numerically specific but high levels by type of violence
64	Silva et al.	2017	Brazil	To analyze factors associated with physical violence against pregnant women using structural modeling	Not exactly reported; cited studies range 0.9–57.1%
65	Sønderlund et al.	2022	Multinational	To systematically review the association between IPV and postpartum depression incidence	Varies by study; many found significant association between IPV and postpartum depression
66	Stiller et al.	2022	Kenya	To estimate prevalence and associated factors of IPV in pregnant women using national survey data	9.2% general; physical 78.6%, emotional 67.8%, and sexual 34.8%
67	Taft and Watson	2007	Australia	To examine the associations between termination, reproductive events, sociodemographic characteristics, and violence experience among young Australian women	4% IPV during pregnancy
68	Thompson et al.	2022	Ghana	To determine the association between IPV and maternal and perinatal outcomes	31.1% IPV during pregnancy; 42% before pregnancy

(continued)

Table 4.1 (continued)

Item	Authors	Year	Country	Study objective	Reported IPV-P prevalence (pregnancy)
69	Mossie et al. [46]	2023	Ethiopia	To fill the information gap by providing numerical evidence on the impact of IPV on birth outcomes and designing a strong intervention to improve maternal and neonatal health outcomes in Ethiopia	42.5% women exposed to IPV
70	Velasco et al.	2014	Spain	To estimate prevalence and risk factors of IPV in pregnant women using two screening instruments	7.7% (AAS); 21% nonphysical and 3.6% physical (ISA)
71	Wong et al.	2023	Various	Umbrella review on P-DV: prevalence, risk factors, consequences, and strategies	Emotional P-DV 28.4%, physical 13.8%, and sexual 8%
72	Woofter et al.	2024	Kenya	To evaluate the association between IPV and postpartum health access and family planning during COVID-19	36% IPV overall; increase or persistence during the pandemic in 33%
73	Yaya et al.	2021	Zimbabwe	To explore the association between IPV during pregnancy and preterm birth	8.9% of women exposed to IPV during pregnancy had preterm birth (vs. 3% without)
74	Yüksel-Kaptanoğlu et al.	2021	Turkey	To determine risk and protective factors for IPV during pregnancy using national surveys	7% physical violence during pregnancy (Turkey 2014 national survey)
75	Ramsubramani	2024	India	To identify the association between domestic violence and undesirable pregnancy events	Prevalence of undesirable pregnancy events: 25.0% (95% CI: 24.4–25.7%) among women aged 18–49

Source: Prepared by the authors

Particularly noteworthy are the high prevalence rates reported in sub-Saharan Africa, where some studies indicate that IPV may even increase during pregnancy [12, 20, 27, 32, 36]. Psychological, emotional, and controlling behaviors appear to be the forms of violence that increase most during this period [25, 41]. However, a study based on routine epidemiological surveillance in Colombia found that sexual violence was the most prevalent form of IPV during pregnancy [31, 45]. Overall, the evidence reveals that multiple forms of violence often co-occur, and the combination of different types is a common and recurrent pattern across the contexts studied [8, 23, 50].

A clear example is the meta-analysis by Bifftu and Guracho [16], which focused on Ethiopia and found a combined IPV prevalence of 37% during pregnancy, with 24% experiencing physical IPV, 21% sexual IPV, and 27% psychological IPV. This study also emphasizes the influence of structural factors such as low education, alcohol consumption, and a history of childhood violence, which increase the likelihood of IPV during pregnancy [16].

From a historical standpoint, Nasir and Hyder [49] provided one of the earliest analyses of IPV during pregnancy in developing countries, estimating prevalence rates between 4% and 29%. Their study highlighted the role of low educational attainment, poverty, and unintended pregnancies as key social determinants of IPV risk [49]. Similarly, a study by Barzola in Peru associated the presence of IPV with precarious living conditions [13].

In South Asia, Nepal et al. [50] documented an overall IPV prevalence of 23.4% among pregnant women, with 13.6% experiencing physical IPV, 8.5% sexual IPV, and 20.2% emotional IPV. These findings reinforce the notion that in settings marked by severe gender inequality, emotional and psychological violence may be even more prevalent than physical violence.

Special attention must also be given to vulnerable populations. For example, among pregnant adolescents in sub-Saharan Africa, [51] reported prevalence rates ranging from 8.3% to 41%. This review identifies poverty, early marriage, and childhood trauma as critical intersecting factors that compound the risk of IPV during pregnancy. In the case of pregnant women with disabilities, the study by Laughon et al. [33] found that they likely face higher IPV incidence and prevalence yet experience lower screening and inadequate prenatal care compared to women without disabilities. Among displaced pregnant women in Iraq, Mishkin et al. [44] reported a prevalence of 13%, which was comparable to rates observed in non-refugee populations.

It is also important to note that two systematic reviews identified the COVID-19 pandemic as a significant amplifier of IPV during pregnancy [30, 47]. Huldani et al. [30] estimated a combined prevalence of 22% during the pandemic, with psychological IPV being the most common form (24%). This increase was attributed to social isolation, financial stress, and disruptions in healthcare services. Similarly, Savvoudi et al. [58] confirmed that IPV-P rates increased during the pandemic, even though they did not report aggregated figures. These authors emphasized how confinement, loss of income, and limited access to healthcare intensified IPV exposure among pregnant women.

4.4 Factors Associated with Partner Violence During the Perinatal Period and Postpartum

Theoretical frameworks that seek to explain and understand violence broadly have established its multicausal nature and its deep interrelation with multiple social, economic, and health-related determinants. Many of the studies included in this review analyzed the contributing and associated factors of perinatal IPV (IPV-P), identifying a range of risks at different levels.

At the individual level, high-risk factors for IPV exposure during pregnancy include low educational attainment, unemployment, low income, unintended pregnancies, and a history of childhood abuse or exposure to violence [17, 66, 70]. Early age at pregnancy [12, 60] and lack of social support [1, 21] have also emerged as strong predictors. Women with a prior history of mental health conditions, particularly depression or anxiety, are more likely to be victims of IPV during the perinatal period [18].

Several studies further emphasize how socioeconomic vulnerability increases the risk of IPV during pregnancy [8, 23, 36]. Other associated risk factors include early sexual debut (before age 14), the desire to terminate the pregnancy, illness during pregnancy, and having multiple recent sexual partners [60].

At the relational level, couple dynamics are consistently identified as a central dimension in the onset of IPV. The most commonly cited risk factors include frequent alcohol consumption by the partner [2, 12, 60, 63], the partner's unemployment [25, 57, 61], rejection of condom use, and not being the biological father of the fetus [61]. IPV was more frequently reported among women cohabiting with their partners, or those in noncommitted or unsupported relationships [12, 64]. Additional factors include infidelity, power imbalances, emotional detachment [65], and unilateral decision-making within the relationship [17, 66]. Coercive control and isolation were also frequently reported as mechanisms that exacerbate partner violence.

At the community level, lack of support networks and social isolation [32, 64] were important factors. Additionally, cultural norms that tolerate or normalize violence [10] and inadequate access to confidential, comprehensive health services during pregnancy further hinder timely detection and intervention.

At the structural level, gender inequalities, structural poverty, and economic instability were consistently identified as underlying conditions that increase IPV-P risk [22, 70]. These risks were often exacerbated during crises such as the COVID-19 pandemic, which acted as a trigger or amplifier of violence [10, 58, 63, 67]. The study by Atilla et al. [10] emphasizes that economic hardship and the deterioration of relationship quality during lockdowns significantly contributed to the increase in IPV risk.

4.5 Consequences of Perinatal Partner Violence

The evidence gathered demonstrates that IPV-P has multifaceted and far-reaching consequences for women during pregnancy and postpartum, as well as for the fetus and newborn. This form of violence is now recognized as a key determinant of adverse maternal and perinatal health outcomes. Across different geographical contexts, studies consistently show a robust association between IPV exposure and negative outcomes such as preterm birth, low birth weight, premature rupture of membranes [55], admission to neonatal intensive care units, and increased neonatal morbidity [59].

Among pregnant women, the most consistent and well-documented effect of IPV is its association with depression during pregnancy and the postpartum period [8, 14, 26, 28, 29, 38, 42, 48].

In Saudi Arabia, Al-Marhabi et al. [7] found that IPV-exposed pregnant women were more likely to experience preterm labor, low birth weight, and neonatal ICU admissions, with contributing factors including the husband's low education level, poverty, tobacco use, and forced marriage. In Australia, Lockington et al. [37], analyzing over 45,000 births, reported a higher likelihood of small-for-gestational-age births, preterm delivery, premature rupture of membranes, and serious neonatal complications among IPV victims. The same study also identified elevated postpartum depression rates (EPDS ≥12) and acute obstetric presentations. Similarly, Aslam et al. [9] in Pakistan documented significant fetal health complications among IPV-exposed mothers.

In the USA, Alhusen et al. [6] found that women with disabilities were 2.5 times more likely to experience IPV during pregnancy, placing them at higher risk for adverse maternal, neonatal, and child health outcomes. These include increased risks of depression, suicidal ideation, substance use, inadequate prenatal care, and unplanned pregnancies. IPV was also linked to preterm birth and low birth weight, both strong predictors of neonatal morbidity and mortality.

In Taiwan, Lin et al. [34] showed that IPV during pregnancy significantly increased the likelihood of low birth weight in full-term infants (OR = 1.37), although no effect was found for preterm infants—highlighting the importance of considering gestational age when studying the effects of abuse.

A meta-analysis performed by Pastor-Moreno et al. [53] reported significant impacts on maternal mental health and perinatal health, including stress, anxiety, depressive symptoms, disruptions in mother-infant bonding, obstetric complications, and difficulties in accessing health services [11, 53]. Similarly, Maruyama et al. [39] in Japan found a prevalence of 13.4%, with comparable patterns of mental health consequences.

The longitudinal study by Taft and Watson [62] in young Australian women found a strong association between IPV and increased likelihood of abortion (pregnancy termination). IPV-exposed women were also more likely to report unintended pregnancies, preterm births, and gestational losses, suggesting a pattern of cumulative reproductive risk linked to violence [53, 62].

Finally, although Ankerstjerne et al. [8] did not report prevalence figures, their review reinforces the strong link between IPV and postpartum depression, underscoring that this association persists in both high- and low-income countries. This finding reinforces the importance of IPV during pregnancy as a critical determinant of maternal mental health.

4.6 Implications for Clinical Practice and Health Policies

The findings of this review, along with the conclusions drawn from the included studies, reinforce the need for the systematic and sustained implementation of screening strategies for intimate partner violence (IPV) during pregnancy. Such screening is among the most effective strategies, as early identification and intervention could reduce adverse outcomes for both the mother and the fetus [22, 24, 64]. Continuous monitoring of the social and health conditions to which pregnant women are exposed becomes a key tool for health professionals working in maternal and perinatal care to identify IPV [46], particularly given the numerous barriers to detection and self-reporting, especially in settings where gender-based violence and inequality are normalized [57].

The role of healthcare services in the prevention and early detection of IPV can significantly shape both the short- and long-term health trajectories of pregnant women. Accordingly, it is essential to train healthcare professionals to screen for and respond to IPV effectively [40]. This training should be incorporated into professional education and aim to promote awareness, sensitivity, and preparedness to act.

In line with these efforts, it is crucial to implement routine indicators within epidemiological surveillance systems to measure IPV exposure during pregnancy. One of the main limitations in understanding the true magnitude and impact of IPV is the widespread underreporting, heterogeneous measurement, and limited availability of data to track and compare IPV trends globally.

Moreover, findings such as those presented in this chapter support the imperative to integrate an intersectional approach into public health policies. Intersectionality, understood as the interaction of multiple forms of inequality—such as gender, socioeconomic status, ethnicity, age, disability, sexual orientation, migration status, and displacement—offers a powerful lens to understand how certain groups of pregnant women face compounded vulnerabilities to violence. Public health policies must acknowledge that not all women experience perinatal IPV in the same way, nor do they have equal access to protection, care, or justice.

4.7 Conclusions

Evidence on perinatal IPV supports the conclusion that intimate partner violence during pregnancy is a global public health issue, with reported prevalence rates ranging from 4% to 65%, depending on the country, population group, and time of measurement. While some studies suggest a slight decline in IPV during pregnancy, this does not reflect a resolution of the problem, as many women remain exposed to chronic or subtler forms of violence, particularly emotional abuse and controlling behaviors. Pregnancy, far from being a universal protective factor, should instead be seen as a critical window for identifying, addressing, and preventing the continuation of violence against women.

Structural, socioeconomic, and cultural disparities must be central considerations in the design of context-sensitive screening systems, policies, and intervention programs. The prevalence rates of perinatal IPV found in this review are, in most cases, higher than those reported by the WHO for the general female population aged 18–49 [68], highlighting the critical and urgent need to incorporate IPV detection and response into prenatal care systems.

Exposure to violence not only compromises the pregnant person's physical and mental health but also has measurable consequences for neonatal outcomes, including increased risk of preterm birth, low birth weight, severe neonatal morbidity, and even perinatal mortality. The evidence also emphasizes that certain subgroups—such as women with disabilities, Indigenous populations, and those from low-income backgrounds—face even higher risks, thus calling for differentiated and equity-driven responses in both public policy and clinical practice.

From a structural perspective, gender inequality, ethnic or linguistic discrimination, and the absence of effective public health policies to prevent and respond to IPV during pregnancy were reported in several studies as key structural drivers of violence. These findings underscore the urgency of adopting intersectional and multisectoral approaches to confront this pressing health issue, with interventions at the personal, community, social, and systemic levels, addressing not only the victim but the broader sociocultural environment in which IPV occurs.

Collectively, the studies included in this review highlight that methodological heterogeneity, lack of longitudinal frameworks, and non-standardized measures limit the ability to robustly synthesize the evidence on IPV during pregnancy. Nevertheless, the consistent recognition of this issue as an urgent global problem provides a strong foundation for advancing improved screening practices, rigorous research, and effective interventions.

References

1. Abujilban S, Mrayan L, Damra JK. Intimate partner violence among Jordanian pregnant women and its predictors. Nurs Open. 2022;9(1):267–76. https://doi.org/10.1002/nop2.1060.
2. Adebowale O, James B. The association between intimate partner violence, psychiatric morbidity amongst pregnant women and partner alcohol use in southern Nigeria. Afr J Prim Health Care Fam Med. 2020;12(1):e1–7. https://doi.org/10.4102/phcfm.v12i1.2226.
3. Agyemang-Duah W, Asare BYA, Adu C, Agyekum AK, Peprah P. Intimate partner violence as a determinant of pregnancy termination among women in unions: evidence from the 2016–2018 Papua New Guinea Demographic and Health Survey. J Biosoc Sci. 2024;56(1):141–54. https://doi.org/10.1017/S002193202300007X.
4. Albini PT, Zakhary B, Edwards SB, Coimbra R, Brenner ML. Intimate partner violence and pregnancy: nationwide analysis of injury patterns and risk factors. J Am Coll Surg. 2023;236(1):198–207. https://doi.org/10.1097/XCS.0000000000000421.

5. Alhusen JL, Ray E, Sharps P, Bullock L. Intimate partner violence during pregnancy: maternal and neonatal outcomes. J Women's Health. 2015;24(1):100–6. https://doi.org/10.1089/jwh.2014.4872.
6. Alhusen JL, Lyons G, Laughon K, Hughes RB. Intimate partner violence during the perinatal period by disability status: findings from a United States population-based analysis. J Adv Nurs. 2023;79(4):1493–502. https://doi.org/10.1111/jan.15340.
7. Al-Marhabi BD, Fahim WA, Katooa NE, Al-Nujaydi AA. Maternal and fetal outcomes among pregnant women exposed to violence. Cureus. 2023;15:e44715. https://doi.org/10.7759/cureus.44715.
8. Ankerstjerne LBS, Laizer SN, Andreasen K, Normann AK, Wu C, Linde DS, Rasch V. Landscaping the evidence of intimate partner violence and postpartum depression: a systematic review. BMJ Open. 2022;12(5):e051426. BMJ Publishing Group. https://doi.org/10.1136/bmjopen-2021-051426.
9. Aslam S, Farooq N, Ain QU, Khalid L, Siraj N, Mushtaq N. Exploring factors associated with domestic violence among pregnant women in Pakistan and its implications for maternal and perinatal health. Women Health. 2024;64:819–28. https://doi.org/10.1080/03630242.2024.2419055.
10. Atilla R, Yavuz A, Kocaöz S. Exposure of pregnant women to intimate partner violence during the pandemic in Turkey and influencing factors. J Community Health Nurs. 2023;40(1):1–13. https://doi.org/10.1080/07370016.2022.2094708.
11. Atsbaha M, Alemayehu M, Mekango DE, Moges S, Ejajo T, Erkalo D, Tamrat H. Prevalence and associated factors of intimate partner violence among pregnant women attending health care facilities, Northern Ethiopia: comparative cross-sectional study. J Obstet Gynaecol. 2022;42(5):1155–62. https://doi.org/10.1080/01443615.2022.2026900.
12. Azene ZN, Merid MW, Taddese AA, Andualem Z, Amare NS, Taye BT. Intimate partner sexual violence during pregnancy and its associated factors in Northwest Ethiopian women. Front Sociol. 2023;8:797098. https://doi.org/10.3389/fsoc.2023.797098.
13. Barzola Macha M, Moquillaza Alcántara V, Diaz Tinoco C. Violencia doméstica durante el embarazo en un hospital especializado del Perú: Prevalencia y factores asociado. Rev Chil Obstet Ginecol. 2020;85(6):641–53. https://doi.org/10.4067/S0717-75262020000600641.
14. Belay S, Astatkie A, Emmelin M, Hinderaker SG. Intimate partner violence and maternal depression during pregnancy: a community-based cross-sectional study in Ethiopia. PLoS One. 2019;14(7):e0220003. https://doi.org/10.1371/journal.pone.0220003.
15. Biagio LD, Devakumar D, Da Silva PL, López RVM, Argentato PP, Luzia LA, Rondó PHC. Violence, mental health and nutritional status in pregnant women: the Araraquara Cohort Study. Public Health Nutr. 2024:1–29. https://doi.org/10.1017/S1368980024002295.
16. Bifftu BB, Guracho YD. Determinants of intimate partner violence against pregnant women in Ethiopia: a systematic review and meta-analysis. Biomed Res Int. 2022;2022:4641343. Hindawi Limited. https://doi.org/10.1155/2022/4641343.
17. Boyacioğlu NE, Günaydın S, Özcan NK, Dinç Kaya H. Intimate partner violence during pregnancy in Turkey: a systematic review and meta-analysis. Perspect Psychiatr Care. 2021;57(3):1515–27. https://doi.org/10.1111/ppc.12879.
18. Chen XY, Lo CKM, Ho FK, Leung WC, Ip P, Chan KL. Changing patterns of intimate partner violence against pregnant women: a three-year longitudinal study. Int J Environ Res Public Health. 2022;19(21):14397. https://doi.org/10.3390/ijerph192114397.
19. Chen XY, Lo CKM, Chen Q, Gao S, Ho FK, Brownridge DA, Leung WC, Ip P, Ling Chan K. Intimate partner violence against women before, during, and after pregnancy: a meta-analysis. Trauma Violence Abuse. 2024;25:2768–80. SAGE Publications Ltd. https://doi.org/10.1177/15248380241226631.
20. Damtew SA, Shiferaw S, Seme A, Kassa BA, Fantaye FT, Armdie AZ, Berhe SY, Nerisho DG, Amogne A, Gidey MY, Atnafu NT. Intimate Partner Violence during the Index Pregnancy and its correlates among a panel of pregnant women in Ethiopia, evidence from performance, and monitoring for action (PMA) 2021 cohort two baseline survey. BMC Pregnancy Childbirth. 2024;24(1):759. https://doi.org/10.1186/s12884-024-06947-5.

21. Eikemo R, Barimani M, Elvin-Nowak Y, Eriksson J, Vikström A, Nyman V, Backman-Enelius M, Jonas W. Intimate partner violence during pregnancy – prevalence and associations with women's health: a cross-sectional study. Sex Reprod Healthc. 2023;36:100843. https://doi.org/10.1016/j.srhc.2023.100843.
22. Eikemo R, Elvin-Nowak Y, Åhlund S, Vikström A, Nyman V, Jonas W, Barimani M. I had to tell to survive"– a cross-sectional study on exposure to intimate partner violence in pregnant women and the importance of screening. Sex Reprod Healthc. 2024;42:101045. https://doi.org/10.1016/j.srhc.2024.101045.
23. Fan XM, Kim HW. The status of intimate partner violence against pregnant women in contemporary China: a scoping review. Korean J Women Health Nurs. 2024;30(1):41–55). Korean Society of Women Health Nursing. https://doi.org/10.4069/whn.2024.03.16.
24. Fernández-López R, Andreasen K, Ankerstjerne L, Martín-de-las-Heras S, Rasch V, Megías JL, Linde DS, de-León-de-León S, Schei B, Wu C, Oviedo-Gutiérrez A, Zapata-Calvente AL. Prevalence and associated factors of intimate partner violence against pregnant women who attend antenatal care in Denmark and Spain: a digital screening approach. Acta Obstet Gynecol Scand. 2024;104:139–50. https://doi.org/10.1111/aogs.15000.
25. Ferrari CA, Ana AI, Segall-Corrêa M, Silvia I, Santiago M, Maria da Graça I, Andrade G, Rafael I, Ii P-E, Aparecida C, Audi F. Violence against pregnant women: prevalence and associated factors. Rev Saúde Pública. 2008;42(5):877–85.
26. Galbally M, Watson S, MacMillan K, Sevar K, Howard LM. Intimate partner violence across pregnancy and the postpartum and the relationship to depression and perinatal wellbeing: findings from a pregnancy cohort study. Arch Womens Ment Health. 2024;27(5):807–15. https://doi.org/10.1007/s00737-024-01455-z.
27. Gebreslasie KZ, Gebre G, Zenebe D, Nardos R, Birhane A. Intimate partner violence during pregnancy and its association with birth asphyxia in hospitals of Tigray region, Ethiopia. BMC Pediatr. 2024;24(1):113. https://doi.org/10.1186/s12887-024-04585-6.
28. Ghoneim HM, Elprince M, Ali TYM, Gharieb WF, Ahmed AA. Violence and depression among pregnant women in Egypt. BMC Pregnancy Childbirth. 2021;21(1):502. https://doi.org/10.1186/s12884-021-03932-0.
29. Hou F, Zhang X, Cerulli C, He W, Mo Y, Gong W. The impact of intimate partner violence on the trajectory of perinatal depression: a cohort study in a Chinese sample. Epidemiol Psychiatr Sci. 2020;29:e133. https://doi.org/10.1017/S2045796020000463.
30. Huldani H, Kamal Abdelbasset W, Abdalkareem Jasim S, Suksatan W, Turki Jalil A, Thangavelu L, Fakri Mustafa Y, Karami M. Intimate partner violence against pregnant women during the COVID-19 pandemic: a systematic review and meta-analysis. Women Health. 2022;62(6):556–64. https://doi.org/10.1080/03630242.2022.2096755.
31. Instituto Nacional de Salud. Informe quincenal epidemiológico nacional. 2018. https://www.ins.gov.co/buscador-eventos/IQEN/IQEN%20vol%2023%202018%20num%207.pdf.
32. Kebede AA, Aklil MB, Gessesse DN, Tsega NT, Temesgan WZ, Abegaz MY, Anteneh TA, Tibebu NS, Alemu HN, Haile TT, Seyoum AT, Tiguh AE, Yismaw AE, Nenko G, Wondie KY, Taye BT, Mihret MS. Nearly half of women have experienced intimate partner violence during pregnancy in northwest Ethiopia, 2021; the role of social support and decision-making power. Front Public Health. 2022;10:904792. https://doi.org/10.3389/fpubh.2022.904792.
33. Laughon K, Hughes RB, Lyons G, Roarty K, Alhusen J. Disability-related disparities in screening for intimate partner violence during the perinatal period: a population-based study. Womens Health Issues. 2025;35:97–104. https://doi.org/10.1016/j.whi.2024.12.001.
34. Lin CH, Lin WS, Chang HY, Wu SI. Domestic violence against pregnant women is a potential risk factor for low birthweight in full-term neonates: a population-based retrospective cohort study. PLoS One. 2022;17:e0279469. https://doi.org/10.1371/journal.pone.0279469.
35. Lin CL, Sun JC, Lin CP, Chung CH, Chien WC. Associations between domestic violence and poor pregnancy outcomes in Taiwanese women: a nested case–control study. BMC Womens Health. 2023;23(1):465. https://doi.org/10.1186/s12905-023-02602-x.
36. Liyew AM, Alem AZ, Ayalew HG. Magnitude and factors associated with intimate partner violence against pregnant women in Ethiopia: a multilevel analysis of 2016 Ethiopian demo-

graphic and health survey. BMC Public Health. 2022;22(1):284. https://doi.org/10.1186/s12889-022-12720-0.
37. Lockington EP, Sherrell HC, Crawford K, Rae K, Kumar S. Intimate partner violence is a significant risk factor for adverse pregnancy outcomes. AJOG Glob Rep. 2023;3(4):100283. https://doi.org/10.1016/j.xagr.2023.100283.
38. Manongi R, Rogathi J, Sigalla G, Mushi D, Rasch V, Gammeltoft T, Meyrowitsch DW. The association between intimate partner violence and signs of depression during pregnancy in Kilimanjaro region, northern Tanzania. J Interpers Violence. 2020;35(23–24):5797–811. https://doi.org/10.1177/0886260517724256.
39. Maruyama N, Horiuchi S, Kataoka Y. Prevalence and associated factors of intimate partner violence against pregnant women in urban areas of Japan: a cross-sectional study. BMC Public Health. 2023;23(1):1168. https://doi.org/10.1186/s12889-023-16105-9.
40. McGing M, Ashbrook M, Cheng V, Matsuo K, Schellenberg M, Martin M, Inaba K, Matsushima K. Identifying pregnant patients with suspected intimate partner violence. Am Surg. 2024;90:2398–402. https://doi.org/10.1177/00031348241248799.
41. Mekuriaw Liyew AM, Alem AZ, Ayalew HG. Magnitude and factors associated with intimate partner violence against pregnant women in Ethiopia: a multilevel analysis of 2016 Ethiopian demographic and health survey. BMC Public Health. 2022;22(1):284. https://doi.org/10.1186/s12889-022-12720-0. PMID: 35148725; PMCID: PMC8840032.
42. Melby TC, Sørensen NB, Henriksen L, Lukasse M, Flaathen EME. Antenatal depression and the association of intimate partner violence among a culturally diverse population in south-eastern Norway: a cross-sectional study. Eur J Midwifery. 2022;6:44. https://doi.org/10.18332/ejm/150009.
43. Mella M, Binfa L, Carrasco A, Cornejo C, Cavada G, Pantoja L. Violencia contra la mujer durante la gestación y postparto infligida por su pareja en Centros de Atención Primaria de la zona norte de Santiago, Chile. Rev Med Chile. 2021;149:543.
44. Mishkin KE, Ahmed HM, Maqsood SS. Factors associated with experiencing lifetime intimate partner violence among pregnant displaced women living in refugee camps in Erbil, Iraq. Glob Public Health. 2022;17(12):3455–64. https://doi.org/10.1080/17441692.2022.2048409.
45. Monterrosa-Castro Á, Arteta-Acosta C, Ulloque-Caamaño L. Violência doméstica em adolescentes grávidas: caracterização do casal e prevalência das formas de expressão. Iatreia. 2017;30(1):34–46. https://doi.org/10.17533/udea.iatreia.v30n1a03.
46. Mossie TB, Mekonnen FH, Tadesse M, Tadele A. Mapping the disparities in intimate partner violence prevalence and determinants across Sub-Saharan Africa. Front Public Health. 2023;11:1188718. https://doi.org/10.3389/fpubh.2023.1188718. PMID: 37448663; PMCID: PMC10337829.
47. Muldoon KA, Denize KM, Talarico R, Boisvert C, Frank O, Harvey ALJ, Rennicks White R, Fell DB, O'Hare-Gordon MA, Guo Y, Murphy MSQ, Corsi DJ, Sampsel K, Wen SW, Walker MC, El-Chaar D. COVID-19 and perinatal intimate partner violence: a cross-sectional survey of pregnant and postpartum individuals in the early stages of the COVID-19 pandemic. BMJ Open. 2021;11(5):e049295. https://doi.org/10.1136/bmjopen-2021-049295.
48. Narayanan S, Abd Rahman FN, Sutan R, Kumarasuriar GK, Leong AKS. Prevalence and determinants of antenatal depression and its association with intimate partner violence: a cross-sectional study at Hospital Melaka, Malaysia. Front Psych. 2024;15:1466074. https://doi.org/10.3389/fpsyt.2024.1466074.
49. Nasir K, Hyder AA. Violence against pregnant women in developing countries review of evidence. Eur J Pub Health. 2003;13:105–7.
50. Nepal S, Atreya A, Shrestha DB, Budhathoki P, Lamichhane S, Nepal S, Marahatta A, Dhital R. Intimate partner violence during pregnancy in South Asia: systematic review and meta-analysis. J Nepal Health Res Counc. 2023;20(3):562–9. https://doi.org/10.33314/jnhrc.v20i3.3983.
51. Nyemgah AC, Ranganathan M, Stöckl H. Intimate partner violence during pregnancy against adolescents in sub-Saharan Africa: a systematic review. Inj Prev. 2024;30(3):177–182. https://doi.org/10.1136/ip-2023-044985. PMID: 38195654; PMCID: PMC11137446.

52. ONU Mujeres. ODS 5: lograr la igualdad entre los géneros y empoderar a todas las mujeres y las niñas. 2022. https://www.unwomen.org/es/news/in-focus/women-and-the-sdgs/sdg-5-gender-equality#:~:text=Lograr%20la%20igualdad%20de%20g%C3%A9nero,la%20esfera%20p%C3%BAblica%20como%20privada.
53. Pastor-Moreno G, Ruiz-Pérez I, Henares-Montiel J, Petrova D. Intimate partner violence during pregnancy and risk of fetal and neonatal death: a meta-analysis with socioeconomic context indicators. Am J Obstet Gynecol. 2020;222(2):123–133.e5. https://doi.org/10.1016/j.ajog.2019.07.045.
54. Pollock D, Evans C, Menghao Jia R, Alexander L, Pieper D, Brandão de Moraes É, Peters MDJ, Tricco AC, Khalil H, Godfrey CM, Saran A, Campbell F, Munn Z. "How-to": scoping review? J Clin Epidemiol. 2024;176:111572. https://doi.org/10.1016/j.jclinepi.2024.111572.
55. Ramasubramani P, Krishnamoorthy Y, Ganesh K, Kathiresan L, Kadir V. Association between domestic violence and unintended, terminated pregnancy and complications during pregnancy among Indian women: findings from nationally representative survey: domestic violence and pregnancy outcomes in India. Heliyon. 2024;10(5):e27158. https://doi.org/10.1016/j.heliyon.2024.e27158.
56. Rivara F, Adhia A, Lyons V, Massey A, Mills B, Morgan E, Simckes M, Rowhani-Rahbar A. The effects of violence on health. Health Aff. 2019;38(10):1622–9. https://doi.org/10.1377/hlthaff.2019.00480.
57. Santos SMB, Oliveira ZM, Coqueiro RDS, Santos VC, Anjos KFD, Casotti CA. Prevalência e fatores associados à violência física contra mulheres grávidas. Rev Baiana Saude Publica. 2017;40(1):1881. https://doi.org/10.22278/2318-2660.2016.v40.n1.a1881.
58. Savvoudi D-M, Orovou E, Dagla M, Kirkou G, Iatrakis G, Antoniou E. Domestic violence in pregnancy during the pandemic era: a systematic review. Maedica. 2024;19(2):400–9. https://doi.org/10.26574/maedica.2024.19.2.400.
59. Shidhani NAA, Kendi AAA, Kiyumi MHA. Prevalence, risk factors and effects of domestic violence before and during pregnancy on birth outcomes: an observational study of literate Omani women. Int J Women's Health. 2020;12:911–25. https://doi.org/10.2147/IJWH.S272419.
60. Silva RDP, Leite FMC. Intimate partner violence during pregnancy: prevalence and associated factors. Rev Saude Publica. 2019;54(97):1–11. https://doi.org/10.11606/s1518-8787.2020054002103.
61. Silva RDP, Leite FMC, Dos Santos Netto ET, Deslandes SF. Intimate partner violence during pregnancy: a focus on partner characteristics. Cienc Saude Coletiva. 2022;27(5):1873–82). Associacao Brasileira de Pos – Graduacao em Saude Coletiva. https://doi.org/10.1590/1413-81232022275.06542021EN.
62. Taft AJ, Watson LF. Termination of pregnancy: associations with partner violence and other factors in a national cohort of young Australian women. Aust N Z J Public Health. 2007;31(2):135–42. https://doi.org/10.1111/j.1753-6405.2007.00031.x.
63. Thompson NN, Mumuni K, Oppong SA, Sefogah PE, Nuamah MA, Nkyekyer K. Effect of intimate partner violence in pregnancy on maternal and perinatal outcomes at the Korle Bu teaching hospital, Ghana: an observational cross sectional study. Int J Gynecol Obstet. 2023;160(1):297–305. https://doi.org/10.1002/ijgo.14375.
64. Velasco C, Luna JD, Martin A, Caño A, Martin-De-las-heras S. Intimate partner violence against Spanish pregnant women: application of two screening instruments to assess prevalence and associated factors. Acta Obstet Gynecol Scand. 2014;93(10):1050–8. https://doi.org/10.1111/aogs.12459.
65. Wassie ST, Ejigu AG, Tilahun AG, Lambyo SHM. The impact of intimate partner violence on adverse birth outcomes in public health facilities. A prospective cohort study. Midwifery. 2023;126:103815. https://doi.org/10.1016/j.midw.2023.103815.
66. Wong SC, Do PH, Eisner M, Hughes C, Valdebenito S, Murray AL. An umbrella review of the literature on perinatal domestic violence: prevalence, risk factors, possible outcomes and

interventions. Trauma Violence Abuse. 2023;24(3):1712–26). SAGE Publications Ltd. https://doi.org/10.1177/15248380221080455.

67. Woofter R, Mboya J, Golub G, Sudhinaraset M. Intimate partner violence and postpartum healthcare access in Kenya: a cross-sectional study. BMC Pregnancy Childbirth. 2024;24(1):168. https://doi.org/10.1186/s12884-024-06342-0.
68. World Health Organization. Violence against women prevalence estimates, 2018: global, regional and national prevalence estimates for intimate partner violence against women and global and regional prevalence estimates for non-partner sexual violence against women. WHO, on behalf of the United Nations Inter-Agency Working Group on Violence Against Women Estimation and Data (VAW-IAWGED). 2021. https://www.who.int/publications/i/item/9789240022256.
69. Yaya S, Odusina EK, Adjei NK, Uthman OA. Association between intimate partner violence during pregnancy and risk of preterm birth. BMC Public Health. 2021;21(1):1610. https://doi.org/10.1186/s12889-021-11625-8.
70. Yüksel-Kaptanoğlu İ, Adalı T. Intimate partner violence during pregnancy in Turkey: determinants from nationwide surveys. J Interpers Violence. 2021;36(15–16):7802–31. https://doi.org/10.1177/0886260519837652.

5 Optimizing Research on Stress in Pregnancy: Development and Evolution of the Prenatal Distress Questionnaire

Marci Lobel

Abstract

Studies measuring stress by the occurrence of life events or anxiety during pregnancy have produced inconsistent findings about the impact of prenatal maternal stress on birth outcomes. More robust approaches conceptualize and measure prenatal stress as the confluence of conditions or events (stimuli), appraisals of these, and resulting emotions (responses). These approaches are improved by including pregnancy-specific stress, which results from women's appraisals and responses to the specific aspects of pregnancy that they find stressful. Pregnancy-specific stress has been shown to be a particularly harmful type of stress, predicting poorer maternal health, unhealthy behaviors, and adverse birth outcomes. The Prenatal Distress Questionnaire (PDQ) and its successor, the NuPDQ, are well-tested instruments that measure pregnancy-specific stress with strong reliability and validity. Using these instruments to assess pregnancy-specific stress enhances our ability to identify and quantify the difficulties faced by pregnant women and can help us provide the supports and resources that promote healthy birth outcomes.

Keywords

Pregnancy · Stress · Prenatal distress questionnaire · Maternal health · Women

M. Lobel (✉)
Department of Psychology, Stony Brook University, Stony Brook, NY, USA
e-mail: marci.lobel@stonybrook.edu

R. A. Caparros-Gonzalez (ed.), *Maternal Stress during Pregnancy and Postpartum*, https://doi.org/10.1007/978-3-032-09245-8_5

The potentially harmful impact of stress on a pregnant woman and her developing child has been a long-standing topic of concern. Rigorous studies of prenatal stress were initiated in the 1970s with mounting evidence that stress affects various aspects of health. The focus on prenatal maternal stress also resulted from growing recognition that medical risk factors alone are poor predictors of pregnancy outcomes such as low birthweight and preterm birth. A number of early studies examined the possibility that experiencing major, stressful life events during pregnancy could adversely affect the course of pregnancy and was harmful to a pregnant woman and her baby [1–4]. Stressful life events were defined as events that require substantial adjustment, with events presumed to require the most adjustment (such as the death of a spouse) assigned a higher "life change unit" score. Typical studies counted the number of major life events that occurred during the study period or the total life change units that accrued from these. Other studies focused on negative maternal emotions, especially anxiety, as a risk factor during pregnancy. Implicit in these studies was the presumed equivalence of anxiety and stress.

Many studies of prenatal maternal stress (hereafter, PNMS) in the ensuing decades have continued to operationalize this variable either as the occurrence of life events or as high anxiety (usually state anxiety) during the prenatal period. Studies using these measurement approaches have produced inconsistent findings about the impact of PNMS on birth outcomes [5–8]: Some find associations of PNMS with poorer outcomes, and others do not. Given that the published literature overrepresents studies with confirmatory findings, it is likely that an even larger number of studies fail to find effects of PNMS on birth outcomes when operationalized with measures of life events or anxiety.

A major limitation of this literature has been the absence of theory to undergird and guide the measurement of PNMS. In the 1990s, my colleagues and I [8, 9] drew from well-elaborated theories of stress, especially the influential work of Richard Lazarus [10–12], to highlight the flaws inherent in measuring PNMS through life events or state anxiety. We emphasized that life events represent *potentially* stressful occurrences. Differences in the impact of life events exist because people respond to them differently. People have different intrapersonal, interpersonal, and tangible resources that affect the way they appraise, experience, and react to life events [10–13]. Thus, there is likely to be great interindividual variability in the extent to which women are taxed or distressed by the life events that occur during their pregnancy. Because the same events do not produce distress for all individuals who experience them, my colleagues and I proposed that prenatal life events be viewed as *stimuli* that may or may not evoke stress [8, 9].

Additionally, we maintained that measuring PNMS as state anxiety is also inadequate because this approach overlooks the conditions or reasons why a pregnant woman is experiencing anxiety [8]. State anxiety is an emotional response to stressors or stimuli, which may include life events, that are perceived as dangerous, threatening, aversive, or stressful. However, anxiety may also reflect a pregnant woman's tendency or disposition to experience this negative emotion, irrespective of events or prevailing conditions. Furthermore, pregnant women with low state anxiety may be managing stressful life events and conditions well and not be made anxious by them. Thus, I argued that state anxiety should be viewed as a *response* to stress but not as stress itself [8].

Apart from Lazarus, other theorists also recognized the multidirectional associations among stress stimuli, appraisals, and responses [e.g., 14–16], providing a strong basis for considering them to be components of a multidimensional stress construct. This perspective views conditions or discrete events such as major life events as stress stimuli, and it recognizes the variability in the extent to which people subjected to these stimuli evaluate, perceive, or appraise them as stressful. Stressful appraisals, in turn, can elicit stress responses. The responses to conditions or events that individuals find stressful may be physiological, cognitive, behavioral, or emotional. Applying this theoretically guided approach, our team suggested that PNMS should be defined as the confluence of stress stimuli (e.g., life events) that occur during pregnancy, women's appraisals of their stressfulness, and their responses [8, 9]. Combining indicators of stress in this manner, we suggested, would enable a more reliable and conceptually powerful test of the relationship of PNMS with adverse birth outcomes than had been attempted previously.

In one of our first tests of this approach to PNMS conceptualization and operationalization, Dunkel-Schetter and I [9] used structural equation modeling to construct a latent factor comprised of the number of life events that occurred during study participants' pregnancy, their appraisals of the distress engendered by the life events that they experienced (how "undesirable or negative" was each event), appraisals of the stressfulness of chronic conditions across pregnancy ("perceived stress"), and state anxiety scores averaged across pregnancy. We selected state anxiety as the emotional stress response to examine in this study because of its prominence in prior research on PNMS, although other emotions, such as anger or sadness, may also occur as a response to stress.

We found that the best fitting model was a latent factor measured by appraisals of life events, appraised conditions (perceived stress), and state anxiety [9]. Number of life events did not load on the latent factor, indicating that the latent factor was comprised exclusively of stress-related perception and emotion but not stressors. The latter was the objective indicator of stress stimuli represented by the occurrence of major life events during pregnancy. This finding reinforced the idea that stressors are not equivalent to stress-related perception and emotion. Study results underscored the inadequacy of measuring PNMS exclusively through stress stimuli such as life events or through stress responses such as anxiety, which was the common approach in other studies. Instead, the results suggested that PNMS could be conceptualized and operationally defined by integrating the appraisals and emotions of pregnant women. This type of PNMS, we suggested, might be considered and labeled *distress*.

Our research team then examined whether the latent PNMS factor and the separate objective stressor variable (number of prenatal life events) predicted birthweight and gestational age at delivery [17]. Number of prenatal life events was not associated with birth outcomes. The latent PNMS factor, however, was a powerful predictor of lower birthweight ($\beta = -0.18$) and earlier birth ($\beta = -0.23$), over and above the impact of obstetric medical risk on these outcomes. The latent PNMS factor also predicted the additional variability in birthweight beyond that explained by the timing of birth, an important finding because higher birthweight even within normal range (2500–4500 g) is linked to better long-term health and development [18–20]. Logistic regression analyses corroborated study findings using clinically defined outcomes. That is, low birthweight and preterm delivery were also predicted by the latent PNMS factor.

This study provided a strong test of the impact of PNMS on birth outcomes, rigorous because of its inclusion and statistical control for obstetric risk factors to verify the independent impact of PNMS, and its use of a multidimensional stress factor. Studies from other teams also corroborated the predictive validity of multidimensional PNMS measures, confirming the value of this approach [21–23].

5.1 Development of the Prenatal Distress Questionnaire

Although our findings demonstrated the reliability and predictive validity of a multidimensional PNMS factor [17], my collaborators and I recognized an important limitation of this research. This limitation, we suggested, also applied to the many prior studies that had assessed PNMS exclusively as the occurrence of life events or anxiety during pregnancy. These studies focused on general, nonspecific stress or distress, not stress that women experience because of pregnancy itself. Yet qualitative studies and descriptive research demonstrated that pregnant women are distressed by specific aspects of their pregnancy including their physical symptoms or obstetric complications, their bodily changes, the health of the fetus, impending childbirth, and the care of a newborn [24, 25]. Our team raised the possibility that failing to assess *pregnancy-specific* stress may have resulted in inaccurate estimates of the magnitude of stress that pregnant women experience and may underestimate the extent to which PNMS affects outcomes.

This realization led us to create the Prenatal Distress Questionnaire (PDQ), an instrument assessing distress that may emanate from pregnancy-specific circumstances. We generated PDQ items from the descriptive and qualitative literature, revised them through structured interviews with a sample of pregnant women, and then pilot tested them in an additional pregnant sample. This process produced 12 items that were administered in midpregnancy to a sample of 167 women [26]. The PDQ queried how worried or upset a respondent was about each item on a scale ranging from 0 (not at all) to 4 (extremely). In one of the first tests of this instrument, the internal consistency of the PDQ was high (Cronbach's alpha 0.81), confirming the appropriateness of summing responses to create a total pregnancy-specific stress score for each woman. Scores ranged from 3 to 47 out of a 0 to 48 possible range, indicating broad interindividual differences in pregnancy-specific stress and lending support for its ecological validity. The mean PDQ score was 14.9 (±7.2). Participants in this study were recruited from a high-risk prenatal care practice, which was reflected in the items they found most distressing, bolstering confidence in the construct validity of the instrument. Items most frequently endorsed as causing moderate to extreme distress were concerns about premature delivery (53%), physical symptoms (53%), labor and delivery (52%), weight gain (47%), and the baby's health (40%). Few women were distressed about changes in their relationship with the baby's father (12%). Even fewer were distressed about forming an emotional attachment to the baby (5%). As would be expected, PDQ scores were correlated ($r = 0.53$, $p < 0.01$) with a nonspecific, global distress variable constructed by aggregating scores on a measure of general perceived stress (the Perceived Stress Scale [27]) with scores on a measure of state anxiety (the State Anxiety Inventory [28]). The moderate magnitude of this correlation confirmed that while related, pregnancy-specific stress and nonspecific, global stress are distinct constructs.

In a subsequent analysis, we [29] included the PDQ in a multidimensional PNMS factor that also included measures of life events (number and distress), state anxiety, and perceived chronic stress. This PNMS factor indirectly predicted lower birthweight and earlier delivery via an association of PNMS with lower dispositional optimism and poorer prenatal health behaviors, particularly lack of physical activity. We attributed the absence of direct PNMS associations with birth outcomes to characteristics of the sample, which was comprised of highly educated and well-resourced women, likely offering some protection from the impact of stress. Nevertheless, study results confirmed that pregnancy-specific stress as measured by the PDQ was a significant component of a well-fitting, multidimensional PNMS factor that affected birth outcomes, indirectly in this sample through their health behaviors and in conjunction with a negative outlook on life.

Because the PDQ had been developed for use in midpregnancy [26], it was necessary to expand the instrument to enable its application across pregnancy for stressors that are more pertinent in early pregnancy (e.g., nausea and vomiting) and late pregnancy (e.g., the approaching birth). To incorporate these additional sources of stress, we expanded the PDQ and eventually renamed it the Revised Prenatal Distress Questionnaire, or NuPDQ (pronounced "New-PDQ") [30, 31]. The initial version of the NuPDQ included nine core items representing pregnancy stressors pertinent at any time point in pregnancy with additional items added in midpregnancy (three items) and late pregnancy (five items) for stressors that become more relevant as pregnancy progresses. The response scale for the NuPDQ was also reduced for greater ease and speed of administration, using a scale from 0 (not at all) to 2 (very much) for respondents to indicate the extent to which they are feeling "bothered, upset, or worried" about each item.

5.2 Applications and Tests of the NuPDQ

My collaborators and I were interested in determining whether the NuPDQ could predict birth outcomes as well as or possibly better than measures of general, global PNMS. Research from other studies was suggestive that pregnancy-specific stress may be a more powerful contributor to birth outcomes than stress that originates from sources unrelated to a woman's pregnancy [32–35]. Roesch et al., for example, had found that a "pregnancy anxiety" variable predicted earlier birth, whereas its correlate, general anxiety, did not (general perceived stress and life events also did not predict earlier birth in the Roesch et al. study) [35]. Similarly, DiPietro et al. found that fetal activity was better predicted by scores on their measure of pregnancy-specific hassles and uplifts than by general stress [33]. However, neither DiPietro et al. nor Roesch et al. directly compared the predictive validity of their pregnancy-specific measure to a multivariable aggregate of general, nonspecific stress. Therefore, our team undertook a test of the NuPDQ's ability to predict birth outcomes compared with that of general stress, operationalized multidimensionally.

We compared the sole predictive validity of the NuPDQ against a latent stress factor that included the NuPDQ as well as general stress measures: state anxiety, perceived stress, and life events [30]. Additionally, we compared the predictive power of the NuPDQ against each of the individual, general stress measures. These comparisons offered a direct test of the independent contribution of pregnancy-specific stress and an opportunity to determine whether it was a stronger contributor to birth outcome than general stress.

Results of this study indicated that pregnancy-specific stress measured with the NuPDQ was a stronger predictor of lower birthweight and earlier birth than was state anxiety, perceived stress, or life event stress [30]. Moreover, the NuPDQ alone predicted birth outcomes better than a latent factor constructed from all of the stress variables. Delivery was 9 days earlier for those with high obstetric risk scores and high NuPDQ scores than for women with low scores on these measures. Pregnancy-specific stress was also associated with a variety of health behaviors including eating, exercise, and cigarette smoking. Associations of NuPDQ scores with birth outcomes persisted after controlling for obstetric risk, illustrating the independent impact of pregnancy-specific stress. Clinically defined outcomes, namely, low birthweight and preterm birth, were also predicted by pregnancy-specific stress (and by cigarette smoking).

A limitation of the NuPDQ was that it contained different items at early, mid-, and late pregnancy and therefore could not be used to compare the impact of pregnancy-specific stress at these different points in pregnancy. Yet growing evidence from other teams suggested that the consequences of PNMS might differ depending upon when it occurred in pregnancy [36, 37]. Our team was eager to create a single instrument optimized for use with women at any point in pregnancy. For these reasons, in subsequent research with the NuPDQ, all 17 items were included, regardless of when the instrument was administered in pregnancy.

Over time, the growth of research using the PDQ or NuPDQ supported a need for thorough analysis of the psychometric soundness of these instruments. The breadth of evidence that had been collected with the PDQ and NuPDQ also provided an opportunity to summarize what was known about pregnancy-specific stress. Ibrahim and I [38] conducted an extensive review of studies that had used the PDQ (45 studies) or the NuPDQ (37 studies). Our review confirmed that pregnancy-specific stress is common in pregnancy and that this type of stress is associated with distinct sociodemographic and obstetric characteristics. For example, across studies, younger pregnant women, those with less education, and nulliparous women reported greater pregnancy-specific stress. Scores on the PDQ or NuPDQ were also shown across studies to be associated with poorer maternal health and health behaviors and predicted adverse birth outcomes in the studies that examined these variables. Based on our review, Ibrahim and I concluded that the NuPDQ is an especially robust instrument with well-demonstrated reliability, convergent validity, concurrent validity, and predictive validity, and we recommended its use over the PDQ. Some teams continue to use the 12-item PDQ successfully, however [e.g., 39–41].

Pregnancy-specific stress was particularly relevant to women who became pregnant during the recent COVID-19 pandemic. This was especially true at the onset of the pandemic when impacts of the virus were poorly understood, and prenatal care and birthing practices were altered to mitigate infection risks, creating great uncertainty and worry for many pregnant women. Collaborating with researchers in the USA and six other Western nations (Germany, Israel, Italy, Poland, Spain, and Switzerland), we documented high levels of stress among pregnant women residing in each of the participating countries [42]. Across the seven countries, women experienced high pregnancy-specific stress resulting from pandemic stressors, and they also experienced high pregnancy-specific stress irrespective of those stressors, measured with the NuPDQ (or in Spain, the PDQ). Pregnancy-specific stress predicted levels of maternal anxiety and depressive symptoms above clinically defined thresholds. Furthermore, in a study conducted with more than 1300 pregnant women in the USA during the pandemic, my collaborators and I found that high NuPDQ scores were significant predictors of preterm birth [43, 44]. In this US sample, pregnancy-specific stress was highest among women of color and women who experienced greatest socioeconomic disadvantage [44, 45]. Taken together, studies conducted in the pandemic context with the NuPDQ extended the body of evidence establishing the validity of pregnancy-specific stress as measured with this instrument, demonstrating its harmful impact on physical and mental health in pregnant women, including during a global crisis.

5.3 Pregnancy-Specific Stress Instruments

Several other instruments assessing pregnancy-specific constructs similar to those measured by the PDQ and NuPDQ exist. Some of these instruments are quite lengthy and therefore may not be appropriate for use in clinical settings. For example, an instrument adapted by Glazer [46] and Lederman's Prenatal Self-Evaluation Scale [24, 47] include 62 and 78 items, respectively. The Pregnancy Anxiety Scale [25] purportedly assesses pregnancy-specific stress and is designed for retrospective reporting, administered in the third trimester. The Pregnancy-Related Anxiety Questionnaire [48] has been widely used [49] and collects ratings of how relevant or true are specific worries, concerns, or fears about pregnancy and birth. Although labeled an anxiety instrument, it does not assess anxiety per se. In contrast, Dunkel-Schetter and colleagues created a four-item measure that directly assesses anxiety, or what these researchers label pregnancy anxiety [35]. Respondents report how anxious, concerned, afraid, and panicky they have felt about being pregnant over the past week.

In 2012, Alderdice, Lynn, and I evaluated pregnancy-specific instruments with varying item content and response scales [50]. We found that many of the instruments designed to measure pregnancy-specific stress or pregnancy anxiety have methodological or conceptual weaknesses, including poor internal consistency, lack of predictive validity, or use of conceptually inappropriate items. Despite these weaknesses, we concluded that there is sufficient evidence to confirm that pregnancy-specific stress and pregnancy-specific emotional states are correlated with global stress but that the pregnancy-specific constructs are distinct and in some cases exhibit stronger independent prediction of birth outcomes. Alderdice et al. concluded that the PDQ was the strongest measure of pregnancy-specific stress available at the time (our analysis was conducted prior to creation of the NuPDQ, successor to the PDQ).

5.4 Lessons Learned About Pregnancy-Specific Stress

Pregnancy-specific stress instruments offer a variety of strengths for research on PNMS. These instruments often have greater predictive power than general measures of prenatal stress. In part, this may be because pregnancy-specific stress instruments include explicit references to pregnancy, birth, and parenting that facilitate recall and reporting. Additionally, pregnancy-specific instruments are often completed during prenatal care appointments, a context which is likely to cue or enhance attention to one's pregnancy experience. Thus, instruments such as the NuPDQ with well-established psychometric properties and a strong conceptual foundation are valuable tools for researchers. They also offer practical advantages. Using a single, reliable, and valid instrument to assess prenatal maternal stress reduces burden on respondents. A brief measure can also be administered repeatedly across pregnancy to examine change in levels of stress and responses to different sources of stress. Common contributors to stress in early pregnancy, such as uncomfortable symptoms, may differ from those that emerge later in pregnancy, as childbirth approaches, although some stressors and threats such as the threat of miscarriage, have been shown to persist in women with a previous poor pregnancy outcome [51]. Studies utilizing repeated measurement of prenatal stress can also advance our understanding of whether women are more vulnerable to the impact of stress during particular periods of their pregnancy. Prior studies of this issue have produced conflicting evidence [e.g., 36, 52, 53].

The NuPDQ may also offer value to health-care providers, including obstetricians and midwives. The total score can be examined by a clinician to assess a pregnant patient's overall level of stress but also, examining responses to specific items, might be used to identify the particular factors that are most stressful for her. This can be a basis for tailoring patient care and targeting appropriate interventions. The NuPDQ was not designed to be used as a clinical screening tool, however, so should be used for this purpose cautiously.

5.5 Conclusions

As indicated by systematic reviews and multiple individual studies, pregnancy-specific stress measures predict adverse birth outcomes more powerfully than do measures of general or global stress, distress, or anxiety. These findings indicate that pregnancy-specific stress is a particularly harmful type of stress. Both behavioral and physiological mechanisms have been shown to explain the impacts of pregnancy-specific stress. For example, higher levels trigger greater fetal arousal than does general stress [32–34], and pregnancy-specific stress is associated with poorer health behaviors among pregnant women [30]. Unlike general stress, pregnancy-specific stress involves stressors that are often immediate and concrete. Therefore, pregnancy-specific stress may be especially potent. Women may lack experience managing or coping with this type of stress, especially if they are pregnant for the first time or if they are encountering problems that they did not experience in a prior pregnancy [54]. Improving our ability to identify and measure pregnancy-specific stress will enable researchers and clinicians to better understand and address the needs of pregnant women so that we can provide the supports and resources that promote healthy birth outcomes.

References

1. Berkowitz GS, Kasl SV. The role of psychosocial factors in spontaneous preterm delivery. J Psychosom Res. 1983;27(4):283–90. https://doi.org/10.1016/0022-3999(83)90050-8.
2. Boyce WT, Schaefer C, Harrison HR, Haffner WH, Lewis M, Wright AL. Social and cultural factors in pregnancy complications among Navajo women. Am J Epidemiol. 1986;124(2):242–53. https://doi.org/10.1093/oxfordjournals.aje.a114382.
3. Gorsuch RL, Key MK. Abnormalities of pregnancy as a function of anxiety and life stress. Psychosom Med. 1974;36(4):352–62. https://doi.org/10.1097/00006842-197407000-00009.
4. Newton RW, Webster PA, Binu PS, Maskrey N, Phillips AB. Psychosocial stress in pregnancy and its relation to the onset of premature labour. Br Med J. 1979;2(6187):411–3. https://doi.org/10.1136/bmj.2.6187.411.
5. Littleton HL, Breitkopf CR, Berenson AB. Correlates of anxiety symptoms during pregnancy and association with perinatal outcomes: a meta-analysis. Am J Obstet Gynecol. 2007;196(5):424–32. https://doi.org/10.1016/j.ajog.2007.03.042.
6. Littleton HL, Bye K, Buck K, Amacker A. Psychosocial stress during pregnancy and perinatal outcomes: a meta-analytic review. J Psychosom Obstet Gynaecol. 2010;31(4):219–28. https://doi.org/10.3109/0167482X.2010.518776.
7. Beydoun H, Saftlas AF. Physical and mental health outcomes of prenatal maternal stress in human and animal studies: a review of recent evidence. Paediatr Perinat Epidemiol. 2008;22(5):438–66. https://doi.org/10.1111/j.1365-3016.2008.00951.x.
8. Lobel M. Conceptualizations, measurement, and effects of prenatal maternal stress on birth outcomes. J Behav Med. 1994;17(3):225–72. https://doi.org/10.1007/bf01857952.
9. Lobel M, Dunkel-Schetter C. Conceptualizing stress to study effects on health: environmental, perceptual, and emotional components. Anxiety Res. 1990;3(3):213–30. https://doi.org/10.1080/08917779008248754.
10. Lazarus RS. Psychological stress and the coping process. New York: McGraw-Hill; 1966.

11. Lazarus RS, Launier R. Stress-related transactions between person and environment. In: Pervin LA, Lewis M, editors. Perspectives in interactional psychology. Boston: Springer US; 1978. p. 287–327.
12. Lazarus RS, Folkman S. Stress, appraisal, and coping. Springer Publishing Company; 1984.
13. Hobfoll SE. Conservation of resources. A new attempt at conceptualizing stress. Am Psychol. 1989;44(3):513–24. https://doi.org/10.1037/0003-066X.44.3.513.
14. Monroe SM. Major and minor life events as predictors of psychological distress: further issues and findings. J Behav Med. 1983;6(2):189–205. https://doi.org/10.1007/BF00845380.
15. Billings AG, Moos RH. Stressful life events and symptoms: a longitudinal model. Health Psychol. 1982;1(2):99–117. https://doi.org/10.1037/0278-6133.1.2.99.
16. Baum A, Davidson LM, Singer JE, Street SW. Stress as a psychophysiological process. In: Handbook of psychology and health: stress, vol. 5. Hillsdale: Lawrence Erlbaum Associates, Inc; 1987. p. 1–24.
17. Lobel M, Dunkel-Schetter C, Scrimshaw SC. Prenatal maternal stress and prematurity: a prospective study of socioeconomically disadvantaged women. Health Psychol. 1992;11(1):32–40. https://doi.org/10.1037/0278-6133.11.1.32.
18. Raznahan A, Greenstein D, Lee NR, Clasen LS, Giedd JN. Prenatal growth in humans and postnatal brain maturation into late adolescence. Proc Natl Acad Sci USA. 2012;109(28):11366–71. https://doi.org/10.1073/pnas.1203350109.
19. Abel KM, Wicks S, Susser ES, Dalman C, Pedersen MG, Mortensen PB, et al. Birth weight, schizophrenia, and adult mental disorder: is risk confined to the smallest babies? Arch Gen Psychiatry. 2010;67(9):923–30. https://doi.org/10.1001/archgenpsychiatry.2010.100.
20. Shenkin SD, Starr JM, Deary IJ. Birth weight and cognitive ability in childhood: a systematic review. Psychol Bull. 2004;130(6):989–1013. https://doi.org/10.1037/0033-2909.130.6.989.
21. Molfese VJ, Bricker MC, Manion LG, Beadnell B, Yaple K, Moires KA. Anxiety, depression and stress in pregnancy: a multivariate model of intra-partum risks and pregnancy outcomes. J Psychosom Obstet Gynecol. 1987;7(2):77–92. https://doi.org/10.3109/01674828709019593.
22. Norbeck JS, Tilden VP. Life stress, social support, and emotional disequilibrium in complications of pregnancy: a prospective, multivariate study. J Health Soc Behav. 1983;24(1):30–46.
23. Molfese VJBM, Manion L, Beadnell B, Yaple K, Moires KA. Anxiety, depression and stress in pregnancy: a multivariate model of intra-partum risks and pregnancy outcomes. J Psychosom Obstet Gynaecol. 1987;7:77–92.
24. Halman LJ, Oakley D, Lederman R. Adaptation to pregnancy and motherhood among subfecund and fecund primiparous women. Matern Child Nurs J. 1995;23(3):90–100.
25. Levin JS. The factor structure of the pregnancy anxiety scale. J Health Soc Behav. 1991;32(4):368–81.
26. Yali AM, Lobel M. Coping and distress in pregnancy: an investigation of medically high risk women. J Psychosom Obstet Gynaecol. 1999;20(1):39–52. https://doi.org/10.3109/01674829909075575.
27. Cohen S, Kamarck T, Mermelstein R. A global measure of perceived stress. J Health Soc Behav. 1983;24(4):385–96. https://doi.org/10.2307/2136404.
28. Spielberger CD. Manual for the state-trait anxiety inventory. Palo Alto: Consulting Psychologists Press; 1983.
29. Lobel M, DeVincent CJ, Kaminer A, Meyer BA. The impact of prenatal maternal stress and optimistic disposition on birth outcomes in medically high-risk women. Health Psychol. 2000;19(6):544–53. https://doi.org/10.1037/0278-6133.19.6.544.
30. Lobel M, Cannella DL, Graham JE, DeVincent C, Schneider J, Meyer BA. Pregnancy-specific stress, prenatal health behaviors, and birth outcomes. Health Psychol. 2008;27(5):604–15. https://doi.org/10.1037/a0013242.
31. Yali AM, Lobel M. Stress-resistance resources and coping in pregnancy. Anxiety Stress Coping. 2002;15(3):289–309. https://doi.org/10.1080/1061580021000020743.
32. DiPietro JA, Ghera MM, Costigan K, Hawkins M. Measuring the ups and downs of pregnancy stress. J Psychosom Obstet Gynaecol. 2004;25(3–4):189–201. https://doi.org/10.1080/01674820400017830.

33. DiPietro JA, Hilton SC, Hawkins M, Costigan KA, Pressman EK. Maternal stress and affect influence fetal neurobehavioral development. Dev Psychol. 2002;38(5):659–68.
34. Huizink AC, Mulder EJ, Robles de Medina PG, Visser GH, Buitelaar JK. Is pregnancy anxiety a distinctive syndrome? Early Hum Dev. 2004;79(2):81–91. https://doi.org/10.1016/j.earlhumdev.2004.04.014.
35. Roesch SC, Dunkel SC, Grace W, Hobel CJ. Modeling the types and timing of stress in pregnancy. Anxiety Stress Coping. 2004;17(1):87–102. https://doi.org/10.1080/1061580031000123667.
36. Glynn LM, Wadhwa PD, Dunkel-Schetter C, Chicz-Demet A, Sandman CA. When stress happens matters: effects of earthquake timing on stress responsivity in pregnancy. Am J Obstet Gynecol. 2001;184(4):637–42. https://doi.org/10.1067/mob.2001.111066.
37. Glynn LM, Schetter CD, Wadhwa PD, Sandman CA. Pregnancy affects appraisal of negative life events. J Psychosom Res. 2004;56(1):47–52. https://doi.org/10.1016/s0022-3999(03)00133-8.
38. Ibrahim SM, Lobel M. Conceptualization, measurement, and effects of pregnancy-specific stress: review of research using the original and revised prenatal distress questionnaire. J Behav Med. 2020;43(1):16–33. https://doi.org/10.1007/s10865-019-00068-7.
39. Romero-Gonzalez B, Caparros-Gonzalez RA, Gonzalez-Perez R, Delgado-Puertas P, Peralta-Ramirez MI. Newborn infants' hair cortisol levels reflect chronic maternal stress during pregnancy. PLoS One. 2018;13(7):e0200279. https://doi.org/10.1371/journal.pone.0200279.
40. Xie W, Wang M, Ng S, Lu S, Yeung A, Chan KP, et al. Effects of a mindfulness-based intervention delivered by Mobile phone on perinatal-specific stress and neonatal outcomes: a randomized controlled trial. Mindfulness. 2024;15(10):2595–608. https://doi.org/10.1007/s12671-024-02457-9.
41. Mariño-Narvaez C, Puertas-Gonzalez JA, Romero-Gonzalez B, Cruz-Martinez M, Gonzalez-Perez R, Juncosa-Castro Y, et al. High-risk pregnancy and its relationship with the neurodevelopment and behavior of 2-year-old children. Dev Psychopathol. 2024:1–8. https://doi.org/10.1017/S0954579424000786.
42. Lobel M, Preis H, Mahaffey B, Schaal NK, Yirmiya K, Atzil S, et al. Common model of stress, anxiety, and depressive symptoms in pregnant women from seven high-income Western countries at the COVID-19 pandemic onset. Soc Sci Med. 2022;315:115499. https://doi.org/10.1016/j.socscimed.2022.115499.
43. Preis H, Mahaffey B, Pati S, Heiselman C, Lobel M. Adverse perinatal outcomes predicted by prenatal maternal stress among U.S. women at the COVID-19 pandemic onset. Ann Behav Med. 2021;55(3):179–91. https://doi.org/10.1093/abm/kaab005.
44. Preis H, Wang WH, Zhu W, Mahaffey B, Lobel M. Social determinants of health, prenatal maternal stress, and earlier birth during the COVID-19 pandemic. Soc Personal Psychol Compass. 2023;17(7):9. https://doi.org/10.1111/spc3.12751.
45. Rehbein E, Levinson A, Preis H, Mahaffey B, Lobel M. Gendered racism in pregnancy and stress among women in the United States during the COVID-19 pandemic. Int Perspect Psychol. 2024;13(3):119–27. https://doi.org/10.1027/2157-3891/a000104.
46. Glazer G. Anxiety levels and concerns among pregnant women. Res Nurs Health. 1980;3(3):107–13. https://doi.org/10.1002/nur.4770030305.
47. Lederman RP, Lederman E, Work BA, McCann DS. Relationship of psychological factors in pregnancy to progress in labor. Nurs Res. 1979;28(2):94–7. https://doi.org/10.1097/00006199-197903000-00012.
48. Van den Bergh BR. The influence of maternal emotions during pregnancy on fetal and neonatal behavior. J Prenat Perinat Psychol Health. 1990;5(2):119–30.
49. Hadfield K, Akyirem S, Sartori L, Abdul-Latif A-M, Akaateba D, Bayrampour H, et al. Measurement of pregnancy-related anxiety worldwide: a systematic review. BMC Pregnancy Childbirth. 2022;22(1):331. https://doi.org/10.1186/s12884-022-04661-8.
50. Alderdice F, Lynn F, Lobel M. A review and psychometric evaluation of pregnancy-specific stress measures. J Psychosom Obstet Gynaecol. 2012;33(2):62–77. https://doi.org/10.3109/0167482X.2012.673040.

51. Côté-Arsenault D. Threat appraisal, coping, and emotions across pregnancy subsequent to perinatal loss. Nurs Res. 2007;56(2):108–16. https://doi.org/10.1097/01.Nnr.0000263970.08878.87.
52. Bergeron J, Avraam D, Calas L, Fraser W, Harris JR, Heude B, et al. Stress and anxiety during pregnancy and length of gestation: a federated study using data from five Canadian and European birth cohorts. Eur J Epidemiol. 2024;39(7):773–83. https://doi.org/10.1007/s10654-024-01126-4.
53. Collins JM, Keane JM, Deady C, Khashan AS, McCarthy FP, O'Keeffe GW, et al. Prenatal stress impacts foetal neurodevelopment: temporal windows of gestational vulnerability. Neurosci Biobehav Rev. 2024;164:105793. https://doi.org/10.1016/j.neubiorev.2024.105793.
54. Mahaffey BL, Tilley JL, Molina LK, Gonzalez A, Park E, Lobel M. "How am I going to make it through pregnancy?" A qualitative examination of prenatal maternal stress. Birth. 2022;49(2):253–60. https://doi.org/10.1111/birt.12598.

6 Wars as a Source of Maternal Stress During Pregnancy and Postpartum

Maria F. Rodríguez-Muñoz, Magdalena Chrzan-Dętkoś, Ana Uka, and Gracia Fellmeth

Abstract

In this chapter, the most relevant data from the literature on the impact of war on perinatal mothers and their children are presented. From the maternal perspective, post-traumatic stress disorder (PTSD) in mothers will be analyzed. Regarding the children, different sections address the impact of war on the mother-infant bond, cognitive development, and the presence of psychopathology. Finally, the interventions established by the literature are compiled, along with suggestions for best practices based on evidence.

Keywords

War · Maternal stress · Infant

6.1 Introduction

Armed conflict poses significant challenges for civilians. According to the Institute for Research on International Conflicts, Heidelberg's Conflict Barometer identified 54 wars in 2022. According to the Conflict Intensity Index (CII) developed by

M. F. Rodríguez-Muñoz (✉)
Department of Psychology, Universidad Nacional de Educación a Distancia, Madrid, Spain
e-mail: mfrodriguez@psi.uned.es

M. Chrzan-Dętkoś
Institute of Psychology, University of Gdańsk, Gdańsk, Poland

A. Uka
Department of Nursing and Physiotherapy, Western Balkans University, Tirana, Albania

G. Fellmeth
National Perinatal Epidemiology Unit, University of Oxford, Oxford, UK

R. A. Caparros-Gonzalez (ed.), *Maternal Stress during Pregnancy and Postpartum*, https://doi.org/10.1007/978-3-032-09245-8_6

Maplecrof [1], geographical areas affected by conflict have expanded by 65% since 2021 to include 4.6% of the entire globe. This is the equivalent of 6.15 million km^2, nearly double the size of India, the second largest country in the world.

Situations of conflict can include numerous stressful and traumatic events including explosions, sexual assault, imprisonment, kidnapping, forced displacement, torture, sieges, and the loss of loved ones [2]. Alongside these, a lack of access to clean water, overcrowded living conditions (for example in refugee camps and bomb shelters), limited food access, and poverty create challenging environments that contribute to the spread of infectious diseases and widespread malnutrition. Additionally, the collateral effects of war can severely impact mental health [3].

These conflicts leave lasting impacts on societies, but their effects are not evenly distributed. Women, newborns, and children are among the most vulnerable groups, bearing the brunt of these negative impacts [4]. Pregnant and postpartum (perinatal) women are particularly vulnerable in war situations [5], facing extraordinary challenges in parenting that are compounded by the constant stress of poverty and lack of basic resources. For example, in Palestine, women face uncertainty and delays when access to hospitals is impeded, for instance because of the presence of military checkpoints. The reality of being unable to reach a hospital to access safe delivery care means that many women have to deliver in nonhospital settings with reduced standards of care, increased risks to themselves and their babies, and increased risk of mortality [6].

These issues affect both physical and mental health, leading to increased maternal mortality [7] and low birth in newborns [8]. Furthermore, war can disrupt parenting patterns and attachment [9], increasing the likelihood of trauma [10, 11]. Exposure to stress is hypothesized to lead to a depletion of resources. Resources that would typically support the child's growth or the parent's ability to co-regulate the dyadic interaction are diverted, oriented toward regulating the parent and survival. When stress exposure becomes chronic, which is frequent in war-affected areas and among refugees, this reduction in resources can have long-lasting effects on the quality of dyadic interaction and infant development. This will be further developed later in this chapter.

According to the United Nations' Global Humanitarian Overview 2025 [12], civilians are bearing the effect of a record number of armed conflicts marked by deliberate indifference to international humanitarian and human rights law. The year 2024 was among the most brutal and violent in recent history for civilians trapped in conflict zones, and without immediate interventions, may prove even worse. In 2024, nearly 123 million people were forcibly displaced by conflict and violence [12]. The number of United Nations-verified cases of conflict-related sexual violence was 50% higher in 2023 than the year before. In the meantime, global military costs have surged, reaching US$2.4 trillion in 2023 [12]. Today, more than 78 million children in war-scarred areas are out of school. For example, in countries such as Syria, a generation of children has grown up knowing only war, ruining their education and future opportunities [12]. The report emphasizes that crises are lasting longer, with an average duration of 10 years, leading to increased maternal mortality and plummeting vaccination rates [12]. Severe violations against children have increased to extraordinary levels in multiple conflicts, with Sudan alone observing a 480% rise from 2022 to 2023. Over the past year, more women and children were killed in Gaza than in any other conflict over the past two decades [12].

A number of sources have highlighted that in Ukraine, an average of 16 children have been killed or injured every week since Russia's invasion in February 2022 [12]. Reports suggest a 12% increase in birth complications, including higher rates of Cesarean sections and premature deliveries. Many women are forced to give birth in makeshift shelters with limited medical support [12]. According to the Ukrainian Ministry of Health, Russian forces destroyed 174 medical facilities in Ukraine and drastically damaged another 1106 during the first year of the full-scale invasion [13].

In Gaza, the situation is equally dire. As of November 2023, according to data from the Ministry of Health, 2326 women and 3760 children have been killed since the start of the conflict in Gaza, corresponding to 67% of all casualties [14, 15]. Thousands more have been injured. Estimates suggest as many as 420 children are killed or injured each day, some of whom are only a few months old [16]. An estimated 60,000 of pregnant women in Gaza lack access to adequate prenatal healthcare. At least 183 women give birth in Gaza every day, and most do not have access to midwives, doctors, or healthcare. According to the International Rescue Committee, only two of the 12 partially operating hospitals in Gaza are able to provide maternity services, out of a total of 36 hospitals that were functioning before October 7 [17]. As of December 2024, over 155,000 pregnant and breastfeeding women were at high risk of malnutrition, and this number has likely risen exponentially since then [17].

In Sudan, over 2 million babies are estimated to have been born in 18 months of destructive war, and all are at high risk from a reduced healthcare system and crisis levels of deprivation [18]. In Somalia, only 31.9% of women give birth with the assistance of a doctor, midwife, or nurse, the lowest rate of skilled birth attendance in the world [19].

In Myanmar, civil conflict has persisted in one form or another for almost eight decades and has intensified since the military coup of February 2021. According to Amnesty International, an estimated 6000 civilians have been killed and 3.5 million have been internally displaced in the last 4 years [20, 21]. Many more have been displaced to neighboring countries including Bangladesh and Thailand. The conflict has had a devastating impact on Myanmar's economy and healthcare infrastructure, sending many into extreme poverty and with little or no access to health services. For displaced populations from Myanmar living in Thailand, access to maternity care is limited due to their precarious legal status, fear of authorities, long distances to healthcare facilities, and the prohibitive cost of transport to access these facilities. A number of nongovernmental organizations provide community-based antenatal care and birthing facilities, funded by international organizations such as UNICEF, the Global Fund, the European Union, and USAID. The recent decision by the current US government to freeze foreign aid has led to the abrupt closing down of many of these maternal health clinics along the border with devastating impacts on women who are unable to access safe delivery [20, 21].

6.1.1 Born into Hell

If parenting is complex and exhausting for many mothers, having an infant and raising a child in the midst of war is an extremely challenging and traumatic experience. Nothing can compare to the horrors of giving birth and bringing up a child in situations of conflict. Violence, destruction, bombings, and the use of chemical and biological weapons render motherhood extremely difficult and tragic in this context.

Pregnancy and childbirth in war zones can compromise the life of the mother and the fetus or newborn due to the lack of hospitals, medical personnel, and essential supplies. Many mothers give birth in precarious conditions in shelters, without pain relief or anesthesia, without professional care, and with a high risk of complications or premature delivery. Lack of vaccinations and neonatal care also increases infant mortality.

In addition, wars often cause food shortages that affect both mother and child. Maternal malnutrition affects breastfeeding, putting the health of the newborn at risk. Extreme stress can also affect breastmilk production, creating even more hardship for mothers who rely on breastfeeding to feed their babies. For those who use formula, finding clean, safe water to prepare bottles becomes a daily challenge. In the most extreme cases, mothers may be forced to feed their babies with dirty water or inadequate substitutes. This is particularly acute when humanitarian access is blocked, resulting in severe shortages of food, clean water, formula, and diapers.

The war-related challenges faced by new mothers and the helplessness of their relatives are illustrated by the case vignettes below:

> … It became really terrifying when my milk started to disappear due to nerves in the second month postpartum. We lived (or rather existed) in constant fear and tension and were prepared for the worst. We ate and slept in our clothes. A bag with documents and diapers under our heads. I trembled incessantly. At home, because of constant sirens and explosions we followed the rule of four walls (a room without windows). During an air raid alarm, we were either in the bathroom or the corridor. In these rooms, there was a chance of staying intact during a shock wave or explosion (in rooms with windows, there was a high probability of death from shrapnel). I was so stressed with getting the formula milk: pharmacies and stores were not working, and there was no way to order the milk and food online, the courier service was not working. Realizing that I had nothing to feed my infant drove me crazy. It seemed to me that it was the end. My husband, despite the risk, went to look for some stores, negotiated with relatives and friends (someone gave a bottle, someone shared food), and we survived … (Olya Bondarenko, Mykolaiv, frontline city citizen)

> … February 25, 2022. I woke up in hospital due to a powerful explosion. It seemed that in the next second, the hospital walls would collapse like dominoes. At 10 a.m., I was taken to the delivery room. At the same time, I was informed that the doctor who was supposed to deliver the infant did not come to work. As I was told, he sent an SMS with apologies. (We are all human. Fear for one's own life and the lives of family members. Now I understand and do not judge him. At that moment, this news crushed me even more.) Nerves were on edge. Due to stress and endless explosions, I didn't understand what was happening. I was given anesthesia and didn't notice when I started giving birth. Exactly at 1 p.m., everything began. The infant was born at 13:41. Throughout this time, my husband was in contact with me. He was present at the birth of our child via phone. He calmed me, joked, and cheered me on. Without his support, I wouldn't have been able to endure it all. But… at 20:00, nurse

> ran in and informed us that patients and staff should immediately evacuate to the basement. But after giving birth, I couldn't move on my own. For safety, the power was turned off. The windows were tightly covered. To move around in the dark, we used pocket flashlights and phones. Of course, the elevator was out of the question. Two paramedics lifted me and literally carried me to the basement. I can't give the exact number now, but there were many people. Patients, women in labor, their relatives, medical staff. They laid out beds for us, covered the floor with blankets and pillows. The basement was very small. People were everywhere. Girls with babies crowded three in one bed. Newborns were fed and changed on the floor. Another girl gave birth in the basement (she has healthy twins). Due to the large number of people, there was a severe lack of oxygen. It was hell. Mothers after childbirth were crying, babies were screaming, the staff was nervous. The thought wouldn't leave my mind: if a bomb hits the hospital, we will all be buried alive. A great mass grave. I was after birth with my healthy son but I couldn't think about anything else" ... (Olya Bondarenko, 28 years, Mykolaiv citizen, giving birth on the second day of war)

> After seven months, I was forced to leave my home and live in a tent. I cried a lot, feeling that my brave infant would never see the walls of his room that I had always dreamed of preparing for him. It was a cry from the depths of my heart that I had to give birth out of my home. (…). We are here, starting from nothing—no shelter, no home, not even a destiny. We built a tent again, and we promised each other again that we must survive, whatever happens ... (Ala Al Akhras from Palestine, in a letter of thanks to United Nations)

6.2 Theoretical Model and Outcomes

In situations of conflict and war, the Fetal Programming Hypothesis becomes particularly relevant. This hypothesis suggests that exposure to trauma—including war-related stress—during development, especially in the womb, has long-term effects on both physical and mental health throughout a child's life. It posits that periods of intense stress during pregnancy can influence fetal development, as environmental factors such as dietary changes, infections, and most notably, maternal stress impact the formation of the unborn child's essential biological systems [22].

This is especially critical in wartime, as mothers often face food shortages, the psychological trauma of life-threatening situations, and harsh environmental conditions that contribute to poor living standards with a high impact of stress. In fact, some authors prefer the term *toxic war stress* over *general stress* [23]. Various studies have examined the effects of fetal programming on the health and development of the unborn child. The central nervous system and the autonomic nervous system are among the most affected; even minor disruptions can alter fetal development, increasing the risk of cognitive and language impairments as well as susceptibility to mental disorders such as autism [22].

6.2.1 PTSD in Mothers

Psychological trauma refers to the adverse effects of highly stressful events on an individual's life [24]. According to DSM-5, diagnoses related to such stressful situations fall under the category of "trauma and stressor-related disorders" [25]. With the DSM-5 update to DSM5-TR [26], some clinical descriptors have been refined to improve diagnostic accuracy, although the overall structure of PTSD remains significantly unchanged. Within this framework, two significant disorders affecting adults are acute stress disorder (ASD) and post-traumatic stress disorder (PTSD). ASD symptoms can emerge within 3 days and last up to 1 month. Both ASD and PTSD share symptom clusters such as re-experiencing, avoidance, and negative cognitions and mood. The following citation relates an example of war-related re-experiencing:

> … I flinch at every rustle. I'm terribly afraid of loud, sharp sounds, and I have trouble sleeping. One day, I woke up during a storm; there was heavy rain with thunder and lightning. It seemed to me that shells were flying at us from all sides, I felt it was so real. My subconscious already reacts, and my imagination draws its own pictures. My husband calmed me down for a long time. I don't know if we will ever be able to calm our nerves. I think it will take a lot of time … (Ukrainian mother, internally displaced to Central Ukraine)

However, ASD includes an additional cluster: dissociation. Common dissociative symptoms include emotional blunting, dazedness, depersonalization, a sense of unreality, and an inability to recall significant aspects of the traumatic event [25]. Understanding as well as identifying and treating PTSD and its symptoms in individuals affected by war who are caring for young children is very important. It not only helps alleviate the suffering of mothers themselves but also supports them in caring for and regulating the emotions of young children, who are particularly dependent on the mental state of their primary caregiver.

Indeed, PTSD is one of the most common mental health disorders among individuals affected by war. Studies show that the prevalence of PTSD in war-affected populations can be high, with some estimates indicating a point prevalence of 23.7% for PTSD symptoms and 25.6% for depressive features among war-afflicted civilians [27]. Additionally, individuals affected by war often face multiple types of trauma. Mothers and caregivers may experience premigration trauma associated with war exposure as well as peri-migration displacement trauma and acculturation trauma [28]. Refugee families and children may develop complex post-traumatic stress disorder (C-PTSD) as a result of their experiences of multiple traumatic events [29]. These experiences impact maternal mental health and predict child development including PTSD symptoms, behavioral problems, and somatic complaints [30]. A systematic review of the effects of armed conflict and terrorism on children aged 0–6 years found that maternal depression and post-traumatic stress (PTS) were predictors of children's development, and according to Ahmed et al. [27], one in four war-affected mothers may develop the disorder. ASD, PTSD, C-PTSD, and depression can reduce mothers' levels of sensitivity to the infant's needs [31, 32].

Below are two case vignettes of refugee mothers from Ukraine during the first two months of the Russian invasion. The mothers were living with Polish host families, and it was the host families rather than the mothers themselves who asked midwives to refer the mothers for psychological care.

Case vignette illustrating acute stress disorder:

> … According to the Polish host family, the mother does not touch the infant but only provides regular care such as feeding and changing diapers. The mother is constantly watching reports on her phone from her village, where intense military actions are taking place. She doesn't want to go for walks, is often sad and absent, and prefers to be alone. She gave birth in a Polish hospital just a few weeks after the war outbreak; her daughter was 1 month old. The Polish host family tried to chat with her and offer help with the infant, but the mother seemed sad or absent when asked.
>
> Another referral to the midwife focused on a new mother with a 3-month-old infant who cried a lot. The mother watched TV and talked on the phone in Ukrainian with her relatives. She seemed very distressed, especially when she could not contact her partner, who could not leave Ukraine. The infant cried a lot. The host family suggested avoiding watching too much "war news," but the mother wanted to continue.
>
> Although the mothers were referred to a psychologist, they did not take up the offer of support. However, the host family still benefited: they were encouraged to accompany the mothers, for example, to watch the news together and to talk about their village using Google Translate to facilitate communication. In short, they were encouraged not to distract the mothers but to be with them during their moments of distress. This advice was helpful to the host families and made them feel that the mothers were less detached and alone …

As the number of wars increases and the growing body of research highlights the importance of caregiver mental health in predicting the developmental outcomes of war-affected children [33], the question of support is vital. However, in war situations, fear, anger, sadness, and stress associated with constant mobilization may also play an important, adaptive role in being vigilant to possible threats while also being a natural part of the grief reaction. Additionally, there has been an important paradigm shift in war-related studies. The emphasis has moved away from the "war exposure" model on children and families to the impact of "daily stressors": the chronically stressful conditions of daily life that are caused or exacerbated by wars and armed conflict, such as poverty, overcrowded and unsafe housing, lack of electricity, impaired parenting due to parental distress, heightened risk of family violence, and lack of or changed access to education [34]. This is exemplified in the following case vignette, where the mother of a 10-month-old infant describes the daily burden she faced while living in a Ukrainian city under attack:

> … In Mykolaiv, the situation with electricity and water was critical. The Russians blew up the main artery supplying water to the city. The city command and volunteers installed mobile water trucks from neighboring areas. People carried water in buckets and bottles. Three years have passed, and due to continuous shelling, only technical water (the quality of the water is disgusting—color, smell) has been restored to the homes of Mykolaiv residents. My husband carried water from supply points—clean water is so much needed, when you have an infant. There was no power for 4–6–8 hours a day. Water was boiled on a gas stove. Above all, we prepared infant formula and washed the infant's clothes by hand … (Olga Bodnarowa, citizen of Mykolaiv city, Ukraine)

Among pregnant and postpartum women and their infants, an important additional challenge is access to healthcare. Armed conflicts often target healthcare facilities, despite this being against international humanitarian law, leading to the destruction of infrastructure such as hospitals and the loss of essential medical personnel. This has a profound detrimental effect on the health of pregnant women and babies. Pregnant women are left without skilled birth attendants, increasing the risk of complications during childbirth and without access to essential services such as vaccinations and emergency obstetric care [35, 36]. As a result, families and children are not only exposed to war-related violence but also have to cope with many additional challenges under conditions of diminished interpersonal resources observed in families. These stressors can result in changes in parenting style. Associations between parental traumatization and harsh parenting have been demonstrated across multiple war-affected contexts, including Sri Lanka [11], northern Uganda [37], Israel [38], and resettled refugees in the Netherlands [39].

Returning to the clinical vignettes presented, the support provided by host families in accompanying mothers during their bereavement did not directly affect ASD symptoms in women, but it may have mitigated the impact of daily stressors. By being accompanied and supported during their grief, the women were not alone in facing daily challenges. They received not only material support in the form of infant supplies, which the families were able to organize, but also emotional support, ensuring they were not alone in dealing with difficult information.

This change in paradigm has impacted the scope of interventions, shifting the focus from PTSD to interventions targeting issues such as harsh parenting. The overall aim of interventions has remained similar: to decrease parental PTSD symptoms and the impact of parental traumatization on offspring. However, the specific goal of interventions has changed.

6.2.2 Infant

In the 50 most fragile states in the world that have displaced populations (including South Sudan, Somalia, Yemen, Syria, Central African Republic, Congo Democratic Republic, Sudan, Chad, Afghanistan, and Zimbabwe) [40], 60% and 53% of deaths among mothers and young children were reported to be preventable, respectively [40]. The trauma of displacement and the stress of migration increase the risk of premature birth [41] and fetal growth failure among pregnant women [42], which is a strong predictor of neonatal mortality as well as future child development including cognition, emotional development, and psychopathology.

6.2.2.1 The Impact of War on Mother-Infant Bonding

Taking care of infants in the context of armed conflict is highly demanding. Recent studies show a negative effect of war-related trauma on maternal and infant well-being [28, 43]. Yet, little is known regarding the influence of trauma on mother-infant bonding and the underlying mechanism, especially among refugee women. Ongoing conflict across several countries such as Ukraine, Russia, Israel, the Gaza Strip, and elsewhere have generated extensive fear, anxiety, and traumatic stress among the general population including women giving birth and experiencing the postpartum period concurrently with these events. These women are exposed to collective trauma, which heightens their risk of developing psychological problems and mental health disorders. More significantly, this period is critical for the development of an emotional tie between the infant and the mother, which is referred to as maternal-infant bonding. Such a relationship is defined as a strong emotional connection that the mother develops with the infant [44]. Though there are many studies assessing the impact of war on pregnancy outcomes, such as PTSD, maternal stress, and preterm birth, evidence is scarce on the impact of war on postpartum maternal mental health and especially on maternal-infant bonding. It is well established in the literature that maternal mental health problems may lead to disrupted mother-infant interactions, thus adversely affecting mother-infant bonding [45]. Studies show that if mothers are exposed to war-related trauma, they are more likely to experience mental health problems leading to more disruptions of mother-infant emotional connection [46]. As such, mothers become less sensitive and experience more emotional withdrawal and negative emotions. Another study conducted in Central Africa, Chad, and Cameroon found that mothers who displayed high levels of post-traumatic stress disorder, anxiety, and depression had lower levels of sensitivity, lower levels of social engagement with the infant, more maternal intrusiveness, and higher likelihood of a negative emotional state of the infant. The study suggested that maternal exposure to war-related trauma may negatively influence interaction quality and maternal responsiveness. Additionally, the study indicated that there is a potential transmission of trauma through maternal interactions with the infant during the war [47].

While some studies show that maternal exposure to traumatic events may increase the negative impact of maternal mental health problems on mother-infant bonding, other studies report that social support may act as a buffer, decreasing the impact of trauma on mother-infant interaction [48]. Studies also show that apart from war, there are a number of other mother-related factors that have a negative impact on mother-infant bonding such as younger age of the mother, being a single mother, low socioeconomic status, and maternal psychopathology [49, 50]. In war conditions, mothers who share these characteristics are at a higher risk of raising children with physical, cognitive, and psychosocial developmental issues. Mother experience more instability and stress under war conditions, and they are less likely to display quality parenting toward their babies, leading to less effective and less healthy mother-infant interactions. A meta-analysis conducted by Eltanamly et al. [43] found that higher levels of parental war exposure were associated with decreased warmth and increased harshness toward children. These parenting behaviors partially mediated the link between war exposure and child adjustment outcomes, including post-traumatic stress symptoms, depression, anxiety, social difficulties, externalizing behaviors, and reduced positive outcomes such as overall quality of life. In this context, considering the influential role of the mother on child's social emotional adaptation through quality mother-child interaction and attachment [51, 52], especially under strained conditions such as war, it is paramount to provide these mothers with social support and other resources to decrease the negative impact of war on these domains.

6.2.2.2 Impact of War and Maternal Stress on Infants' Cognitive Development

There is increasing evidence highlighting the associations between maternal mental health and a child's cognitive development. Maternal stress experienced during the perinatal period acts as a significant threat to the quality of mother-infant interactions and subsequently to infants' cognitive development. Even before the birth of the infant, fetal programming theory suggests that antenatal maternal stress is associated with long-lasting impacts on the development of the fetal nervous system and alterations in cognitive development which may persist throughout infancy and into older childhood [53]. Against the backdrop of war, these associations between maternal stress and infant development are intensified. Besides increasing women's likelihood of experiencing severe levels of stress, war in and of itself can disrupt the stability and security of the environment that infants need for the healthy development of their cognitive abilities. Conflict, military violence, gender-based violence and displacement, and the deprivation or precarity of basic needs intensify the negative impact on infants' development.

There is some evidence to suggest that certain factors can diminish the negative associations between maternal stress and infant cognitive development or even act as protective factors. For example, a study of Palestinian women who were in the first trimester of pregnancy during the 2014 Gaza war found that women's exposure to traumatic war events were associated with higher cognitive skills among their infants at 18 months [54]. The authors suggested that trauma-exposed mothers intensified their efforts to maintain protective and loving interactions with their vulnerable infants which in turn conferred a protective effect on their infants' development.

6.2.2.3 Impact on Biological Markers (Infant)

The chaotic and terrifying nature of war fosters an atmosphere of fear, uncertainty, and deprivation. This chronic stress that stems from the unpredictable and frightening situation can profoundly impact neurobiology, hindering brain development during pregnancy as well as in the postpartum period. Research in both humans and animals suggests that early exposure to maternal stress may have long-term consequences on stress reactivity [55] from pregnancy outcome to postpartum emotional regulation.

6.2.2.3.1 Maternal War-Related Stress and Pregnancy Outcome

Experiencing severe and prolonged stress during the prenatal period can also have a detrimental effect on women's obstetric outcomes. Vezhnovets [56] observed an increase in perinatal mortality and preterm births (PTB) among women in war-affected Ukraine. Delays caused by military checkpoints in Palestine were associated with an increase in the proportion of births occurring at home, rising from 8% in 1999 to 33% in 2002 [6]. Ten percent of pregnant Palestinian women were delayed at military checkpoints each year between 2000 and 2007, resulting in 69 deliveries, 35 infant deaths, and 5 maternal deaths occurring at the checkpoints [6]. In a systematic review and meta-analysis by Ding et al. [57], prenatal stressful life events were associated with a 20% increased risk of PTB and a 14% increased risk of infants being born small for gestational age (SGA). Due to damage and destruction of healthcare facilities in conflict-affected areas, PTB and SGA children and their parents may have poorer access to adequate medical care, which may additionally impact their development. Low birth weight and prematurity elevate the risk of long-term adverse outcomes in children including mental health and behavioral problems, eating disorders, lower IQ, and poorer educational attainment. While fleeing to another country can help to ensure safety, better access to medical care, and the fulfillment of basic needs, it may not be enough to prevent preterm births and low birth weight [41, 58]. Research from Ukraine suggests that refugees displaced by war have high rates of PTSD. The prevalence of PTSD was 32.9% among non-displaced persons (NDPs), 39.4% among internally displaced persons (IDP), and 47.2% among refugees. DSM-V criteria for PTSD diagnosis were met by 50.8% of NDPs, 55.4% of IDPs, and 62.2% of refugees [59]. An increased risk of preterm birth was observed in war refugees during the first year of residency in Sweden, with risks for very preterm birth continuing for up to 5 years [41]. Similar trends were observed in a Canadian study [58].

6.2.2.3.2 Maternal Stress and Infant Stress Reactivity

Several studies have focused on the association between maternal stress and infant stress reactivity. A number of biological markers include cortisol reactivity, parasympathetic nervous system (PNS) activity measured by the decrease in heart rate after stress exposure, and infant respiratory sinus arrhythmia (RSA), also a measure of heart rate variability related to respiration, that are crucial for infant regulatory capacities: returning the body to its resting state. They are based on the Still Face (SF) paradigm, in which maternal withdrawal is a potential stressor and returning to joint play allows for the measurement of biological markers after the mother comes back from a state of withdrawal. Enlow et al. [60] found that maternal trauma was associated with a less pronounced heart rate recovery after the SF stressor. Prenatal stress was linked to greater changes in infant respiratory sinus arrhythmia (RSA), a measure of heart rate variability related to respiration, during the SF episode [61]. In line with these studies, Edward Tronick's Mutual Regulation Model theory posits that maternal stress disrupts maternal caregiving abilities, resulting in inconsistencies in dyadic co-regulation, which is hypothesized to be a critical factor in the development of a child's stress response [62]. It can be observed in the postpartum period with the marker of infants' increased cortisol reactivity [63] as well as with increased vulnerability to psychological disorders later in life [64] with difficulties in attention, learning, and emotional regulation [54]. Although the above-cited studies were not conducted on mothers and children with war experience, they help us understand the probable mechanisms of the impact of war on child development and can help to inform the development of potential interventions. Difficulties in the dyadic co-regulation during war and missile alarms are described in the following example:

> … A child senses the mother's behavior, and my condition was very bad. I was and I still am afraid of everything. He didn't sleep well. Sometimes he would predict air raid alarms. He would wake up and cry very loudly. Just a few minutes later, the siren would start to wail. It is very hard to watch my child cry and not be able to help him, I was also so stressed … (Olya Bondarenko, Ukraine)

Also in line with this evidence, Marti-Castaner et al. [65] study found that maternal refugee background increased the risk of regulatory problems in offspring. This effect was partially mediated by maternal postpartum mental health concerns, a finding which aligns with other studies showing that maternal mental health mediates the impact of war on infants [66]. Based on these studies, we assume that sensitive caregiving mitigates the rise of stress hormones and shields the infant's developing brain from the potentially toxic and harmful effects of maternal stress and trauma. However, sensitive caregiving in the context of war, migration, and trauma needs adequate, accessible support for caregivers. In the words of Selma Fraiberg, "When this mother's own cries are heard, she will hear her child's cries" (1980, p. 396) [67]. Possible interventions which focus on maternal mental health are described by the authors in another publication [66].

6.2.2.4 Child Psychopathology

Children exposed to war have a higher prevalence of mental health problems compared to the general population. However, the magnitude of the impact on mental health depends on various factors including the nature of trauma, duration of exposure, and cultural differences [41]. Often, childhood distress following war trauma goes unnoticed because children may have difficulty expressing or communicating their experiences. Adults tend to underestimate symptoms of post-traumatic stress in their children and may even deny the severity of the situation in an initial response to trauma [41]. Evidence from early studies suggested that children did not understand or remember traumatic events, but it is now recognized that, on the contrary, children are highly vulnerable to the stresses of war and terrorism and that these experiences are associated with a variety of psychological problems.

Children living in contexts of war and armed conflict often manifest a wide range of externalizing and internalizing problems. First, they may experience anxiety, reflected in behaviors such as frequent startling, nervousness, intense fear of darkness or noise, prolonged and inconsolable crying, somatic symptoms, and even aggressive behaviors [30]. They may also present symptoms of separation anxiety, anxious attachment, or strong dependence on their caregivers [23, 68]. In addition, the literature has described behaviors such as low frustration tolerance, excessive demands for attention, aggressiveness, and angry outbursts [30]. At the emotional level, the presence of deep sadness and prolonged crying episodes has been identified [69].

Childhood depression is an often-underestimated condition, in part because children express their distress differently from adults. Many children tend to show depressive symptoms with irritability rather than sadness (TCI). It is also common for children to present with prolonged episodes of crying without an apparent cause and a decrease in emotional expression, appearing shut down or disconnected from their environment. In contexts of war and conflict, where exposure to trauma is constant, depressive symptoms may intensify and manifest themselves in a variety of ways and are often difficult to recognize [69].

In relation to sleep patterns, literature has found direct links between war and poor sleep habits such as refusal to go to sleep alone, nightmares, nighttime waking, and wanting to sleep with parents [30]. Patterns in play are also affected; in fact, it has been seen that children who have experienced war or conflict settings tend to have repetitive play including morbid themes related to death, pain, or destruction of war and less fantasy play [30, 70].

Among children, the effects of war are not exclusively centered on specific mental disorders but also have an impact on a broad range of outcomes including family relationships, friendships, and school performance [71]. Contemporary wars almost exclusively affect low-resource settings and are often associated with a range of risk factors at various ecological levels, including extreme poverty, lack of healthcare resources, collapse of the educational system, and increased levels of family and community violence. Children are particularly sensitive to this accumulation of stressors [71].

Family relationships and functioning play a crucial role in the interplay between risk and protective factors related to war-induced stress. War is associated with high levels of family violence against children [72]. Despite these negative outcomes, research has also highlighted that positive parental care can serve as a protective factor, reducing the severity of trauma and internalizing behaviors [37].

6.3 Interventions and Best Practice

As discussed throughout the chapter, perinatal women and children living in conflict zones face extreme challenges that put their physical and mental health at risk, creating situations of severe vulnerability. This section presents a summary of some of the key interventions to support women and children in war and conflict-affected settings that have been described to date (Tables 6.1 and 6.2). Additionally, an analysis will be conducted to determine the best practices for implementing context-appropriate interventions.

Table 6.1 Summary of studies focused on war

Author and year	Main interventions
UNICEF [73]	UNHCR protects children taking care of their basic needs and giving them medical care. They also protect their rights by registering and documenting their identity. For example, after the war outbreak in Ukraine, 11 Ukrainian-speaking obstetric departments were created in Poland with midwife, breastfeeding, and psychological support for postpartum mothers [74, 75]
Ministry of Health, Israel (2024) [75]	Coping with breastfeeding during wartime This program supports mothers so they can continue breastfeeding. It also includes a breast milk donation bank for babies who are not being breastfed due to their mothers' situation caused by the armed conflict https://www.gov.il/en/pages/cd-511494623
Avendaño-Vásquez et al. (2021) [76]	The systematic review describing nursing interventions for children in situations of armed conflict. The results suggest that nursing interventions reduce psychological symptoms and improve health and function in children with longer-standing symptoms

(continued)

Table 6.1 (continued)

Author and year	Main interventions
Ayoya et al. (2013) [77]	Protecting and improving breastfeeding practices during a major emergency: infant tents for mother and babies has shown very promising results. Seventy percent (67,759) of the babies benefiting from the support were exclusively breastfed until 6 months, 10% of the other 30%—those who received "mixed feeding" (i.e., breast milk plus commercial milk formula and/or other foods or liquids)—transitioned to exclusive breastfeeding before the end of their participation in the infant tent program
Romanenko and Shlemkevych (2022) [78] Retrieved: Слайд 1	Information about UNICEF, NGOs, and Ukrainian ministry of hotline telephone number for psychological support and breastfeeding support: For example, UNICEF together with the NGO Milk Rivers of Ukraine prepared a course of 10 video lectures on BF with answers to questions that women have during pregnancy and after the birth of an infant. https://www.youtube.com/playlist?list=PLJ231j4oXT5uMvc_gyE_SyTM6wzM2EWX
WHO (2016) [79]	PTSD prevention Problem management plus (PM+). A brief, low-intensity transdiagnostic psychological intervention that addresses mental health treatment gaps in low- and middle-income countries and populations experiencing adversity
Sperlic et al. (2011) [80]	PTSD intervention/ prevention The survivor moms' Companion is a manualized self-study psychoeducation intervention which addresses the pregnancy-specific needs of traumatic stress-affected abuse survivors
Najavits (2022) [81]	PTSD intervention/prevention Seeking safety is a manualized psychosocial education program designed to improve coping skills among individuals with PTSD and comorbid substance abuse
Upshur et al. (2016) [82]	PTSD intervention/prevention Seeking Safety improves coping skills and medical appointments in pregnant women
Zlotnick et al. (2011) [83]	PTSD intervention/prevention Short-term interpersonal psychotherapy intervention is a manualized preventive intervention, including four sessions and one session 2 weeks after the delivery. The intervention had moderate effects in reducing symptoms of PTSD and depression during pregnancy and a large effect for PTSD symptoms from pregnancy up to 3 months postpartum
Almoshmosh (2016) [84]	PTSD intervention/prevention Provides recommendation of self-management approach in war trauma survivors (general population)
Bass et al. (2020) [85]	PTSD, treatment Systematic review of PTSD treatment for pregnant women: Improvement of PTSD symptoms was reported in 10 of the 13 studies, significant results in four studies: CBT, TF-CBT, survivor moms' companion, and seeking safety
Bright et al. (2020) [86]	PTSD, treatment IPT is an effective intervention for the prevention and treatment of psychological distress in women during the perinatal period. IPT is effective in significantly reducing symptoms of depression and anxiety as well as improving social support, relationship quality/satisfaction, and adjustment

(continued)

Table 6.1 (continued)

Author and year	Main interventions
Tol et al., WHO (2014) [33]	PTSD intervention/prevention Provides recommendations focusing on supporting community-based interventions that promote resilience, skills building, functioning, and a sense of productivity
Sperlich et al. (2017) [87]	PTSD/prevention Trauma-informed care in maternity practice
Practice guideline for the treatment of patients with acute stress disorder and posttraumatic stress disorder, APA (Ursano et al. 2004) [88]	PTSD, ASD, prevention, treatment The sequence of treatment steps: Once stabilization of symptoms such as insomnia, extreme dissociation, rage, or agitation is achieved, supportive psychotherapy, psychoeducation, and assistance in accessing resources can be beneficial

Based on Rodriguez-Muñoz et al. [66]

Table 6.2 Best practice during the perinatal period

Guarantee access to basic needs during the conflict: Guaranteeing access to drinking water, food, and shelter is fundamental. These shelters must guarantee minimum conditions of sanitation, safety, and temperature. Commonly, there is a dependence on humanitarian aid to cover these basic needs of food and hygiene [17]
Breastfeeding: An increase in the number of conflict casualties is associated with a significant decrease in the likelihood that a child will be breastfed [89]. It is therefore essential to provide comprehensive support to mothers, both physically, through the provision of humanitarian assistance to ensure adequate nutrition, and psychologically, through strategies to mitigate the stress of war
Healthcare: Access to medical care is often limited in these situations. Hospitals and healthcare centers are often attacked, which amplifies and expands the damage to the population. In this situation, it is important to convey that hygiene should be monitored to prevent infections (e.g., boiling water) without forgetting vaccinations and checkups whenever possible [90]
Education: During wars and armed conflicts, schools and colleges are often severely affected. Air raids, bombings, and fighting destroy or damage schools, leaving them totally devastated. In some cases, educational facilities are used as military bases, shelters for displaced persons, or detention centers, preventing their use for teaching. In other cases, it is the families themselves who stop sending their children for fear of violence, kidnapping, or forced recruitment by armed groups. This limits opportunities for the future [41]
Safety: Protecting the child/infant from the immediate dangers of conflict, such as shelling and shooting, is crucial. In this regard, families may often have to relocate to safer areas or live in shelters as internal refugees within the country of conflict or externally by moving to other countries [17]

(continued)

Table 6.2 (continued)

Emotional support: The stress of war affects both parents and infants. Maintaining a calm environment, despite the chaos, helps an infant's emotional development. Singing, talking, and playing can provide comfort and a sense of normalcy within the circumstances [91]
Promoting community support and resilience: Creating a support network with other families in similar situations can provide emotional and practical help. Sharing resources and information can help parents cope with challenges more effectively [17]. Early postwar interventions should focus on promoting safety, self-concept and community efficacy, relationships, and hope [41, 80]. Communities, families, and individuals should be given the opportunity to regain confidence in themselves and in the future. The development and implementation of culturally sensitive community-based programs is imperative to effectively address the challenges faced by large groups of children and their families in their natural environments [30]

6.4 Clinical and Research

Research on perinatal women in conflict zones remains severely limited, with existing studies primarily focusing on postpartum depression and anxiety. These narrow investigations fail to capture the multifaceted challenges faced by women in such volatile environments. For instance, broader mental health research in conflict settings often generalizes experiences across genders, overlooking crucial distinctions tied to life stage and maternal responsibilities. This omission neglects pressing concerns such as post-traumatic stress specific to childbirth in war zones, the realities of being a refugee with an infant, and the difficulties of breastfeeding under extreme conditions.

Addressing this research gap is essential, but it also raises significant ethical dilemmas. Conducting studies in these settings involves navigating the delicate balance between gathering vital data and respecting the profound suffering of those affected. The very act of administering surveys and measuring psychological distress in traumatized populations presents moral and logistical challenges. Furthermore, gaining access to displaced mothers and their infants is inherently complex due to security concerns, mobility restrictions, and the unpredictability of conflict zones.

Despite these obstacles, any research—no matter how constrained—sheds much-needed light on this neglected area. Even small-scale studies can inform policies and interventions that improve maternal and infant well-being in war-torn regions, ultimately contributing to a more comprehensive understanding of how to support these vulnerable populations.

When considering psychological interventions, it is essential to acknowledge the challenges that may arise. One of the primary difficulties involves barriers to access and continuity of care. The constant displacement of individuals living in conflict zones makes it difficult to maintain consistent psychological support. Additionally, mental health services in these settings are often scarce or entirely unavailable due to the impact of war.

Furthermore, the violence many women endure—such as abuse, torture, or family separation—can lead to fear, distrust, or reluctance to seek help and share their experiences. Another critical issue is the lack of research in this field, which has resulted in a shortage of culturally sensitive interventions. Many existing psychological approaches have not been specifically designed for war-affected populations and may require significant adaptation to be effective.

War inflicts profound wounds, both visible and unseen, yet it also creates a crucial opportunity to heal and rebuild. Supporting perinatal women and their babies is more than an act of compassion; it is a vital step toward restoring communities, fostering resilience, and ensuring future generations grow up in a world that values life, stability, and hope. By prioritizing maternal and infant well-being, we establish the foundation for societies that can emerge from conflict stronger, united, and determined to break the cycle of war's devastation.

6.5 Conclusion

A deep understanding of how war impacts mothers and infants can lead to better-informed policies on conflict prevention, humanitarian aid, and post-conflict recovery. This insight can help shape decisions on policy priorities including resource allocation, and implementation of prevention and support programs to protect the developmental potential of the most vulnerable. Furthermore, this knowledge could guide post-conflict treatment by emphasizing the importance of addressing the developmental consequences of war across generations [91].

> … We live in the 21st century, can't we really find a way to resolve everything diplomatically? All countries need to unite. But since adults can't agree, and armed conflicts break out around the world from time to time, conditions must be created for a normal life for affected women and babies. Mandatory war child status. Conditions for life and support for development of affected children. Financial help, help from doctors and psychologists …
> (Ukrainian mother, IDP)

References

1. Maplecrof. Political risk. 2024.
2. Morina N, Stam K, Pollet TV, Priebe S. Prevalence of depression and posttraumatic stress disorder in adult civilian survivors of war who stay in war-afflicted regions. A systematic review and meta-analysis of epidemiological studies. J Affect Disord. 2018;239:328–38. https://doi.org/10.1016/j.jad.2018.07.027. Epub 2018 Jul 24. PMID: 30031252.
3. Murthy RS, Lakshminarayana R. Mental health consequences of war: a brief review of research findings. World Psychiatry. 2006;5(1):25. PMID: 16757987; PMCID: PMC1472271.
4. El Bizri M, Langlois EV, Reid A, Khosla R. Women and children first: delivering solutions in conflict-affected settings. PLOS Global Public Health. 2025;5(1):e0004084.
5. Chrzan-Dętkoś M, Rodríguez-Muñoz MF, Krupelnytska L, Morozova-Larina O, Vavilova A, García López H, Murawska N, Nakiš RS. Good practices in perinatal mental health for women during wars and migrations: a narrative synthesis from the COST action Riseup-PPD in the context of the war in Ukraine. Clín Salud. 2022;33(3):127–35. https://doi.org/10.5093/clysa2022a14.
6. Shoaibi H. Response to health in the Occupied Palestinian Territory–Author's reply. The Lancet. 2011;378(9802):e1. Retrieved from: https://www.thelancet.com/pb/assets/raw/Lancet/pdfs/palestine/palestine2011-4.pdf tracts Childbirth at checkpoints in the occupied Palestinian territory.

7. Fatusic Z, Kurjak A, Grgic G, Tulumovic A. The influence of the war on perinatal and material mortality in Bosnia and Herzegovina. J Matern Fetal Neonatal Med. 2005;18(4):259–63. https://doi.org/10.1080/14767050500198501.
8. Skokić F, Bačaj D, Selimović A, Hasanović E, Muratović S, Halilbašić A. Association of low Birth Weight Infants and Maternal Sociodemographic Status in Tuzla Canton during 1992-1995 war period in Bosnia and Herzegovina. Int J Pediatr. 2010;2010:789183. https://doi.org/10.1155/2010/789183. Epub 2011 Mar 28. PMID: 21490700; PMCID: PMC3068307.
9. Keren M, Abdallah G, Tyano S. WAIMH position paper: infants' rights in wartime. Infant Ment Health J. 2019;40(6):763–7. https://doi.org/10.1002/imhj.21813. Epub 2019 Aug 15. PMID: 31415108.
10. Benner AD, Wang Y, Shen Y, Boyle AE, Polk R, Cheng YP. Racial/ethnic discrimination and well-being during adolescence: a meta-analytic review. Am Psychol. 2018;73(7):855–83. https://doi.org/10.1037/amp0000204. Epub 2018 Jul 19. PMID: 30024216; PMCID: PMC6172152.
11. Catani C, Jacob N, Schauer E, Kohila M, Neuner F. Family violence, war, and natural disasters: a study of the effect of extreme stress on children's mental health in Sri Lanka. BMC Psychiatry. 2008;8(1):33. https://doi.org/10.1186/1471-244X-8-33.
12. United Nations. Global Humanitarian Overview 2025. 2024.
13. European Civil Protection and Humanitarian Aid Operations. Born under fire: despite war, new life in Ukraine prevails [Internet]. 2024. Available from: https://civil-protection-humanitarian-aid.ec.europa.eu/news-stories/stories/born-under-fire-despite-war-new-life-ukraine-prevails_en.
14. UNICEF. Violence in Israel and the State of Palestine. https://www.unicef.ch/en/current/statements/2023-10-09/violence-israel-and-state-palestine.
15. United Nations. Gaza: Humanitarians warn of worsening crisis amid renewed hostilities [Internet]. 2024 Jun. Available from: https://news.un.org/en/story/2024/06/1151286.
16. UNICEF, WHO, UNFPA, UNRWA. Joint statement: women and newborns bearing the brunt of conflict [Internet]. 2024. Available from: https://www.unicef.org/press-releases/joint-statement-unicef-who-unfpa-and-unrwa-women-and-newborns-bearing-brunt-conflict.
17. International Rescue Committee. Pregnant women and mothers in Gaza are fighting to keep themselves and their babies alive [Internet]. 2024. Available from: https://www.rescue.org/eu/press-release/pregnant-women-and-mothers-gaza-are-fighting-keep-themselves-and-their-babies-alive.
18. Save the Children. Sudan: over 2 million babies born in 18 months of devastating conflict [Internet]. 2024. Available from: https://www.savethechildren.net/news/sudan-over-2-million-babies-born-18-months-devastating-conflict.
19. Save the Children. The pregnancy and childbirth 'silent emergency' as 24 million mothers worldwide will give birth without a doctor, midwife or nurse in 2024 [Internet]. 2024. Available from: https://www.savethechildren.org.uk/news/media-centre/press-releases/2024/24-million-mothers-will-give-birth-without-doctor-midwife-or-nurse-in-2024#:~:text=Somalia%20is%20grappling%20with%20the,in%20the%20world%20%5B8%5D.
20. Amnesty International. Myanmar: Four years after coup, world must demand accountability for atrocity crimes [Internet]. 2025 Jan. Available from: https://www.amnesty.org/en/latest/news/2025/01/myanmar-four-years-after-coup-world-must-demand-accountability-for-atrocity-crimes/.
21. Amnesty International. Myanmar: Recklessly abrupt US aid stoppage poses existential threat to human rights [Internet]. 2025 Feb. Available from: https://www.amnesty.org/en/latest/news/2025/02/myanmar-recklessly-abrupt-us-aid-stoppage-poses-existential-threat-to-human-rights/.
22. Riquelme-Gallego B, Ramos-Soberbio L, Leno-Duran E, Martínez-Vázquez S, Caparros-Gonzalez RA. Adverse fetal and neonatal impact of war conflicts during pregnancy: a systematic review. IUBMB Life. 2025;77(2):e70006. https://doi.org/10.1002/iub.70006.

23. Samara M, Hammuda S, Vostanis P, El-Khodary B, Al-Dewik N. Children's prolonged exposure to the toxic stress of war trauma in the Middle East. BMJ. 2020;371:m3155. https://doi.org/10.1136/bmj.m3155.
24. Isobel S, Goodyear M, Furness T, Foster K. Preventing intergenerational trauma transmission: a critical interpretive synthesis. J Clin Nurs. 2019;28(7–8):1100–13. https://doi.org/10.1111/jocn.14735.
25. American Psychiatric Association. Desk reference to the diagnostic criteria from DSM-5®. Washington, DC: American Psychiatric Association; 2013.
26. American Psychiatric Association, editor. Diagnostic and statistical manual of mental disorders: DSM-5-TR. 5th ed. American Psychiatric Association Publishing; 2022.
27. Ahmed SH, Zakai A, Zahid M, Jawad MY, Fu R, Chaiton M. Prevalence of post-traumatic stress disorder and depressive symptoms among civilians residing in armed conflict-affected regions: a systematic review and meta-analysis. General Psychiatry. 2024;37(3):e101438. https://doi.org/10.1136/gpsych-2024-101438.
28. Hazer L, Gredebäck G. The effects of war, displacement, and trauma on child development. Humanit Soc Sci Commun. 2023;10(1):1–9. https://doi.org/10.1057/s41599-023-02438-8.
29. Pieloch KA, McCullough MB, Marks AK. Resilience of children with refugee statuses: a research review. Can Psychol. 2016;57(4):330. https://doi.org/10.1037/cap0000073.
30. Slone M, Mann S. Effects of war, terrorism and armed conflict on young children: a systematic review. Child Psychiatry Hum Dev. 2016;47:950–65. https://doi.org/10.1007/s10578-016-0626-7.
31. Mueller I, Snidman N, DiCorcia JA, Tronick E. Acute maternal stress disrupts infant regulation of the autonomic nervous system and behavior: a CASP study. Front Psych. 2021;12:714664. https://doi.org/10.3389/fpsyt.2021.714664.
32. Beebe B, Lachmann F, Jaffe J, Markese S, Buck KA, Chen H, Cohen P, Feldstein S, Andrews H. Maternal postpartum depressive symptoms and 4-month mother–infant interaction. Psychoanal Psychol. 2012;29(4):383. https://doi.org/10.1037/a0029387.
33. Tol WA, Barbui C, Bisson J, Cohen J, Hijazi Z, Jones L, De Jong JT, Magrini N, Omigbodun O, Seedat S, Silove D. World health organization guidelines for management of acute stress, PTSD, and bereavement: key challenges on the road ahead. PLoS Med. 2014;11(12):e1001769. https://doi.org/10.1371/journal.pmed.1001769.
34. Miller KE, Jordans MJ. Determinants of children's mental health in war-torn settings: translating research into action. Curr Psychiatry Rep. 2016;18(6):58. https://doi.org/10.1007/s11920-016-0692-3. PMID: 27091645.
35. Akol AD, Caluwaerts S, Weeks AD. Pregnant women in war zones. BMJ. 2016;353:i2037. https://doi.org/10.1136/bmj.i2037.
36. Jawad M, Hone T, Vamos EP, Cetorelli V, Millett C. Implications of armed conflict for maternal and child health: a regression analysis of data from 181 countries for 2000–2019. PLoS Med. 2021;18(9):e1003810. https://doi.org/10.1371/journal.pmed.1003810.
37. Saile R, Ertl V, Neuner F, Catani C. Does war contribute to family violence against children? Findings from a two-generational multi-informant study in northern Uganda. Child Abuse Negl. 2014;38(1):135–46. https://doi.org/10.1016/j.chiabu.2013.10.007.
38. Halevi G, Djalovski A, Vengrober A, Feldman R. Risk and resilience trajectories in war-exposed children across the first decade of life. J Child Psychol Psychiatry. 2016;57(10):1183–93. https://doi.org/10.1111/jcpp.12622.
39. Van Ee E, Kleber RJ, Mooren TT. War trauma lingers on: associations between maternal posttraumatic stress disorder, parent–child interaction, and child development. Infant Ment Health J. 2012;33(5):459–68. https://doi.org/10.1002/imhj.21324.
40. Messner JJ, Haken N, Taft P, Onyekwere I, Blyth H, Fiertz N, et al. Fragile states index 2018: issues of fragility touch the world's richest and most developed countries in 2018. Washington, DC: The Fund for Peace; 2018.
41. Liu C, Urquia M, Cnattingius S, Hjern A. Migration and preterm birth in war refugees: a Swedish cohort study. Eur J Epidemiol. 2014;29(2):141–3. https://doi.org/10.1007/s10654-013-9877-9. Epub 2014 Jan 14. PMID: 24420703; PMCID: PMC3955479.

42. Sanguanklin N, McFarlin BL, Park CG, Giurgescu C, Finnegan L, White-Traut R, Engstrom JL. Effects of the 2011 flood in Thailand on birth outcomes and perceived social support. J Obstet Gynecol Neonatal Nurs. 2014;43(4):435–44. https://doi.org/10.1111/1552-6909.12466. Epub 2014 Jun 24. PMID: 24956975.
43. Eltanamly H, Leijten P, Jak S, Overbeek G. Parenting in times of war: a meta-analysis and qualitative synthesis of war exposure, parenting, and child adjustment. Trauma Violence Abuse. 2021;22(1):147–60. https://doi.org/10.1177/1524838019833001. Epub 2019 Mar 10. PMID: 30852950; PMCID: PMC7675766.
44. De Falco S, Emer A, Martini L, Rigo P, Pruner S, Venuti P. Predictors of mother-child interaction quality and child attachment security in at-risk families. Front Psychol. 2014;5:898. https://doi.org/10.3389/fpsyg.2014.00898.
45. Parfitt YM, Ayers S. The effect of post-natal symptoms of post-traumatic stress and depression on the couple's relationship and parent-baby bond. J Reprod Infant Psychol. 2009;27(2):127–42. https://doi.org/10.1080/02646830802350831.
46. Tichelman E, Westerneng M, Witteveen AB, van Baar AL, van de Horst HE, de Jonge A, et al. Correlates of prenatal and postnatal mother-to-infant bonding quality: a systematic review. PLoS One. 2019;14(9):e0222998. https://doi.org/10.1371/journal.pone.0222998.
47. Dozio E, Feldman M, Viaux-Savelon S, Bizouerne C, Mansouri M, Moro MR, Radjack R. The transmission mechanisms of war trauma in early mother–child interactions, observed through the Coding Interactive Behaviour Scale. Child Care Pract. 2025:1–20. https://doi.org/10.1080/13575279.2024.2402473.
48. Scharpf F, Mkinga G, Neuner F, Machumu M, Hecker T. Fuel to the fire: the escalating interplay of attachment and maltreatment in the transgenerational transmission of psychopathology in families living in refugee camps. Dev Psychopathol. 2021;33(4):1308–21. https://doi.org/10.1017/S0954579420000516.
49. Svoboda DV, Shaw TV, Barth RP, Bright CL. Pregnancy and parenting among youth in foster care: a review. Child Youth Serv Rev. 2012;34(5):867–75. https://doi.org/10.1016/j.childyouth.2012.01.023.
50. Yoshikawa H, Aber JL, Beardslee WR. The effects of poverty on the mental, emotional, and behavioral health of children and youth: implications for prevention. Am Psychol. 2012;67(4):272. https://doi.org/10.1037/a0028015.
51. Bowlby EJ. Attachment and loss: attachment volume 1. London: Hogarth Press; 1969.
52. Ainsworth MD, Blehar MC, Waters E, Wall SN. Patterns of attachment: a psychological study of the strange situation. London: Psychology Press; 2015.
53. Glover V, O'Donnell KJ, O'Connor TG, Fisher J. Prenatal maternal stress, fetal programming, and mechanisms underlying later psychopathology—a global perspective. Dev Psychopathol. 2018;30(3):843–54. https://doi.org/10.1017/S095457941800038X.
54. Qouta SR, Palosaari E, Diab M, Punamäki RL. Intervention effectiveness among war-affected children: a cluster randomized controlled trial on improving mental health. J Trauma Stress. 2012;25(3):288–98. doi: https://doi.org/10.1002/jts.21707. Epub 2012 May 30. Erratum in: J Trauma Stress 2018;31(1):163–4. doi: 10.1002/jts.22225. PMID: 22648703.
55. Kaufman J, Plotsky PM, Nemeroff CB, Charney DS. Effects of early adverse experiences on brain structure and function: clinical implications. Biol Psychiatry. 2000;48(8):778–90. https://doi.org/10.1016/S0006-3223(00)00998-7.
56. Vezhnovets TA, Korotkyi OV, Gurianov VG, Paryi VD, Orabina TM, Pysariev AO, Marushko YV. Predicting fertility, neonatal and perinatal mortality, and stillbirths for evaluation of the needs for perinatal care in the future post-war reconstruction of Ukraine. Wiad Lek. 2024;77(4):716–23. https://doi.org/10.36740/WLek202404116. PMID: 38865628.
57. Ding X, Liang M, Wu Y, Zhao T, Qu G, Zhang J, Zhang H, Han T, Ma S, Sun Y. The impact of prenatal stressful life events on adverse birth outcomes: a systematic review and meta-analysis. J Affect Disord. 2021;287:406–16. https://doi.org/10.1016/j.jad.2021.03.083.
58. Urquia ML, Frank JW, Moineddin R, Glazier RH. Immigrants' duration of residence and adverse birth outcomes: a population-based study. BJOG Int J Obstet Gynaecol. 2010;117(5):591–601. https://doi.org/10.1111/j.1471-0528.2010.02523.x.
59. Lushchak O, Velykodna M, Bolman S, Strilbytska O, Berezovskyi V, Storey KB. Prevalence of stress, anxiety, and symptoms of post-traumatic stress disorder among Ukrainians after

the first year of Russian invasion: a nationwide cross-sectional study. Lancet Reg Health Eur. 2023;36:100773. https://doi.org/10.1016/j.lanepe.2023.100773. PMID: 38019977; PMCID: PMC10665943.

60. Enlow MB, Kullowatz A, Staudenmayer J, Spasojevic J, Ritz T, Wright RJ. Associations of maternal lifetime trauma and perinatal traumatic stress symptoms with infant cardiorespiratory reactivity to psychological challenge. Biopsychosoc Sci Med. 2009;71(6):607–14. https://doi.org/10.1097/PSY.0b013e3181ad1c8b.
61. Bush NR, Jones-Mason K, Coccia M, Caron Z, Alkon A, Thomas M, Coleman-Phox K, Wadhwa PD, Laraia BA, Adler NE, Epel ES. Effects of pre-and postnatal maternal stress on infant temperament and autonomic nervous system reactivity and regulation in a diverse, low-income population. Dev Psychopathol. 2017;29(5):1553–71. https://doi.org/10.1017/S0954579417001237.
62. Tronick E, Beeghly M. Infants' meaning-making and the development of mental health problems. Am Psychol. 2011;66(2):107–19. https://doi.org/10.1037/a0021631. PMID: 21142336; PMCID: PMC3135310.
63. Zietlow AL, Nonnenmacher N, Reck C, Ditzen B, Müller M. Emotional stress during pregnancy—associations with maternal anxiety disorders, infant cortisol reactivity, and mother-child interaction at pre-school age. Front Psychol. 2019;10:2179. https://doi.org/10.3389/fpsyg.2019.02179. PMID: 31607996; PMCID: PMC6773887.
64. Carr CP, Martins CM, Stingel AM, Lemgruber VB, Juruena MF. The role of early life stress in adult psychiatric disorders: a systematic review according to childhood trauma subtypes. J Nerv Ment Dis. 2013;201(12):1007–20. https://doi.org/10.1097/NMD.0000000000000049.
65. Marti-Castaner M, Hvidtfeldt C, Fredsted Villadsen S, Pagh Pedersen T, Elsenburg LK, Norredam M. Infants born to first-time mothers with a refugee background faced an increased risk of regulatory problems. Acta Paediatr. 2023;112(12):2541–50. https://doi.org/10.1111/apa.16938. Epub 2023 Aug 17. PMID: 37548569.
66. Rodriguez-Muñoz MF, Chrzan-Dętkoś M, Uka A, Garcia-López HS, Bina R, Le HN. A narrative review on emerging issues about war-related trauma in perinatal women: good practice for assessment, prevention, and treatment. Arch Womens Ment Health. 2025;28:201–17. https://doi.org/10.1007/s00737-024-01537-y.
67. Fraiberg S, editor. Clinical studies in infant mental health: the first year of life. New York: Basic Books; 1980.
68. Sadeh A, Hen-Gal S, Tikotzky L. Young children's reactions to war-related stress: a survey and assessment of an innovative intervention. Pediatrics. 2008;121(1):46–53. https://doi.org/10.1542/peds.2007-1348. PMID: 18166556.
69. Dybdahl R. Children and mothers in war: an outcome study of a psychosocial intervention program. Child Dev. 2001;72(4):1214–30. https://doi.org/10.1111/1467-8624.00343. PMID: 11480943.
70. Dr CE, Chazan S, Lerner M, Maimon E. Posttraumatic play in young children exposed to terrorism: an empirical study. Infant Ment Health J. 2010;31(2):159–81. https://doi.org/10.1002/imhj.20250.
71. Catani C. Mental health of children living in war zones: a risk and protection perspective. World Psychiatry. 2018;17(1):104. https://doi.org/10.1002/wps.20496.
72. Clark CJ, Everson-Rose SA, Suglia SF, Btoush R, Alonso A, Haj-Yahia MM. Association between exposure to political violence and intimate-partner violence in the Occupied Palestinian Territory: a cross-sectional study. Lancet. 2010;375(9711):310–6. https://doi.org/10.1016/S0140-6736(09)61827-4. PMID: 20109958.
73. UNICEF USA. Protect children in conflict: UNICEF's call to action for 2025 [Internet]. 2024 Dec 28. Available from: https://www.unicefusa.org/stories/protect-children-conflict-unicefs-call-action-2025.
74. Babiszewska-Aksamit M, Bzikowska-Jura A, Kotlińska A, Aduła A, Chrobak A, Domosud J, Drążkowska I, Gaweł P, Jakimiuk A, Kołodziej J, Królak-Olejnik B. Good practice in lactation counseling for Ukrainian refugee mothers to ensure the health and mental benefits of breastfeeding—an observational study. Arch Womens Ment Health. 2025;28(2):257–69. https://doi.org/10.1007/s00737-024-01538-x.

75. Ministry of Health, Israel. [Internet]. 2024 [cited 2025 03 01]. Available from: https://www.gov.il/en/pages/cd-511494623.
76. Avendaño-Vásquez CJ, Reina-Gamba NC, Daza-Castillo LA, Quarantini L. Nursing interventions in children living under armed conflict situations and quality of life: a scoping review. J Pediatr Nurs. 2021;58:44–52. https://doi.org/10.1016/j.pedn.2020.11.012.
77. Ayoya MA, Golden K, Ngnie-Teta I, Moreaux MD, Mamadoultaibou A, Koo L, Boyd E, Beauliere JM, Lesavre C, Marhone JP. Protecting and improving breastfeeding practices during a major emergency: lessons learnt from the infant tents in Haiti. Bull World Health Organ. 2013;91:612–7. https://doi.org/10.2471/BLT.12.113936.
78. Romanenko L, Shlemkevych O. The emergency in Ukraine, the war: focus on breastfeeding. Rome; 2022. Retrieved from: Слайд 1.
79. World Health Organization. Problem Management Plus (PM+): individual psychological help for adults impaired by distress in communities exposed to adversity. Geneva: WHO; 2018.
80. Sperlich M, Seng JS, Rowe H, Cameron H, Harris A, McCracken A, Rauch SA, Bell SA. The survivor moms' companion: feasibility, safety, and acceptability of a posttraumatic stress specific psychoeducation program for pregnant survivors of childhood maltreatment and sexual trauma. Int J Childbirth. 2011;1(2):122–35. https://doi.org/10.1891/2156-5287.1.2.122.
81. Najavits L. Seeking safety: a treatment manual for PTSD and substance abuse. New York: Guilford Publications; 2002.
82. Upshur CC, Wenz-Gross M, Weinreb L, Moffitt JJ. Using prenatal advocates to implement a psychosocial education intervention for posttraumatic stress disorder during pregnancy: feasibility, care engagement, and predelivery behavioral outcomes. Womens Health Issues. 2016;26(5):537–45. https://doi.org/10.1016/j.whi.2016.06.003.
83. Zlotnick C, Capezza NM, Parker D. An interpersonally based intervention for low-income pregnant women with intimate partner violence: a pilot study. Arch Womens Ment Health. 2011;14:55–65. https://doi.org/10.1007/s00737-010-0195-x.
84. Almoshmosh N. The role of war trauma survivors in managing their own mental conditions, Syria civil war as an example. Avicenna J Med. 2016;6(02):54–9. https://doi.org/10.4103/2231-0770.179554.
85. Baas MA, Van Pampus MG, Stramrood CA, Dijksman LM, Vanhommerig JW, de Jongh A. Treatment of pregnant women with fear of childbirth using EMDR therapy: results of a multi-center randomized controlled trial. Front Psych. 2022;12:798249. https://doi.org/10.3389/fpsyt.2021.798249.
86. Bright KS, Charrois EM, Mughal MK, Wajid A, McNeil D, Stuart S, Hayden KA, Kingston D. Interpersonal psychotherapy to reduce psychological distress in perinatal women: a systematic review. Int J Environ Res Public Health. 2020;17(22):8421. https://doi.org/10.3390/ijerph17228421.
87. Sperlich M, Seng JS, Li Y, Taylor J, Bradbury-Jones C. Integrating trauma-informed care into maternity care practice: conceptual and practical issues. J Midwifery Womens Health. 2017;62(6):661–72. https://doi.org/10.1111/jmwh.12674.
88. Ursano RJ, Bell C, Eth S, Friedman M, Norwood A, Pfefferbaum B, Pynoos JD, Zatzick DF, Benedek DM, McIntyre JS, Charles SC. Practice guideline for the treatment of patients with acute stress disorder and posttraumatic stress disorder. Am J Psychiatry. 2004;161(11 Suppl):3–31.
89. Diwakar V, Malcolm M, Naufal G. Violent conflict and breastfeeding: the case of Iraq. Confl Heal. 2019;13:61. https://doi.org/10.1186/s13031-019-0244-7.
90. Alderman SL. Holding the infant in mind in times of war. American Academy of Pediatrics [Internet]; 2022. Available from: https://www.aap.org/en/news-room/aap-voices/holding-the-baby-in-mind-in-times-of-war/?srsltid=AfmBOooSwQPRM0qFKn4JALANdn6XU63b9ITT29v0cBS2e3yel8VKQp98.
91. Bilewicz M. Traumaland: Polacy w cieniu przeszłości. Mando; 2024.

Natural Disasters Can Increase Maternal Stress

7

Leire Salazar and Nerea Bello-Iglesias

Abstract

This chapter examines the biological pathways through which prenatal maternal stress, triggered by natural disasters, affects maternal and foetal health. Key mechanisms include HPA axis dysregulation and increased cortisol exposure, which may alter foetal development and long-term stress regulation. The chapter also explores epigenetic modifications, particularly DNA methylation, as lasting markers of prenatal stress, as well as emerging evidence on immune and inflammatory responses. Together, these findings highlight how acute stressors during pregnancy may have lasting, systemic impacts on offspring health and development. While biological mechanisms underlie the effects of prenatal maternal stress, social factors—at both individual and contextual levels—also shape how natural disasters affect maternal and child health and contribute to heterogeneity in its impacts. Country-specific conditions like infrastructures and healthcare quality moderate child outcomes. Maternal socioeconomic resources show a moderating role too. Disadvantaged mothers tend to face greater exposure, display more limited coping strategies and overall show higher risk of adverse outcomes. Timing also matters: First trimester exposure is linked to shorter gestation and low birth weight. Sex differences exist too, with varying physiological responses. Long-term effects of these initial disadvantages induced by natural catastrophes include chronic disease and reduced educational attainment.

L. Salazar (✉)
Institute of Public Goods and Policies (IPP), Spanish National Research Council (CSIC), Madrid, Spain
e-mail: leire.salazar@cchs.csic.es

N. Bello-Iglesias
Department of Sociology II (Social Structure), UNED, and Joint Research Institute, UNED-Instituto de Salud Carlos III (IMIENS), Madrid, Spain
e-mail: nerea.bello@poli.uned.es

R. A. Caparros-Gonzalez (ed.), *Maternal Stress during Pregnancy and Postpartum*, https://doi.org/10.1007/978-3-032-09245-8_7

Keywords

Maternal stress · Hypothalamic-pituitary-adrenal (HPA) axis · Cortisol · Pregnancy · Natural disasters · Perinatal health · Child outcomes · Heterogeneity in impacts · Socioeconomic resources

7.1 Introduction

Natural disasters of all kinds constitute exogenous shocks that affect the physical, mental and material well-being of all those who experience them. When pregnant women are affected, they are exposed to an acute, external stressor at a particularly sensitive time, which can have consequences on the development of the foetus, affecting its health, cognitive development, educational and labour outcomes, among others, throughout the life course.

This chapter focuses on the multidimensional relationship between natural disasters and prenatal maternal stress (hereafter, PNMS), and it spells out the biological and psychosocial mechanisms involved. Understanding how these psychosocial and physiological stressors during key periods of pregnancy can impact both maternal and neonatal health outcomes is critically important, especially as their frequency and severity are expected to rise—and as previously unaffected areas become vulnerable—due to climate change. Unprecedented heatwaves on land and in the ocean, torrential rains, devastating floods, prolonged droughts, extreme wildfires and widespread hurricane-induced flooding are some of the events becoming increasingly common across the globe [7, 12].

Although these events originate purely from natural phenomena, their consequences for human populations are shaped entirely by social factors. Not all countries affected experience the same impacts, nor do all individuals exposed, across contexts or within the same context, suffer the same level of harm. As Torche and Nobles point out, environmental exposures during pregnancy are not just random occurrences; rather, "their emergence, allocation, and impact depend on decisions regulated by institutions and power" [56]. The maternal stress caused by a natural disaster triggers a series of mechanisms that initially result in a biological modification, as we will describe later. However, its progression and life-course consequences are shaped by social processes and stratification dynamics [38].

To fully understand the effect of natural catastrophes on maternal health, it is necessary to first single out the various sources of stress. Natural disasters inherently induce psychological distress during the direct traumatic experience of the event itself. However, they may also generate additional severe stressors that may, in some cases, surpass the initial impact, such as the loss of lives and/or vital resources—such as housing—supply shortages (in particular of water, energy and food), property damage or the need to relocate to a different area or to live in temporary lodges for an uncertain period of time.

Faced with this complex combination of stressors induced by natural disasters, studies have begun differentiating between objective and subjective stress. Objective stress refers to the measurable exposure to disaster-related hardships, like the ones mentioned above, while subjective stress encompasses the emotional and psychological response to stressors as experienced by each individual [30]. It would be logical to assume that there is a direct relationship between the two factors, but this is not always the case, as shown by appraisal theory, which posits that objective exposure to a stressor and subjective distress are relatively independent, as emotional responses are shaped by individual perceptions and coping mechanisms at hand [27]. Moreover, the consequences of exposure to these stressors will vary depending on the genetic variability of both the mother (as hormonal responses are not identical in all women) and the foetus, which adds an additional layer of complexity to the analysis [30].

PNMS, in different degrees, will arise because of an imbalance between an environmental stressor and individual characteristics (socioeconomic conditions, lifestyles, personality traits) and contextual resources. This can increase stress perception, anxiety and depression and lead to behavioural changes and increased risk of adverse health outcomes in both the mother and eventually her offspring [3].

7.2 Biological Mechanisms Implied by Natural Disasters

What are the physiological implications of going through these stressful shocks? PNMS caused by an extreme event, such as experiencing a natural disaster, triggers a series of psychosocial and physiological responses that can lead the pregnant woman—who is in a period of heightened sensitivity to external insults—into a state of anxiety, stress or even depression. This detriment to maternal well-being is already a significant epidemiological concern, but it is only the first step in a cascade of potential adverse effects on foetal health.

Women who experience PNMS face an increased risk of transmitting these effects onto their children, potentially leading to adverse perinatal outcomes and emotional problems during early infancy, symptoms of attention deficit hyperactivity disorder (ADHD) or impaired cognitive development. While genetic predispositions of the baby and postnatal environment, including care, play a significant role in these outcomes, there is also substantial evidence supporting a prenatal causal influence. Anxiety and depression in the prenatal stage are estimated to account for 10%–15% of the attributable risk for emotional and behavioural issues in children [18].

From increased foetal exposure to cortisol—driven by both its higher production and lower metabolisation—to the role of biological mediators such as cytokines, serotonin and epigenetic modifications, we will, in what follows, describe some of the underlying biological mechanisms in maternal response to stress. Most of these studies somehow build upon the Foetal Programming Hypothesis and the Developmental Origins of Health and Disease (DOHaD) framework, which highlights the critical impact of prenatal stress on long-term health, a substantive issue covered by the last chapter of this book.

7.2.1 Activation of the Hypothalamic-Pituitary-Adrenal (HPA) Axis

The hypothalamic-pituitary-adrenal (HPA) axis plays a central role in regulating the body's response to stress, as it induces the production of cortisol by the adrenal glands. The HPA undergoes significant modifications throughout pregnancy to support foetal development. During gestation, the foetus and the mother exchange markers of biological stress through the maternal-placental-foetal unit, like the corticotropin-realising hormone (CRH). This peptide regulates events related to foetal growth, maturation and the time of onset of parturition, as well as taking part in the maturation of the foetal HPA axis itself.

During pregnancy, there is a change in the functioning of the HPA axis, as it becomes a positive feedback loop—stimulating its own further production rather than suppressing it—between placental CRH and cortisol from the adrenal cortex of the mother. As a consequence, levels of both CRH and cortisol rise steadily throughout gestation. The body regulates cortisol levels through the enzyme 11β-hydroxysteroid dehydrogenase-2 (11β-HSD2) in the placenta, which converts cortisol into its inactive form, cortisone. Although 11β-HSD-2 mitigates foetal exposure from maternal cortisol, it does not offer complete protection, allowing a share of maternal cortisol to still reach the foetus [15].

Under normal circumstances, this exposure to hormones has both beneficial and detrimental effects on the foetus, depending on the timing and level of exposure [10]. However, when exposed to a sizeable and most often unexpected adverse event like a natural disaster, maternal stress levels suffer a substantial and sudden peak, which disrupts the HPA axis regulation and leads to elevated maternal cortisol levels. This increase in cortisol stimulates placental CRH production, reinforcing a positive feedback loop that accelerates foetal maturation but also heightens the risk of preterm birth [55]. Higher levels of placental CRH can result in decreased utero-placental flow and hypoxemia, which are risk factors for intrauterine growth restriction (IUGR) [17, 20]. Additionally, stress can downregulate 11β-HSD-2, the placental enzyme responsible for converting cortisol into its inactive form, cortisone [25].

As a result, higher amounts of maternal cortisol cross into foetal circulation, influencing foetal neurodevelopment and immune function and leading to worsened birth outcomes such as low birth weight and preterm birth. Excessive prenatal cortisol exposure can also lead to long-term alterations in foetal HPA axis regulation, increasing the offspring's susceptibility to stress-related disorders later in life. A 2015 study in Iowa found that mothers who were affected by floods during pregnancy and who reported higher subjective PNMS had female toddlers with greater cortisol reactivity, suggesting that prenatal stress may contribute to long-term HPA axis dysregulation [58]. Similarly, exposure to the 2011 Queensland floods was linked to altered HPA axis regulation in offspring, specifically a heightened cortisol awakening response (CAR) in toddlers. Higher maternal subjective distress mediated the association between this dysregulated diurnal rhythm and increased anxiety symptoms in children at age four, underscoring the lasting impact of prenatal stress on stress reactivity and emotional development [36]. On the other hand, there is also evidence supporting a potentially adaptative response through increased infant orienting and regulatory capacity [33].

7.2.2 Epigenetic Modifications

Epigenetic modifications, especially DNA methylation (DNAm), are a potential pathway through which natural disasters can become biologically embedded in the mother and impact child health. These modifications can alter gene expression without changing the DNA sequence, potentially influencing long-term stress regulation, neurodevelopment and other health outcomes [11]. Research trying to prove these links has analysed various natural disasters and has looked at child outcomes at different stages of their life course. In some of the studies, measures of objective and subjective distress are differentiated, while in others, a comparison of exposed and non-exposed children is conducted, without explicitly capturing or measuring maternal stress levels.

Several studies have focused on investigating the association between DNAm and child outcomes using exposure to the 1998 Quebec ice storm in a quasi-experimental way. This natural experiment context allowed the researchers to assess the degree of maternal objective hardship experienced_and subjective distress perceived_and to follow their children over time, assessing their main outcomes. Thirteen years after the ice storm, researchers found that higher maternal objective hardship during pregnancy was associated with widespread DNAm modifications in genes primarily related to immune function in offspring. Notably, these effects were observed across multiple tissue types, reinforcing the idea that PNMS induces a lasting and systemic epigenetic change [6].

These scholars also studied body mass index (BMI) and central adiposity in offspring as additional outcomes. They found a positive association with higher maternal objective stress during pregnancy, while maternal subjective stress did not show the same effect. This association was significatively mediated by DNAm of genes involved in type 1 and 2 diabetes mellitus pathways, suggesting that these epigenetic modifications may play an adaptive role in mitigating the negative metabolic consequences of prenatal stress [5]. Additionally, children of mothers who experienced greater objective stress exhibited higher C-peptide secretion at adolescence. This is a marker of endogenous insulin function, with DNAm of diabetes-related genes acting as a mediator [4].

An alternative research team also studied the epigenetic programming of these participants and found that higher prenatal exposure to stress led to alterations in metabolomic pathways involved in energy metabolism and protein biosynthesis (such as branched-chain amino acid synthesis, alanine metabolism and ketone body metabolism). The dysregulation of these metabolic pathways suggests an increased risk of metabolic diseases like insulin resistance, diabetes and obesity [43].

Studies analysing hurricanes have also identified epigenetic modifications linked to prenatal stress. Research conducted using the HELiOS cohort, which examines the effects of Hurricane Maria in Puerto Rico, showed that maternal stress during pregnancy can alter DNAm profiles in children who were exposed while in utero. Significant differences in methylation levels were associated with maternal mental health assessed post-hurricane and the extent of property damage experienced during the event [28]. Research conducted in New York, studying the effects of Hurricane Sandy on the placental transcriptome, suggested that disaster-related stress during pregnancy may reprogram the placental transcriptome, contributing to HPA axis dysfunction, which in turn contributes to heightened anxiety and dysregulated stress hormone responses in offspring [39].

All in all, available evidence clearly suggests that exposure to acute stress in utero during natural catastrophes is associated with epigenetic modifications of various types that underlie maternal immune function, metabolic conditions and mental health outcomes. These effects that occur via epigenetic modifications are systemic, imply changes across different types of tissues, and lasting, are observable at different stages in the life cycle.

7.2.3 Inflammatory Response

A potential intermediary mechanism linking PNMS, physiological dysregulation and adverse perinatal and child outcomes is an altered inflammatory profile. PNMS has been associated with elevated circulating levels of pro-inflammatory cytokines and increased systemic inflammation in both mothers and their children, contributing to HPA axis dysregulation. Given that environmental stressors activate not only the nervous and endocrine systems but also the immune system, inflammatory response plays a critical role in shaping maternal and foetal health [47]. However, studies examining the effects of natural disasters on maternal stress have yet to fully integrate the assessment of maternal and/or foetal inflammatory markers resulting from shock exposure during pregnancy. Investigating these inflammatory pathways is crucial for establishing the relationship between maternal stress, inflammation and offspring outcomes [21].

7.3 Social Factors Help Explain Heterogeneity in Effects

The weight of biological mechanisms described so far may be moderated by social factors. In fact, social factors—at both the individual and contextual levels—are often significant confounders in some of the associations suggested in the medical literature.

According to the European Environment Agency, a natural disaster is a "violent, sudden and destructive change in the environment without cause from human activity, due to phenomena such as floods, earthquakes, fire and hurricanes" [16]. Despite this, and as mentioned in the introduction, much of the damage caused by natural disasters is embedded in human-made structures and institutions. With the data at hand, it is usually difficult to isolate each potential stressor individually, but it is worth trying to characterise the possible aggravating or alleviating factors, in order to gain a better understanding of how stress caused by natural disasters works. Understanding this is essential from the point of view of public health, for designing targeted public policies that effectively mitigate their adverse impact.

7.3.1 The Contextual Level

Natural disasters will have a potentially different harmful effect depending on the country-specific institutions, on the wealth level, on the degree of development of the healthcare system and other factors at the macro level. Some of the most important moderators at the country level are those that affect directly maternal well-being, for instance, whether a robust infrastructure exists to manage the crisis internally and to receive and handle external aid or whether ad hoc resources are quickly allocated to offer physical and psychosocial support to exposed citizens.

The impact of natural disasters on health outcomes of pregnant women and their children varies significantly between low- and high-income countries, reflecting differences in contextual stressors and access to resources. Findings from Nowak-Szczepanska et al. [40] on Cyclone Aila in India indicate that mothers with lower socioeconomic status, and their children, experienced undernutrition and lower relative weight even years after the disaster [40]. This contrasts with high-income countries, where PNMS from natural disasters is more commonly linked, as previously mentioned in this chapter, to an increased risk of diabetes and obesity in offspring [43].

After Hurricanes Irma and Maria hit Puerto Rico, a study assessed the negative experiences reported by women and the extent to which these experiences were related to postpartum depressive symptoms (PDS). Among them, feelings of unsafety due to lack of order, concerns about losing electricity and difficulty in getting food and clean water were the ones most strongly related to PDS [49]. What becomes clear after the revision of these studies is that a major source of distress stems from what is known as secondary stressors: "circumstances, events or policies that are indirectly related or 'non-inherent and consequential' to the index extreme event" [34]. These are situations that tend to persist longer than the events themselves, including circumstances like infrastructure failure, the need to repair structures and buildings, poor healthcare access or insufficient pre-disaster policies that fail to account for the population needs, among others.

Although disasters are often inevitable, secondary stressors can be mitigated or modified through effective preparedness (pre-disaster strong, health-related and other institutions) and timely responses. High-income countries, with their, in principle, more robust infrastructure and physical and psychosocial support systems, tend to address these challenges more efficiently, while in low-income countries, recovery is often more prolonged and complex to handle [22, 34].

7.3.2 Individual Level Moderators: The Key Role of Socioeconomic Resources

Pre-disaster characteristics and resources across population subgroups determine the level of exposure each individual ends up experiencing and often the strategies and resources available to mitigate the potential adverse consequences that exposure entails. Those facing socioeconomic disadvantage or those who are dealing with pre-existing mental and physical health conditions are typically at greater risk [35]. For example, when Hurricane Katrina hit the city of New Orleans, it revealed inequitable patterns in the population affected, with low-income neighbourhoods—and therefore individuals—being especially harmed [26]. These findings contribute to a wider literature pointing at strong racial and class gaps in how disasters cause loss and displacement [14].

The socioeconomic status of individuals can almost completely shape the level of exposure to a hazard such as a natural disaster, from as soon as before the event, determining the perception of risk itself, the level of preparedness for the disaster or the response to warning communications, as sometimes disadvantage people, despite receiving warning communications, are unable to evacuate. Once the disaster has occurred, other factors keep on determining the level of exposure, as mothers with fewer resources are more likely to live in homes that are more vulnerable, to experience greater material losses or destruction of their homes and to live in locations at a higher risk of harm. These disparities are extensively discussed in, for instance, the SAMHSA report *Greater Impact: How Disasters Affect People of Low Socioeconomic Status* [41]. Failing to account for differential exposure levels can lead to biased conclusions by misinterpreting treatment stratification with effect stratification [56].

Subgroups of the population with lower levels of socioeconomic status may also experience different susceptibility to natural catastrophes, conditioned by poorer overall levels of health resulting from different sources of deprivation. Pregnant women with fewer socioeconomic resources, already affected by the cumulative strain of persistent social stressors, such as economic hardship, time constraints or discrimination, may be weakened by chronic disadvantage, making them more vulnerable to additional stressors [56], such as those entailed by natural disasters. Furthermore, a threshold effect is likely to be at play, where a minimum level of health deterioration needs to be reached to start observing an adverse effect of an acute stressor. Given that individuals with fewer resources often start with poorer baseline health, they are likely to cross this threshold relatively more quickly, making them more susceptible to the adverse effects of a natural disaster [31].

Yet another source of heterogeneity in how harmful a natural disaster is according to the family resources lies in differential compensation or mitigation strategies adopted. Parental responses to adversity vary across socioeconomic groups; parents of different backgrounds are more or less able to compensate or on the contrary reinforce what they perceive as early disadvantages in their children. For instance, a qualitative study examined this effect, measuring cognitive ability among children who suffered the effect of a strong earthquake in utero. The findings show how advantaged parents are more capable of assessing their children's strengths and weaknesses and mobilise resources (such as time, financial support and professional assistance) to mitigate any potential initial handicap. Disadvantaged families, on the other hand, "face substantial barriers in terms of time, economic resources, and—equally important—access to social networks and mastery of cultural resources to effectively negotiate with institutions for advantages for their children" [54].

Lastly, a factor that is often overlooked but should be considered is the differential survival of the foetus across social backgrounds. Exposure to extreme events like natural disasters during pregnancy can lead to pregnancy loss and early life mortality for all. However, the impact of exposure during pregnancy varies depending on its timing, the mother's socioeconomic background and the surrounding environment, with no uniform effect across these factors. This implies that observed (realised) births have already undergone an initial stratification process that we most often do not have the means to measure. Since lower-income families face higher risks of both harmful exposures and infant loss, this may reduce, or even reverse, differences in birth outcomes between socioeconomic groups, sometimes leading to counterintuitive patterns [48]. It is important to consider this often-neglected selection process when designing a study; excess pregnancy losses caused by floods have reached up to 107,888 cases annually across 33 developing countries. This risk is pronounced among women with lower income and less education, as well as among women residing in poorer housing conditions and with access to unsafe water sources [23].

There is indeed enough empirical evidence so far on individual (maternal) socioeconomic status moderating the adverse effects of natural disasters on maternal health, particularly stress levels, and child outcomes, in different national contexts. In their research on the effects of the 1998 Quebec Ice Storm on PNMS and subsequent birth outcomes, Dancause et al. propose that the higher socioeconomic status (measured through maternal education) of the mothers affected might have functioned as a buffer, preventing the physiological effects of anxiety [9]. In another high-income context such as Spain, an analysis of the earthquake that took place in 2011 revealed an adverse impact of exposures on birth weight, particularly for exposures in the first trimester of pregnancy, and a more harmful effect for mothers with lower levels of education [45], which is suggestive of stress as a potential mechanism. For a low-income context, like the 2021 study in India, socioeconomic factors (mainly educational level) contributed to a nutritional and relative weight status protection [40].

In contrast, among pregnant women exposed to Chilean earthquakes, researchers found that their main outcome, an increment in the number of large-for-gestational-age (LGA) babies, was more pronounced among mothers with a low socioeconomic status. The study further revealed that mothers with more resources had a lower incidence of diabetes. Pregnant women exposed to the earthquake but with higher levels of socioeconomic resources were less likely to develop diabetes compared to pregnant exposed women with lower levels of resources. Additionally, mothers with more resources were more likely to use antenatal care control, a response that may cancel out the potential negative effects of PNMS on birth outcomes [1]. This aligns with broader evidence suggesting that parents with higher socioeconomic status tend to adopt compensatory strategies later in life to mitigate adverse perinatal outcomes.

There are more socially induced stressors that can aggravate the impact of natural disasters on PNMS. Single motherhood, in particular, can increase vulnerability to stress. A study on the 1994 Northridge earthquake in Los Angeles found that infants born closest to the epicentre were more likely to have low birth weight, but the effect was even more pronounced among first-time, single mothers, highlighting their greater susceptibility to stress. The combined burden of social and disaster-related stressors may account for the stronger impact observed in this group [29].

In any event, designs allowing for a more accurate representation of individual-level characteristics and therefore more granularity depicting biological-social interactions in exposure levels to natural disasters, susceptibility to them and mitigation strategies deployed should be aimed at. This calls for an intensification of research efforts with multidisciplinary approaches.

7.3.3 Heterogeneity by Trimester of Exposure

PNMS caused by a natural disaster can differentially distress mothers depending on the trimester of pregnancy in which it is experienced, since different susceptibility to various sorts of insults is at work over the gestation, which means that the consequences on perinatal outcomes may also vary accordingly.

A study examined the effects of an earthquake in California on stress depending on the timing of the gestation. It revealed that the earthquake caused the highest stress levels during earlier stages of pregnancy. As pregnancy progressed, the researchers argued, women became increasingly less sensitive to the effects of stress, suggesting a potential protective effect [19].

Other available pieces of evidence suggest a heightened susceptibility to the effects of PNMS induced by natural disasters on the placenta specifically from the third to the sixth month of pregnancy [52]. The biological mechanism underlying this process may involve elevated maternal cortisol levels at 15 weeks of gestation, which has been linked to increased placental corticotropin-releasing hormone (CRH) at 31 weeks. This, in turn, is associated with preterm delivery. These findings suggest that stress signals early in pregnancy could prime the placenta to activate labour-inducing mechanisms later in gestation [46].

Most of the studies about natural disasters that explore trimester-specific effects in fact point at the relevance of exposures in the first trimester of pregnancy. First trimester exposure seems to lead to lower birth weight [53], mostly mediated through a shortened gestational age, as shown in several studies focusing on the impact of earthquakes [29, 37, 55]. A quasi-experimental study on an earthquake that took place in Chile highlights the second and third months of pregnancy as critical periods for the observed decline in gestational age [57]. Exposure to other extreme weather events like floods also decreased gestational age [50], so did the 1998 Canadian ice storm, which affected gestational length and predicted birth weights [9]. When focusing on more sensitive indicators of newborn health, hurricane exposure during the first (and also the third) trimester of pregnancy increased the probability of requiring assisted ventilation for over 30 min [8].

Evidence clearly suggesting the importance of exposure during the second trimester is less abundant, but the work of R. Álvarez-Aranda et al. is relevant in this regard as it points to an alternative mechanism of harm. In their research, earthquake exposure was shown to increase the number of large-for-gestational-age (LGA) babies, especially among mothers with low socioeconomic status. The underlying mechanism proposed by the researchers is an increase in the rates of diabetes and hypertension among the affected population [1].

As regards exposures over the third trimester of gestation, most of the effects found are in line with those discussed for the first trimester, but they are less consistently present throughout the literature. A decrease in birth weight and in gestational age has been reported for exposures to earthquakes in the last trimester [29, 37]. An increase in the probability of requiring assisted ventilation for over 30 min when exposed to severe storms and hurricanes has been shown too [8]. Additionally, babies exposed to earthquakes during the second and third trimesters were shorter at birth [42]. More recent findings also indicate that children whose mothers were exposed to natural disasters during the second half of the pregnancy had higher methylation levels in the promoter region of the LLRC39 gene, which is involved in the development of the sarcomeric M-band and may be linked to cardiac function [28].

Regarding foetal survival, an analysis of 33 developing countries found that flood exposure during gestation is associated with an increased risk of pregnancy loss, with a higher risk during mid to late stages of pregnancy, possibly due to heightened difficulties in mobility and relocation as pregnancy progresses [23].

7.4 Sex-Specific Differences in the Impacts of Stress on Child Outcomes

Stress response in the placenta can differ depending on foetal sex, as different placental glucocorticoid and glucose systems adaptation to PNMS take place. In particular, reduced placental NR3C1-β mRNA levels have been generally found in males, encoding a glucocorticoid receptor. Lower levels of this mRNA suggest a reduced capacity to regulate glucocorticoid signalling, which can increase their sensitivity to maternal stress, while females promoted normal growth [52].

When turning to the empirical evidence of child outcomes, by sex, after a natural disaster, some opposing patterns emerge. Some studies have found an overall negative effect on birth outcomes, but when exploring deeper into these, a differential effect depending on the sex of the foetus has been brought about. For instance, when comparing births that were and were not exposed to the strong 2010 earthquake in Chile, male babies exposed to the earthquake experienced shorter gestational age, with no significant association for females [42]. However, another study revealed the opposite trend, with second- and third-month exposure resulting in a decline in gestational age (and an increase in preterm delivery) that was much larger for females. They also found a decline in the male-to-female birth ratio for exposures during the third month of exposure [57]. This evidence suggests that early stress may influence not only gestational outcomes but also the viability of male pregnancies under specific adverse conditions. Depending on the level of exposure, some male babies may experience adverse perinatal outcomes, while stronger exposures might result in the direct loss of the foetus.

In line with this, male foetuses exposed to PNMS in the second trimester had smaller head circumferences, while female foetuses tended to show this effect when exposed in the third trimester [42]. When examining this same outcome, other researchers alternatively reported that high-objective PNMS levels in early pregnancy predicted smaller head circumferences. However, a sparing effect was found only among male babies, with an alteration in the head circumference to birth length ratios that suggested prioritisation of brain development during gestation. These protective effects diminished in later stages of pregnancy [9].

There is also evidence suggesting a differential adaptation of the hormones regulated by the HPA axis. For instance, a study showed greater cortisol reactivity in female toddlers whose mother experienced floods during pregnancy, while little effect was observed in male counterparts [58]. A study on metabolic profiles found that prenatal maternal stress led to sex-specific modifications in metabolomic pathways, with males showing downregulation and females upregulation in energy metabolism and protein biosynthesis [43].

7.5 Long(er)-Term Consequences of Natural Disasters

The impacts of natural disasters are not limited to maternal stress and the subsequent birth or infant health outcomes. Long-term effects of foetal exposure to stress induced by natural catastrophes remain to be appropriately assessed. We highlight here a few instances of studies that have addressed this matter using quasi-experimental approaches. The first study analysed the long-term consequences of two powerful tropical storms that struck Puerto Rico in 1928 and in 1932. The main finding suggested that diabetes and other cardiovascular disease factors, such as hypertension and high cholesterol, were markedly higher among those in the womb or in their early infancy in the aftermath of both storms. Hurricanes also led to a heightened share of individuals without any formal schooling, an effect that could, in turn, negatively impact subsequent health, given the well-documented link between socioeconomic status, education and health outcomes [51].

The 1930 American Dust Bowl similarly entailed long-term consequences for the human capital of the children who lived through it. The Dust Bowl was a prolonged natural event characterised by drought and severe dust storms that affected the United States Great Plains throughout the 1930s. Exposure in utero to the Dust Bowl increased, according to existing evidence, poverty and disability rates later in life and decreased fertility and college completion rates in affected areas. Public investments associated with the New Deal mitigated some of these negative impacts.

In particular, they showed a reduced need for welfare subsidies, including disability benefits, a relative improvement of college completion and lower rates of work-related disability [2].

The violent outbreak of tornadoes that hit the United States in 1974 also left long-term consequences among those who were exposed in utero, particularly during later stages of pregnancy, as it raised the probability of having at least one physical or cognitive difficulty. However, the impact on adult socioeconomic status was relatively weak, likely due to greater parental investment in education for affected children. This explicit compensatory behaviour through human capital reinforcement may have helped mitigate some of the disaster's adverse effects [24].

Causally assessing long-term consequences, in health and other relevant outcomes such as educational attainment, of exposure to maternal stress during natural disasters is a demanding enterprise. It requires high-quality data over a very long period of life—notably, longitudinal data at the individual level, and/or linked mother-baby information over the life-course. Alternatively, it needs creative research designs trying to come up with innovative identification strategies. This explains the relative lack of studies accomplishing this research objective.

7.6 Limitations of Available Evidence and Ways Forward

Our reading of the literature on natural disasters, maternal stress and child outcomes has identified several limitations that in turn suggest where to focus research efforts in the near future to maximise the quality and external validity of the evidence produced. Some of the shortcoming refer to measurement issues, while others have to do with the external validity of the results.

The first area where there is room for improvement is the quantification of stress levels. The way exposed women evaluate the stress experienced is a factor that can distort the relationship between the actual magnitude of the event and its consequences, introducing heterogeneity into the assessment. While self-reported measures of stress are relevant, as they help us to get closer to the subjective experience of each individual, which will ultimately determine to a large extent the consequences on the well-being of the mother and her child, they also carry limitations. Cognitive biases, recall inaccuracies, and social desirability factors can lead to overestimation or underestimation of the extent of actual exposure and their implications.

To enhance the accuracy of stress assessment, a multifaceted approach is needed. Objective exposure, for instance, measured through geospatial data and/or official records, establishes a standard reference for populations affected by a given disaster. In contrast, self-reported exposure captures the perceived threat and psychological impact, which may differ from objective measures. This discrepancy offers insight into the socioeconomic factors and psychological traits that shape individual responses to disaster-related stress, as self-reported measures can reflect additional fears and concerns beyond the objective exposure, helping to explain differences between the two assessments.

Incorporating objective biomarkers from biological samples, such as cortisol levels, would allow for a physiological assessment of stress responses, offering a more precise understanding of how disasters impact maternal health. By integrating objective exposure data, subjective assessments and biological markers, we can obtain a more comprehensive picture of the true impact of natural disasters on maternal stress and the potential consequences for their offspring [13, 32].

Some data collections have started pursuing this objective. The PERIFACT Study [44], for instance, gathers prospective information on pregnant women and their babies in four municipalities in Spain, two of them exposed to earthquakes and two not exposed but otherwise very similar in terms of population composition, wealth levels, access to healthcare and other relevant contextual attributes. The study collects, stores and analyses biological samples (saliva, hair) to measure acute and chronic stress levels in pregnant mothers, and it also includes a wealth of information on socioeconomic position of women and their relatives, health conditions, lifestyles, subjective distress experienced during the earthquakes, overall perception of stress in their daily lives, birth outcomes and child health and cognitive and socioemotional development over the first year, among others.

The second area where research efforts should be intensified is increasing the external validity of studies. This involves at least three issues. First, studies sometimes differ in their substantive findings, but often the reasons for such inconsistencies are unknown and impossible to ascertain. Natural disasters are rare phenomena, even if increasingly more frequent with climate change, and the data at hand to analyse their effects are usually constructed *ex post*, making the most of existing sources or reconstructing the effects of events well after they have happened. Moreover, these events tend not be distributed at random. This implies that oftentimes the information available is far from the ideal research design that one would aspire to and contains biases of several kinds. In addition, these data are different from event to event, and so findings refer to events, populations and contexts that are difficult to compare. Second, sometimes the samples at hand are very reduced in size, particularly in studies in the clinical domain, and concerns about lack of representativeness are not truly problematised. This hinders comparability with other studies and of course impedes searching for heterogeneity across subgroups of mothers, babies or stages of gestation. Third, conclusions on the role of stress stemming from natural disasters might not be immediately applicable to other settings. More contributions dealing with ordinary stressful life event, which are likely to stir chronic rather than acute types of stress, and on the theoretical foundations on the interaction between acute stress and various baseline levels of chronic stress, are needed. Still, evidence gathered on stress due to natural disasters and other events that potentially generate acute stress are crucial for a deeper understanding of the mechanisms at play.

More intense and candid collaboration between researchers from different disciplines should be aimed at. Biological and psychosocial materials alike need to be collected in order to appropriately capture the complex processes underlying the relationship between environmental events, stress experienced during pregnancy and adverse maternal and child health. Designs should in addition systematically compare events and types of empirical approaches to try and single out macro factors—most notably, institutions affecting the potential harm induced by natural disasters, but also their capacity to mitigate the adverse effects once they occur. Incorporating the comparative logic would allow producing more rigorous evidence to suggest effective policy interventions to partially or fully mitigate early-life disadvantage, whether it comes from the adverse impact of a natural disaster or from other types of shocks.

7.7 Concluding Remarks

Understanding how prenatal maternal stress (PNMS) induced by natural disasters affects maternal and child health is a crucial yet complex task. The evidence reviewed in this chapter points to a compelling association between environmental shocks and a range of outcomes in mothers and their children, from birth weight and gestational age to cognitive and socioemotional development. Natural disasters offer a particularly valuable context for studying these effects, as they allow researchers to approximate experimental conditions in real-world settings. Yet despite the promise of this field, current research remains limited in several important ways.

A clearer understanding of the biological mechanisms linking maternal stress during pregnancy to child health outcomes is essential for advancing this field. Central to this relationship is the functioning of the maternal hypothalamic-pituitary-adrenal (HPA) axis, which responds to stress by increasing the production of cortisol and other glucocorticoids. These hormones, when elevated for prolonged periods or at critical stages of foetal development, can cross the placenta and alter the in utero environment, potentially affecting foetal brain development, immune function and stress regulation systems. The degree to which the placenta buffers or transmits these stress signals—through mechanisms such as the activity of the enzyme 11β-HSD2—adds a further layer of complexity, as does the possibility of sex-specific responses that has been suggested in the literature. More research on these mechanisms is needed in contexts of natural disasters but also when stressors of other kinds are considered.

Measurement remains a central challenge to the topic. While self-reported stress captures meaningful dimensions of individual psychological experiences, it is subject to biases and should be complemented with objective indicators of intensity of disaster exposure and biological stress responses. The integration of these multiple levels of analysis is not just methodologically more rigorous but essential for capturing the nuanced pathways through which disasters affect health. Encouragingly, some initiatives like the PERIFACT Study are moving in this direction, offering a promising format for future data collection efforts.

At the same time, questions of external validity persist. Studies often draw on idiosyncratic events with non-exportable contexts, limiting the generalisability of their findings. Sample sizes are frequently small, and differences across studies are difficult to reconcile due to divergent designs. To build a more cumulative approach to scientific knowledge, research must prioritise larger and more diverse samples, systematic comparisons across events and explicit consideration of how social, economic and institutional contexts shape both exposure and heterogeneous impacts of disasters. Multi-way interactions between the biological, the social and the institutional should increasingly be aimed at in this type of research.

Finally, a more integrated and interdisciplinary approach is clearly needed. Collaboration across medicine, epidemiology, psychology, sociology, demography and public health is essential to develop more robust theoretical models, improve empirical strategies and interpret findings in an integrated manner. This aim includes moving beyond acute stress events to consider how disaster-induced stress interacts with chronic stress linked to structural disadvantage. By embedding research within a comparative and policy-meaningful framework, scholars can contribute not only to academic debates but also to the design of interventions that minimise stress-inducing exposures and buffer the negative effects of early-life adversity.

Acknowledgments This work was supported by the Spanish Ministry of Science and Innovation, grants PID2019-111564RB-I00/AEI/10.13039/501100011033, PRE2020-094473 and PID2023-151383OA-100, funded by MICIU/AEI/10.13039/501100011033 and by ERDF/EU. Beyond funding, this institution had no involvement in the research and/or preparation of the chapter.

References

1. Álvarez-Aranda R, Chirkova S, Romero JG. Growing in the womb: the effect of seismic activity on fetal growth. Econ Hum Biol. 2020;36:100815. https://doi.org/10.1016/j.ehb.2019.100815.
2. Arthi V. "The dust was long in settling": human capital and the lasting impact of the American dust bowl. J Econ Hist. 2018;78(1):196–230. https://doi.org/10.1017/S0022050718000074.
3. Beydoun H, Saftlas AF. Physical and mental health outcomes of prenatal maternal stress in human and animal studies: a review of recent evidence. Paediatr Perinat Epidemiol. 2008;22(5):438–66. https://doi.org/10.1111/j.1365-3016.2008.00951.x.
4. Cao-Lei L, Dancause KN, Elgbeili G, Laplante DP, Szyf M, King S. DNA methylation mediates the effect of maternal cognitive appraisal of a disaster in pregnancy on the child's C-peptide secretion in adolescence: project ice storm. PLoS One. 2018;13(2):e0192199. https://doi.org/10.1371/journal.pone.0192199.
5. Cao-Lei L, Dancause KN, Elgbeili G, Massart R, Szyf M, Liu A, Laplante DP, King S. DNA methylation mediates the impact of exposure to prenatal maternal stress on BMI and central adiposity in children at age 13 1/2 years: project ice storm. Epigenetics. 2015;10(8):749–61. https://doi.org/10.1080/15592294.2015.1063771.
6. Cao-Lei L, Massart R, Suderman MJ, Machnes Z, Elgbeili G, Laplante DP, Szyf M, King S. DNA methylation signatures triggered by prenatal maternal stress exposure to a natural disaster: project ice storm. PLoS One. 2014;9(9):e107653. https://doi.org/10.1371/journal.pone.0107653.
7. Copernicus Climate Change Service (C3S). Global Climate Highlights 2023. 9 Jan 2024 [Online]. Available: https://climate.copernicus.eu/global-climate-highlights-2023. Accessed 29 Jan 2025.
8. Currie J, Rossin-Slater M. Weathering the storm: hurricanes and birth outcomes. J Health Econ. 2013;32(3):487–503. https://doi.org/10.1016/j.jhealeco.2013.01.004.

9. Dancause KN, Laplante DP, Oremus C, Fraser S, Brunet A, King S. Disaster-related prenatal maternal stress influences birth outcomes: project ice storm. Early Hum Dev. 2011;87(12):813–20. https://doi.org/10.1016/j.earlhumdev.2011.06.007.
10. Davis EP, Sandman CA. The timing of prenatal exposure to maternal cortisol and psychosocial stress is associated with human infant cognitive development. Child Dev. 2010;81(1):131–48. https://doi.org/10.1111/j.1467-8624.2009.01385.x.
11. Dieckmann L, Czamara D. Epigenetics of prenatal stress in humans: the current research landscape. Clin Epigenetics. 2024;16(Issue 1):20. https://doi.org/10.1186/s13148-024-01635-9.
12. Ebi KL, Vanos J, Baldwin JW, Bell JE, Hondula DM, Errett NA, Hayes K, Reid CE, Saha S, Spector J, Berry P. Extreme weather and climate change: population health and health system implications. Annu Rev Public Health. 2020;42:293–315. https://doi.org/10.1146/annurev-publhealth-012420-105026.
13. Edwards B, Gray M, Borja JB. Measuring natural Hazard-related disasters through self-reports. Int J Disaster Risk Sci. 2021;12(4):540–52. https://doi.org/10.1007/s13753-021-00359-1.
14. Elliott JR, Pais J. Race, class, and hurricane Katrina: social differences in human responses to disaster. Soc Sci Res. 2006;35(2):295–321. https://doi.org/10.1016/j.ssresearch.2006.02.003.
15. Ellman LM, Schetter CD, Hobel CJ, Chicz-DeMet A, Glynn LM, Sandman CA. Timing of fetal exposure to stress hormones: effects on newborn physical and neuromuscular maturation. Dev Psychobiol. 2008;50(3):232–41. https://doi.org/10.1002/dev.20293.
16. European Environment Agency (EEA). Natural disaster – EEA glossary [Online]. Available: https://www.eea.europa.eu/help/glossary/eea-glossary/natural-disaster. Accessed 5 Feb 2025.
17. Giles WB, McLean M, Davies JJ, Smith R. Abnormal umbilical artery Doppler waveforms and cord blood corticotropin-releasing hormone. Obstet Gynecol. 1996;87(1):107–11. https://doi.org/10.1016/0029-7844(95)00338-X.
18. Glover V. Prenatal stress and its effects on the fetus and the child: possible underlying biological mechanisms. In: Antonelli M, editor. Perinatal programming of neurodevelopment. Advances in neurobiology, vol. 10. New York, NY: Springer; 2015. https://doi.org/10.1007/978-1-4939-1372-5_13.
19. Glynn LM, Wadhwa PD, Dunkel-Schetter C, Chicz-DeMet A, Sandman CA. When stress happens matters: effects of earthquake timing on stress responsivity in pregnancy. Am J Obstet Gynecol. 2001;184(4):637–42. https://doi.org/10.1067/mob.2001.111066.
20. Goland RS, Jozak S, Warren WB, Conwell IM, Stark RI, Tropper PJ. Elevated levels of umbilical cord plasma corticotropin-releasing hormone in growth-retarded fetuses. J Clin Endocrinol Metabol. 1993;77(5):1174–9. https://doi.org/10.1210/jcem.77.5.8077309.
21. Hantsoo L, Kornfield S, Anguera MC, Epperson CN. Inflammation: a proposed intermediary between maternal stress and offspring neuropsychiatric risk. Biol Psychiatry. 2019;85(2):97–106. https://doi.org/10.1016/j.biopsych.2018.08.018.
22. Harville EW, Beitsch L, Uejio CK, Sherchan S, Lichtveld MY. Assessing the effects of disasters and their aftermath on pregnancy and infant outcomes: a conceptual model. Int J Disaster Risk Reduct. 2021;62:102415. https://doi.org/10.1016/j.ijdrr.2021.102415.
23. He C, Zhu Y, Zhou L, Bachwenkizi J, Schneider A, Chen R, Kan H. Flood exposure and pregnancy loss in 33 developing countries. Nat Commun. 2024;15(1):20. https://doi.org/10.1038/s41467-023-44508-0.
24. Hong SC, Kim D, Lee E. The long-term human toll of natural disasters: a study of fetal exposure to the 1974 tornado super outbreak. Appl Econ. 2021;53(4):469–81. https://doi.org/10.1080/00036846.2020.1808181.
25. Jahnke JR, Terán E, Murgueitio F, Cabrera H, Thompson AL. Maternal stress, placental 11β-hydroxysteroid dehydrogenase type 2, and infant HPA axis development in humans: psychosocial and physiological pathways. Placenta. 2021;104:179–87. https://doi.org/10.1016/j.placenta.2020.12.008.
26. Kates RW, Colten CE, Laska S, Leatherman SP. Reconstruction of New Orleans after Hurricane Katrina: a research perspective. Proc Natl Acad Sci U S A. 2006;103:14653. https://doi.org/10.1073/pnas.0605726103.

27. Keller C, Bostrom A, Kuttschreuter M, Savadori L, Spence A, White M. Bringing appraisal theory to environmental risk perception: a review of conceptual approaches of the past 40years and suggestions for future research. J Risk Res. 2012;15(3):237–56. https://doi.org/10.1080/13669877.2011.634523.
28. Kello E, Vieira AR, Rivas-Tumanyan S, Campos-Rivera M, Martinez-Gonzalez KG, Buxó CJ, Morou-Bermúdez E. Pre- and peri-natal hurricane exposure alters DNA methylation patterns in children. Sci Rep. 2023;13(1):3875. https://doi.org/10.1038/s41598-023-30645-5.
29. Kim B, Carruthers CK, Harris MC. Maternal stress and birth outcomes: evidence from the 1994 Northridge earthquake. J Econ Behav Organ. 2017;140:354–73. https://doi.org/10.1016/j.jebo.2017.05.014.
30. King S, Laplante DP. Using natural disasters to study prenatal maternal stress in humans. In: Advances in neurobiology, vol. 10. New York: Springer New York LLC; 2015. p. 285–313. https://doi.org/10.1007/978-1-4939-1372-5_14.
31. Kondo N. Socioeconomic disparities and health: impacts and pathways. J Epidemiol. 2012;22(1):2–6. https://doi.org/10.2188/jea.JE20110116.
32. Lieberman-Cribbin W, Liu B, Schneider S, Schwartz R, Taioli E. Self-reported and FEMA flood exposure assessment after hurricane sandy: association with mental health outcomes. PLoS One. 2017;12(1):e0170965. https://doi.org/10.1371/journal.pone.0170965.
33. Lipschutz R, Kulesz PA, Elgbeili G, Biekman B, Laplante DP, Olson DM, King S, Bick J. Maternal mental health mediates the effect of prenatal stress on infant temperament: the Harvey Mom Study. Dev Psychopathol. 2024;36(2):893–907. https://doi.org/10.1017/S0954579423000160.
34. Lock S, Rubin GJ, Murray V, Rogers MB, Amlôt R, Williams R. Secondary stressors and extreme events and disasters: a systematic review of primary research from 2010-2011. PLoS Curr. 2012;4:20121029. https://doi.org/10.1371/currents.dis.a9b76fed1b2dd5c5bfcfc13c87a2f24f.
35. Lowe SR, Raker EJ, Zacher ML. Extremes in context: a life-course approach to disaster mental health. One Earth. 2020;2(6):497–9. https://doi.org/10.1016/j.oneear.2020.05.022.
36. McLean MA, Simcock G, Elgbeili G, Laplante DP, Kildea S, Hurrion E, Lequertier B, Cobham VE, King S. Disaster-related prenatal maternal stress, and childhood HPA-axis regulation and anxiety: the QF2011 Queensland Flood Study. Psychoneuroendocrinology. 2020;118:104716. https://doi.org/10.1016/j.psyneuen.2020.104716.
37. Menclova AK, Stillman S. Maternal stress and birth outcomes: evidence from an unexpected earthquake swarm. Health Econ. 2020;29(12):1705–20. https://doi.org/10.1002/hec.4162.
38. Muller C, Sampson RJ, Winter AS. Environmental inequality: the social causes and consequences of lead exposure. Annu Rev Sociol. 2018;44:263–82. https://doi.org/10.1146/annurev-soc-073117.
39. Nomura Y, Rompala G, Pritchett L, Aushev V, Chen J, Hurd YL. Natural disaster stress during pregnancy is linked to reprogramming of the placenta transcriptome in relation to anxiety and stress hormones in young offspring. Mol Psychiatry. 2021;26(11):6520–30. https://doi.org/10.1038/s41380-021-01123-z.
40. Nowak-Szczepanska N, Gomula A, Chakraborty R, Koziel S. Nutritional and weight status of Indian mother-child dyads experienced by a natural disaster. Matern Child Nutr. 2021;17(3):e13164. https://doi.org/10.1111/mcn.13164.
41. Office of Public Health and Science, Health and Human Services Department. Greater impact: how disasters affect people of low socioeconomic status. [Government] Health and Human Services Department; 2017. https://www.govinfo.gov/app/details/GOVPUB-HE20-PURL-gpo106714.
42. Palmeiro-Silva YK, Orellana P, Venegas P, Monteiro L, Varas-Godoy M, Norwitz E, Rice G, Osorio E, Illanes SE. Effects of earthquake on perinatal outcomes: a Chilean register-based study. PLoS One. 2018;13(2):1–11. https://doi.org/10.1371/journal.pone.0191340.
43. Paxman EJ, Boora NS, Kiss D, Laplante DP, King S, Montina T, Metz GAS. Prenatal maternal stress from a natural disaster alters urinary metabolomic profiles in project ice storm participants. Sci Rep. 2018;8(1):12932. https://doi.org/10.1038/s41598-018-31230-x.

44. Salazar L, Bello-Iglesias N, Seiz M, Eremenko T. PERIFACT Study. Pending registration. 2025.
45. Salazar L. The interaction between maternal resources and environmental stressors: social inequality in birth outcomes in Spain. Mimeo. n.d.
46. Sandman CA, Glynn L, Schetter CD, Wadhwa P, Garite T, Chicz-DeMet A, Hobel C. Elevated maternal cortisol early in pregnancy predicts third trimester levels of placental corticotropin releasing hormone (CRH): priming the placental clock. Peptides. 2006;27(6):1457–63. https://doi.org/10.1016/j.peptides.2005.10.002.
47. Segerstrom SC, Miller GE. Psychological stress and the human immune system: a meta-analytic study of 30 years of inquiry NIH` public access. Psychol Bull. 2004;130(4):601.
48. Seiz M, Salazar L, Eremenko T. Perinatal health in Spain during and after the great recession: educational selection into fertility as a protective factor in high unemployment contexts. Soc Sci Med. 2024;340:116439. https://doi.org/10.1016/J.SOCSCIMED.2023.116439.
49. Simeone RM, House LD, Salvesen von Essen B, Kortsmit K, Hernandez Virella W, Vargas Bernal MI, Galang RR, D'Angelo DV, Shapiro-Mendoza CK, Ellington SR. Pregnant women's experiences during and after hurricanes Irma and Maria, pregnancy risk assessment monitoring system, Puerto Rico, 2018. Public Health Rep. 2023;138(6):916–24. https://doi.org/10.1177/00333549221142571.
50. Simeonova E. Out of sight, out of mind? Natural disasters and pregnancy outcomes in the USA. CESifo Econ Stud. 2011;57(3):403–31. https://doi.org/10.1093/cesifo/ifr005.
51. Sotomayor O. Fetal and infant origins of diabetes and ill health: evidence from Puerto Rico's 1928 and 1932 hurricanes. Econ Hum Biol. 2013;11(3):281–93. https://doi.org/10.1016/j.ehb.2012.02.009.
52. St-Pierre J, Laplante DP, Elgbeili G, Dawson PA, Kildea S, King S, Vaillancourt C. Natural disaster-related prenatal maternal stress is associated with alterations in placental glucocorticoid system: the QF2011 Queensland Flood Study. Psychoneuroendocrinology. 2018;94:38–48. https://doi.org/10.1016/j.psyneuen.2018.04.027.
53. Tan CE, Li HJ, Zhang XG, Zhang H, Han PY, An Q, Ding WJ, Wang MQ. The impact of the Wenchuan earthquake on birth outcomes. PLoS One. 2009;4(12):e8200. https://doi.org/10.1371/journal.pone.0008200.
54. Torche F. Prenatal exposure to an acute stressor and children's cognitive outcomes. Demography. 2018;55(5):1611–39. https://doi.org/10.1007/s13524-018-0700-9.
55. Torche F. The effect of maternal stress on birth outcomes: exploiting a natural experiment. Demography. 2011;48(4):1473–91. https://doi.org/10.1007/s13524-011-0054-z.
56. Torche F, Nobles J. Early-life exposures and social stratification. Annu Rev Sociol. 2025;04:34. https://doi.org/10.1146/annurev-soc-091523.
57. Torche F, Kleinhaus K. Prenatal stress, gestational age and secondary sex ratio: the sex-specific effects of exposure to a natural disaster in early pregnancy. Hum Reprod. 2012;27(2):558–67. https://doi.org/10.1093/humrep/der390.
58. Yong Ping E, Laplante DP, Elgbeili G, Hillerer KM, Brunet A, O'Hara MW, King S. Prenatal maternal stress predicts stress reactivity at 21/2 years of age: the Iowa Flood Study. Psychoneuroendocrinology. 2015;56:62–78. https://doi.org/10.1016/j.psyneuen.2015.02.015.

Advancing Knowledge on Assisted Reproductive Techniques and Stress

8

Jean Calleja-Agius, Olga Gouni, and Neville Calleja

Abstract

It is paramount to recognize that the infertility journey extends far beyond its medical definition, encompassing significant psychological, emotional, and social dimensions that profoundly impact individuals and couples. Understanding and addressing these nonmedical aspects is not merely supportive but crucial for the overall well-being and potentially even the reproductive outcomes of those experiencing infertility. The experience of infertility is frequently accompanied by a range of negative emotions, including stress, anxiety, and depression. The uncertainty surrounding the ability to conceive can be a significant source of anxiety. Each unsuccessful attempt to conceive can lead to feelings of disappointment, sadness, and even grief.

Infertility can be perceived as an invisible loss and a mourning of a longed-for future. The process of assisted reproductive technology (ART), particularly in vitro fertilization (IVF), is frequently described as an "emotional roller coaster" characterized by volatility and intense emotions. In addition, infertility carries a significant social burden. The stigma associated with infertility can lead to feelings of shame and reluctance to disclose their struggles, resulting in loneli-

J. Calleja-Agius (✉)
Department of Anatomy, Faculty of Medicine and Surgery, University of Malta, Tal-Qroqq, Msida, Malta
e-mail: jean.calleja-agius@um.edu.mt

O. Gouni
Prenatal Sciences Research Institute SOPHIA, Volos, Greece

N. Calleja
Department of Public Health, Faculty of Medicine and Surgery, University of Malta, Msida, Malta

Directorate for Health Information and Research, Ministry of Health and Active Ageing, Msida, Malta

R. A. Caparros-Gonzalez (ed.), *Maternal Stress during Pregnancy and Postpartum*, https://doi.org/10.1007/978-3-032-09245-8_8

ness and isolation. Relationships with partners, family, and friends can be strained due to a lack of understanding or social pressure to have children. While infertility can sometimes strengthen couple bonds through mutual support, it can also be a source of conflict.

The infertility treatment process itself adds to this burden. Invasive physical procedures, hormonal fluctuations, and the constant hope followed by potential disappointment create ongoing stress. The significant financial costs of treatments like IVF can lead to additional stress and limit access to care. Many individuals, particularly women, report feeling dehumanized and failed by the healthcare system due to a perceived lack of adequate support, holistic care, and empathetic understanding. It is crucial to acknowledge the gendered nature of this burden, with women often facing greater social and psychological pressure due to societal expectations around motherhood. However, it is equally important to recognize that men also experience significant psychological, social, and sexual challenges during infertility and its treatment, including stress, depression, grief, impacts on self-esteem and relationship difficulties.

Therefore, a holistic approach to infertility care is essential, one that recognizes infertility not just as a medical condition but as a biopsychosocial crisis. Addressing the psychological needs of couples is a crucial aspect of successful infertility treatment. Numerous studies have shown that psychological interventions can effectively reduce mental health disorders, depression, and anxiety in individuals undergoing infertility treatments. Stress management, incorporating skills like positive thinking and cognitive reconstruction, becomes a vital component of counseling. This is especially important since, even in case of a live birth following IVF, there is the potential of peripartum stress and its transmission to the offspring.

Healthcare systems and providers have a responsibility to provide adequate information, time, and empathetic support to maintain the quality of life and well-being of those experiencing infertility. Routine psychosocial screening should be considered, and mental health services should be a standard component of infertility care.

This chapter will explore the emotional and psychological challenges faced by individuals and couples undergoing infertility, with a focus on IVF. It will delve into stress, coping mechanisms, dyadic relationships, gender differences, the role of support, and psychological interventions.

Keywords

Infertility · Assisted reproduction techniques · Psychology · Social · Self-esteem · Relationship · Stressors · Emotion · Coping · Support

8.1 Introduction

8.1.1 Overview of Infertility

Worldwide, infertility affects approximately one in every six people of reproductive age in their lifetime. It has an impact on millions of people, together with their families and communities [1]. Infertility is a disease of the male or female reproductive system defined by the failure to achieve a pregnancy after 12 months or more of regular unprotected sexual intercourse [2]. This may occur due many different causes but is usually classified as being due to female, male, or unexplained factors. In females, infertility may be caused by a range of abnormalities of the ovaries, uterus, fallopian tubes, and the endocrine system. In the male reproductive system, infertility is most commonly caused by difficulties in ejaculation, absence or low levels of sperm, or abnormal sperm morphology and/or motility. Infertility can be primary, when a pregnancy has never been achieved by a person, or secondary, when at least one prior pregnancy has been achieved.

Fertility care encompasses the prevention, diagnosis, and treatment of infertility. Some causes of infertility are preventable. For many, assisted reproductive technologies (ART), such as in vitro fertilization (IVF) and intracytoplasmic sperm injection (ICSI), offer hope for achieving parenthood. IVF involves retrieving eggs from the woman's ovaries, fertilizing them with sperm in a laboratory, and then transferring the resulting embryos into the woman's uterus. ICSI is a specific technique used in conjunction with IVF where a single sperm is directly injected into an egg to facilitate fertilization. The utilization of IVF has increased significantly particularly in developed countries, reflecting its growing role in addressing infertility [3, 4].

8.1.2 The Psychosocial Impact

Beyond its medical definition, infertility carries a profound psychological, emotional, and social burden for those experiencing it. Infertility is a profound life stressor that can trigger a cascade of emotional, psychological, and social challenges [5]. The desire to have children is deeply ingrained in many individuals, and societal expectations often place significant value on parenthood. Consequently, the inability to conceive can lead to substantial emotional distress, impacting an individual's well-being and their relationships [6]. Each unsuccessful attempt to conceive, and particularly failed IVF treatments, can trigger significant emotional vulnerability. Individuals may experience a wide array of negative emotions, including stress, grief, sadness, anger, and frustration. Infertility can be perceived as an invisible loss and mourning of a longed-for future. Feelings of hopelessness, guilt, and shame are also commonly reported. Women, in particular, may feel the weight of social and psychological pressure due to the importance placed on motherhood in many societies. They may internalize the inability to conceive, attributing fault to themselves and experiencing a greater spiritual burden. However, it is equally important to recognize that men also experience significant psychological, social, and sexual challenges during infertility and its treatment [7].

Psychological distress, such as anxiety, insomnia, irritability, and depression, is prevalent among infertile individuals and can be exacerbated by the drugs and hormones used in ART treatment. Up to 70% of infertile patients report psychological issues during the course of IVF treatment [8]. The process of infertility treatment, especially IVF, is often described as an "emotional roller coaster" characterized by volatility, instability, and susceptibility to intense emotions. Furthermore, the uncertainty of treatment outcomes adds to the psychological burden, with patients often rating the anxiety of undergoing IVF as greater than any other important life event. Infertility can also deeply impact an individual's self-esteem, self-confidence, and sense of control. The inability to conceive can disrupt one's personal identity and the narrative they carry about parenthood. This can lead to an existential crisis alongside grief, pain, and loss.

The social burden of infertility is significant. The stigma associated with infertility can lead to feelings of shame and a reluctance to disclose their struggles. This often results in loneliness and isolation as individuals withdraw from others due to fear of judgment and feeling misunderstood. Relationships with partners, family, and friends can be strained. While infertility can sometimes strengthen couple bonds through mutual support, it can also cause conflicts. Social pressure to have children, particularly in cultures with strong pronatalist views, further intensifies the stress.

Infertility treatment itself adds to the burden. Invasive physical procedures, hormonal imbalances, and the constant hope followed by potential disappointment create ongoing stress [9, 10]. The significant financial costs of treatments like IVF can lead to additional stress and limit access to care for some couples. Moreover, some women report feeling dehumanized and failed by the healthcare system due to a perceived lack of adequate support, holistic care, and empathetic understanding. The focus on the medical aspects of infertility can sometimes overshadow the profound emotional and psychological needs of patients. The experience of going through repeated unsuccessful IVF cycles can be particularly traumatic. The stress related to infertility and its treatment can become a vicious cycle, where psychological distress may even impact fertility outcomes. There is evidence of increased risk of postpartum depressive symptoms among women who conceived with infertility treatment [11]. This peripartum stress can potentially adversely affect the offspring.

Given the profound psychological, emotional, and social burdens associated with infertility and its treatment, the need for psychological support and counseling is crucial. Providing a safe space for individuals and couples to express their emotions, develop coping mechanisms, and explore all available options is essential throughout the infertility journey. Mental health professionals with expertise in reproductive issues can play a vital role in alleviating psychosocial stressors and improving the overall well-being of those navigating infertility.

The aim of this chapter is to explore the multifaceted psychological landscape of infertility, examining the emotional impact, the strains it places on relationships, the psychological considerations during infertility treatments, the coping mechanisms employed, available support systems, and the often-overlooked experiences of men.

8.2 The Multifaceted Psychological Burden of Infertility

Research consistently highlights the high prevalence of psychological distress in infertile populations. Up to 70% of infertile patients report psychological issues during the course of IVF treatment [8]. Infertile couples are subject to greater stress and have an increased risk of developing psychological disorders compared with healthy couples. A meta-analysis found that anxiety and depression are the most common negative emotions among infertility patients [12]. These negative emotions can easily lead to the interruption or discontinuation of treatment, potentially affecting pregnancy outcomes. The effect can also impact the peripartum period, and even in case of a successful IVF, meaning there is a live birth, stress can have an effect on the offspring [11].

8.2.1 Emotional Distress

Individuals facing infertility experience a wide range of intense and often debilitating negative emotions, significantly impacting their mental health and overall well-being. These emotions frequently include anxiety, depression, sadness, anger, frustration, guilt, and profound feelings of loss.

Anxiety is a common experience for those struggling with infertility, often linked to the uncertainty of treatment outcomes and the desire to conceive. Patients undergoing IVF, for instance, have rated their anxiety levels as greater than other significant life events. Studies have found that between 25% and 60% of infertile individuals report psychiatric symptoms, with significantly higher levels of anxiety compared to fertile controls. In a study of Korean women undergoing IVF/ICSI, 12.9% experienced clinically significant anxiety [13]. Anxiety can be heightened during specific stages of treatment, such as the period between oocyte pickup and fertilization. Furthermore, the drugs and hormones used in ART can also trigger psychological symptoms, including anxiety.

Depression can also occur during the infertility journey. Infertile women have been shown to experience higher rates of depression compared to the general population. Research indicates that 25% to 60% of infertile individuals report psychiatric symptoms, including significantly higher levels of depression than fertile controls [14]. A study on infertile Turkish women found a significant positive correlation between depression and infertility stigma [15]. Among Korean women seeking fertility treatment, 32.3% exhibited depression [13]. Depression scores have been observed to rise with patient age and the number of infertility treatments undergone.

Sadness and grief are also commonly reported emotions, stemming from the inability to conceive and the loss of the anticipated experience of parenthood. Infertility can be experienced as a silent grief and a mourning of a longed-for future.

Each unsuccessful IVF treatment cycle can trigger emotional vulnerability [9]. The persistent nature of infertility can lead to chronic sadness and a sense of disappointment.

Anger and frustration frequently arise from the perceived injustice of infertility and the difficulties encountered during diagnosis and treatment. Women have reported experiences of frustration and anger related to their infertility. The lack of standardized tools and diagnostic protocols can contribute to these feelings. Furthermore, the often lengthy and complex treatment processes can be a source of significant frustration.

Feelings of guilt and shame can also be profound for individuals facing infertility. In some societies, women are exclusively held responsible for infertility, leading to more significant stress and guilt [16]. Infertility can lead to diminished self-esteem, as well as feelings of shame and guilt, in women who struggle to conceive naturally.

The overarching feeling of loss is central to the emotional burden of infertility. This includes the loss of the ability to have children naturally, the loss of the envisioned family life, and the loss of control over one's own body and future. Infertile women have reported experiencing a sense of loss of control and planning of life.

The infertility journey is marked by a complex interplay of negative emotions, with anxiety, depression, sadness, anger, frustration, guilt, and feelings of loss being particularly prominent. This adverse psychological state has been shown to have an adverse effect on the psycho-neuro-immuno-endocrine network, leading to disruption of immune homeostasis at the mother-fetus interface, the incubation of blastula, and the receptivity of the maternal endometrium. This in turn has a negative impact on the proliferation, invasion, and vascular remodeling of the embryo trophoblast, leading to a reduction of the success rate of embryo transfer [17]. This will further aggravate the psychological pain of infertile patients, leading to a vicious circle. In addition, it can have a direct impact on the development and health of the offspring. The significant prevalence of psychological distress in infertile populations underscores the critical need for comprehensive care that addresses not only the medical aspects but also the profound emotional and psychological challenges faced by these individuals and couples [18].

8.2.2 Impact on Self-Esteem and Identity

Infertility poses a significant challenge to an individual's fundamental sense of self, profoundly impacting their identity, self-worth, and feelings of normality. In many cultures, especially those with strong pronatalist values, motherhood and parenthood are central to a woman's identity [16, 19]. The inability to conceive can disrupt deeply ingrained beliefs about one's role, capabilities, and place in the world. From a young age, socialization often instills the role of mother as a core aspect of female identity and a social obligation in patriarchal societies. Consequently, when faced with infertility, women may experience an existential crisis, questioning their purpose and feeling a sense of uselessness and being defined by their infertility journey.

Some women describe infertility as feeling "unwomanly" and experience a sense of inadequacy and worthlessness. This disruption of one's personal narrative about becoming a parent, a story often carried from childhood, can lead to significant reproductive trauma. Even when male factor infertility is the primary issue, women in many societies are still viewed as responsible for reproduction, further impacting their sense of identity. The gendered nature of this burden is evident, with women often facing greater social and psychological pressure due to societal expectations around motherhood. In patriarchal and traditional societies, a woman's status and value can be inextricably linked to her fertility.

Infertility can severely undermine an individual's self-worth. The inability to conceive can lead to intense feelings of guilt and shame. Women, who are often exclusively held responsible for infertility in some cultures, may experience even more significant stress and guilt. This can lead to diminished self-esteem and a feeling of failure in achieving a fundamental aspect of personal and societal expectations. The persistent nature of infertility, especially with repeated unsuccessful treatments like IVF, can erode self-confidence and self-efficacy perceptions [9].

Feelings of normality are often shattered by the experience of infertility. It is described as an "invisible condition" and an "invisible loss," mourning a future that others may not even perceive [20]. Infertile individuals can feel alienated from the fertile world, experiencing isolation and feeling stigmatized and not understood by friends and family [8]. The social pressure to have children in pronatalist societies exacerbates these feelings of being different and outside the norm. Infertility is sometimes described by women as a "chaos or social disease" that disrupts their relationships. The metaphor of infertility treatment as an "emotional roller coaster" highlights the feeling of a lack of control and instability, further contributing to a sense of lost normality [21].

Therefore, infertility profoundly challenges an individual's sense of self, impacting their identity, self-worth, and feelings of normality. These challenges are significantly amplified within pronatalist societies that place a high value on childbearing and often impose gendered expectations around reproduction. Recognizing and addressing these nonmedical dimensions is crucial for supporting the overall well-being of individuals and couples navigating the infertility journey.

8.2.3 Social and Relationship Strain

Infertility is a dyadic stressor, significantly affecting the relationship between partners. While infertility can bring couples closer through shared adversity, it can also strain their emotional and sexual intimacy. Disagreements about treatment options, differing coping styles, and the emotional toll on each partner can lead to conflict and misunderstandings. The focus on timed intercourse and medical interventions can sometimes detract from the spontaneity and pleasure of sexual intimacy, leading to further relationship difficulties.

Infertility presents significant social challenges and can place considerable strain on an individual's relationships with family, friends, and the broader community.

The inability to conceive can lead to profound feelings of isolation, as individuals may feel disconnected from those around them who can have children seemingly without difficulty. This sense of being on a "lonely road" is often compounded by the fact that the grief associated with infertility is frequently not fully understood by those who have not experienced it. As a result, individuals may withdraw from social interactions, leading to strained relationships with friends and family.

Difficulty in social situations involving children is a common experience for those facing infertility. Encounters with pregnant individuals or families with children can trigger feelings of sadness, envy, and inadequacy. The constant reminders of what they long for but cannot achieve can make otherwise joyful social gatherings painful. This can lead to avoidance of events where children are present, further contributing to feelings of isolation and making it difficult to maintain close relationships with friends who have children. The emotional burden of infertility can permeate various aspects of daily life, potentially affecting work, leisure activities, and overall occupational balance [22].

Societal pressures, particularly in pronatalist societies, exacerbate the social challenges of infertility. In many cultures, "to have a child means living a fulfilled life," and couples unable to conceive may feel "barren and incomplete." This societal emphasis on childbearing can lead to significant stigma associated with infertility. Individuals may feel shame about their infertility and become reluctant to disclose their struggles due to fear of judgment. This reluctance to share can further isolate them from potential sources of support.

The impact on relationships can manifest in various ways. Friends and family, while often well intentioned, may offer unwanted advice or insensitive comments due to a lack of understanding about the complexities of infertility and its treatment. This can lead to frustration and further emotional distancing. Conversely, individuals undergoing infertility treatment often find the most support from others who have had similar experiences.

The healthcare system and society are sometimes perceived as lacking adequate support for individuals experiencing infertility, contributing to feelings of being "failed." The focus on the medical aspects of treatment can inadvertently overlook the significant psychological distress, diminished sense of control, and social stigma associated with infertility.

Addressing these challenges requires greater public awareness, empathetic support from family and friends, and a healthcare system that acknowledges and addresses the psychosocial needs of individuals and couples navigating infertility. Providing counselling and emotional support is crucial to help individuals develop coping strategies, reduce stress, and navigate the social complexities of infertility [8].

8.3 The Stressors Inherent in In Vitro Fertilization (IVF) Treatment

While ART offers the possibility of conception, the treatment process itself can be physically and emotionally demanding. IVF, in particular, involves numerous medical appointments, invasive procedures (such as injections and egg retrieval), and significant financial costs. The hormonal treatments can lead to physical discomfort and mood swings, further adding to the emotional burden.

The period following embryo transfer, often referred to as the "2-week wait," is particularly stressful, as individuals anxiously await the pregnancy test results. The uncertainty of treatment outcomes and the high rates of treatment failure can lead to significant anxiety, disappointment, and grief [23]. The cumulative nature of multiple IVF cycles can also lead to increased emotional vulnerability and higher dropout rates. Studies have shown that anxiety levels in infertile women can significantly impact IVF/ICSI outcomes. Furthermore, the process can feel like a loss of control over one's body and reproductive destiny.

8.3.1 The IVF Process as a Stressor

The IVF treatment process involves several distinct stages, each of which can significantly contribute to stress and anxiety for individuals and couples undergoing the procedure [24].

The first stage typically involves hormone stimulation. This phase aims to stimulate the ovaries to produce multiple eggs and usually involves daily medications, often administered through injections. These injections can be physically demanding and cause discomfort or pain. Furthermore, the hormonal medications themselves can trigger psychological symptoms such as anxiety, insomnia, irritability, and depression. Women have reported experiencing negative emotional and physical tolls from these treatment rounds. The process of administering these injections daily can also be a constant reminder of the ongoing fertility challenges and the medicalized nature of conception.

The next stage involves monitoring, which includes serial transvaginal ultrasounds and blood testing. These frequent appointments can disrupt daily life and work schedules. The results of these monitoring sessions dictate adjustments in medication dosages, adding an element of uncertainty and lack of control to the process. Patients may feel overwhelmed by the amount and type of clinical information provided during this stage and struggle to understand it. Following adequate follicle development, the stage of oocyte retrieval takes place. This is an invasive procedure involving the aspiration of eggs from the ovaries. While typically performed under sedation, it can still be a source of anxiety related to the procedure itself, potential pain or complications, and the anticipation of the number and quality of eggs retrieved.

Once the eggs are retrieved, they are fertilized in the laboratory with sperm. While patients are not directly involved in this stage, the waiting period for fertilization results and embryo development can be a significant source of anxiety. The uncertainty surrounding whether fertilization will occur and the quality of the resulting embryos can trigger feelings of hope and despair. The embryo transfer stage involves the placement of one or more embryos into the woman's uterus. This is generally a less invasive procedure, but it is laden with anxiety about whether the embryos will implant successfully. Patients may experience ambivalent feelings before the embryo transfer, coupled with hope and worry about the new situation.

After the embryo transfer, there is the notorious 2-week waiting period before a pregnancy test can confirm the outcome. This phase is consistently reported as the most stressful part of the entire IVF process [25]. It is a time of intense anticipation, where individuals often experience a roller coaster of emotions, alternating between hope and fear of failure. Women in particular experience high levels of anxiety during this time as they wait to know the outcome. The intense focus on potential pregnancy symptoms, or lack thereof, can be emotionally exhausting. Throughout the entire IVF journey, individuals may also undergo luteal phase support, often involving progesterone supplementation. This continues until the pregnancy test or, if pregnant, for a period afterward. While medically necessary, it adds to the burden of medications and can also have its own side effects, contributing to ongoing physical and emotional strain.

The uncertainty of success is a pervasive stressor throughout all stages of IVF. The lack of guarantees, despite the significant physical, emotional, and financial investment, contributes to high levels of anxiety and can lead to patients feeling unsettled and worried [9]. Each intervention that fails can trigger deep emotions and increase distress, potentially leading to the discontinuation of treatment. The financial burden of ART, the uncertainty regarding pregnancy outcomes, and the time commitment for procedures further compound the stress experienced during each stage.

Hence, each stage of IVF treatment, from the initial hormonal interventions and monitoring to the invasive procedures and the agonizing wait for results, carries its own set of stressors and anxieties. The cumulative effect of these challenges can significantly impact the mental health and well-being of individuals and couples undergoing IVF. Recognizing and addressing these psychological burdens is crucial for providing comprehensive care and support to those navigating the complexities of assisted reproductive technology [26, 27].

8.3.2 Physical Demands and Discomfort

The physical toll of IVF treatment is significant and encompasses side effects from medications, pain associated with procedures, and a general impact on physical health.

The hormone medications used to stimulate egg production can trigger various physical side effects. Synthetic estrogen, such as clomiphene citrate, can cause anxiety, sleep disturbances, and irritability in women. Letrozole, an estrogen receptor blocker, may lead to dizziness, fatigue, headaches, or breast pain. Lupron can also cause physical symptoms like acne. Other commonly used fertility drugs and their side effects include oral contraceptives which can cause weight gain and depression [28]. The medications used in ART can trigger psychological symptoms, and it may be difficult for patients and clinicians to distinguish between psychological responses and medication side effects. Furthermore, the hormonal imbalances caused by these drugs can result in psychosomatic trauma and pain [29].

IVF involves several invasive procedures that can cause physical discomfort and pain. Daily injections of hormone medications are a common part of the stimulation phase and can be physically demanding and cause discomfort or pain. Serial transvaginal ultrasounds are frequently performed for monitoring. The oocyte retrieval is an invasive procedure where eggs are aspirated from the ovaries. While typically done under sedation, it can still be a source of anxiety and potential pain or complications. Even the embryo transfer, though less invasive, is part of the physically demanding process. The constant need for these procedures, including blood testing and providing sperm samples, represents an increased interference with the body. Some women have reported experiencing "rough" care during procedures, leading to increased pain and distress [25]. Many women reported being unprepared for the pain, grief, discomfort, and side effects associated with IVF. Some women have also expressed concerns about the long-term health effects of treatment, including the health impact of ovarian hyperstimulation syndrome and fear of breast and uterine cancer as a result of hormonal treatment. The physical toll can be so significant that the physical demands of ART procedures are a commonly reported stressor [8].

8.3.3 Emotional Roller Coaster

The IVF cycle is often described as an emotional roller coaster, characterized by significant ups and downs throughout the various stages. Couples embarking on this journey typically experience a complex interplay of hope, anticipation, anxiety, and the potential for profound disappointment [9].

Initially, there is often a strong sense of hope. The decision to undergo IVF is usually made with the expectation and desire for a successful pregnancy, representing a helpful step toward success for many. Some research suggests that at the beginning of the first IVF treatment, women may exhibit positive expectations and initial enthusiasm, which can sometimes mask underlying negative emotions. First-time IVF patients, in particular, may show a greater level of hope compared to those undergoing repeated cycles [10, 30]. This initial optimism can be a powerful motivator as individuals prepare for the treatment process.

However, as the IVF cycle progresses, anxiety levels often rise. The stage involving hormone stimulation, with its daily medications, often administered through injections, can be physically demanding and trigger psychological symptoms such as anxiety, insomnia, irritability, and depression. The frequent monitoring, including blood tests and ultrasounds, while necessary, can also contribute to stress due to the disruption of daily life and the constant awareness of the medicalized nature of conception. Patients often report a loss of self-esteem, self-confidence, and sense of control throughout this process, further fueling anxiety.

The period surrounding oocyte retrieval and fertilization is marked by intense anticipation and continued anxiety. There is hope for a good number of retrieved eggs and successful fertilization, but also worry about potential complications or poor results. The waiting period for updates from the laboratory on fertilization and embryo development can be particularly nerve-wracking.

The embryo transfer stage brings a renewed sense of hope that the transferred embryo(s) will implant and lead to a pregnancy. However, this hope is often intertwined with significant anxiety about the outcome. The subsequent 2-week waiting period before the pregnancy test is widely reported as the most stressful phase of the entire IVF process. This is a time of heightened anticipation, where individuals may be hypervigilant to any potential pregnancy symptoms while simultaneously fearing the possibility of failure. The uncertainty of the outcome during this period is a major source of stress.

The arrival of the pregnancy test results can bring either joy and relief or profound disappointment. A failed IVF cycle can trigger deep emotions and increase distress, potentially leading to the discontinuation of treatment. Women may experience grief related to being childless, not being able to reproduce, and not being able to carry forward one's family line. The loss of an embryo can be felt deeply, akin to the loss of a potential child. Each unsuccessful attempt can erode hope and lead to feelings of sadness, anger, and frustration.

Throughout the entire IVF journey, individuals often alternate between states of hope and despair. This cyclical nature of emotions is a key characteristic of the IVF experience. The constant fluctuation between optimism and the fear of failure creates a significant emotional burden. The very thought of failure after such high costs and investments (emotional and physical) inevitably leads to distress.

In conclusion, the IVF cycle is a demanding emotional journey marked by hope, anticipation, anxiety, and the ever-present possibility of disappointment. Understanding these emotional ups and downs is crucial for providing appropriate psychological support to individuals and couples undergoing fertility treatment.

8.3.4 Uncertainty and Lack of Control

The inherent uncertainty of IVF outcomes is a significant factor contributing to stress and anxiety for individuals undergoing treatment. The IVF process, despite advancements in assisted reproductive technologies (ART), does not guarantee pregnancy, leading to a pervasive lack of control for patients.

This lack of control and the uncertainty of success exacerbate stress and anxiety throughout the IVF cycle. During the hormone stimulation and monitoring stages, the unpredictable nature of follicle development and medication adjustments can contribute to a feeling of a lack of control. The waiting period for fertilization results and embryo development is filled with anxiety due to the uncertainty of whether fertilization will occur and the quality of the embryos. The 2-week waiting period after embryo transfer is consistently reported as the most stressful part, characterized by intense anticipation and fear of failure due to the unknown outcome.

Each failed intervention can trigger deep emotions and increase distress, potentially leading to the discontinuation of treatment. The very thought of failure after significant investment inevitably leads to distress. Studies have shown that individuals undergoing ART procedures experience higher stress and pregnancy-specific anxiety than those who conceive spontaneously, reflecting the trauma of potential treatment failure and the indefinite duration of infertility [9].

The stress associated with the uncertainty of ART resulting in pregnancy and/or live birth is a significant psychological demand of the process. The understanding that the outcome does not entirely depend on their efforts can also lead to feelings of helplessness. This emotional burden, stemming from the inherent uncertainty and lack of control in IVF, underscores the need for psychological support for individuals and couples navigating this challenging journey.

8.3.5 Financial Burden

In many European countries, there is a system of partial or full reimbursement for a number of ART cycles [31]. However, equal and equitable access to fertility care is still a challenge especially in low- and middle-income countries, where it is rarely prioritized in national universal health coverage benefit packages [32]. The financial stress of IVF is a major psychological stressor for couples. Individuals undergoing ART report significantly more stress associated with the financial burden compared to those who have not started ART. The mean stress score related to the financial impact of ART is often one of the highest reported stressors. This financial pressure can cause psychological distress and emotional stress for both partners. In the private sector, the economic costs associated with IVF treatment are significant and can impose substantial financial stress on couples. The average cost for a single IVF cycle can range considerably, from $12,400 to $25,000 in the United States [8]. These high costs can prevent some couples from accessing treatment, leading to feelings of hopelessness.

Several factors contribute to the financial burden of IVF. The core procedures of IVF, including ovarian stimulation, oocyte retrieval, fertilization, and embryo transfer, are expensive. The hormone medications used throughout the IVF cycle add to the overall cost. Many couples require more than one IVF cycle to achieve a live birth. In the United States, IVF couples undergo an average of 2.7 cycles, spending an average of $61,377 out of pocket to achieve a live birth. The success rate per cycle is moderate, with only 23% resulting in a live birth in the United States in 2020 [8]. As of 2023, only 21 states in the United States mandated insurance to provide some fertility coverage, and only 15 of these laws covered IVF treatments. Coverage often varies, with limitations based on the type of service, monetary limits, and eligibility criteria such as age [33]. Navigating this variable insurance coverage is itself a source of stress. Some individuals also pay for complementary medical procedures like supplements, acupuncture, and counseling, adding to the financial strain [34].

In order to cover the costs, patients report using credit cards and savings, taking out loans, or even selling belongings. Some may regret their lack of financial preparation for IVF. Stress and financial costs are among the most common reasons for discontinuing IVF treatment. Couples whose first IVF cycle fails may stop treatment due to financial burdens. The significant financial investment, coupled with the uncertainty of success, makes IVF a risky investment [35]. The very thought of failure after incurring such high costs inevitably leads to distress. Stress associated with financial burden is significantly linked to higher stress and depression scores.

The economic challenges of IVF highlight the need for improved access to affordable care, including better insurance coverage and financial support options, to alleviate the significant financial stress experienced by individuals and couples pursuing this treatment [32]. IVF treatment can be time-consuming, requiring frequent appointments and potentially disrupting work and social schedules. Time-off work and paid sick leave to prospective parents receiving IVF treatment is encouraged and already implemented in a number of countries [36].

8.3.6 Impact on Embryo Transfer Outcomes

Research exploring the potential impact of anxiety and depression during the embryo transfer stage on IVF success rates presents conflicting results. Some studies suggest a relationship between psychological distress and IVF outcomes. For instance, a meta-analysis indicated that higher levels of anxiety in infertile women were significantly associated with lower pregnancy following IVF/ICSI treatment [12]. Another study found that elevated levels of a biological stress marker increased the risk of pregnancy failure in couples undergoing IVF. Similarly, some researchers have found a clear relationship between anxiety, depression, and the probability of becoming pregnant after IVF/ICSI treatment. It has also been suggested that stress might reduce the chances of a successful IVF outcome [17, 37]. These adverse psychological states can potentially affect various physiological processes involved in embryo implantation.

However, other research has not found a significant association between psychological factors and IVF outcomes, particularly during the embryo transfer stage. One study showed no significant difference between pregnant and nonpregnant groups in psychological distress (FPI and DASS scores). Similarly, some research did not find any association between IVF clinical pregnancy rates and symptoms of anxiety, depression, and stress. A prospective study also did not indicate any relationship between perceived psychological stress and psychological well-being before or during the first IVF treatment and its outcome. In fact, one study found that anxiety levels in women decreased during the embryo transfer stage compared to the ovarian stimulation stage. This could be because women become more familiar with the treatment process and feel more confident at this stage. Furthermore, a study on women undergoing IVF found that while women undergoing IVF may have been more anxious during the period between oocyte pickup and fertilization, this was not reflected in the overall psychosocial outcomes about IVF. The study suggested that the type of treatment (insemination vs. IVF) did not significantly influence their psychosocial outcomes [17, 38].

It is important to note that the evidence on the relationship between psychological distress and IVF outcomes is contradictory. The influence of anxiety on multicycle IVF treatment was also noted as not affirmative due to the complicated treatment procedures. Factors such as familiarity with the procedure from previous treatments might also lead to reduced anxiety levels, potentially influencing the results of studies.

In conclusion, while some research suggests that anxiety and depression might negatively impact IVF success rates, including around the embryo transfer stage, other studies have not found a significant link. More research is needed to clarify this complex relationship and to understand the specific role of psychological distress at different stages of the IVF process.

8.4 Coping Strategies in the Face of Infertility

Individuals and couples employ various coping mechanisms to navigate the challenges of infertility and its treatment. These strategies can be broadly categorized as problem-focused coping (e.g., seeking information, actively engaging in treatment), emotion-focused coping (e.g., seeking emotional support, using relaxation techniques), and avoidance coping (e.g., denying the problem, withdrawing from social interactions).

Social support from partners, family, friends, and support groups plays a crucial role in psychological adjustment. Feeling understood and validated by others can buffer the negative emotional impact of infertility. However, the effectiveness of coping strategies can vary, and some may be more adaptive than others. For instance, dyadic coping, where partners work together to manage the stress, has been shown to influence marital quality among couples undergoing IVF [39]. Psychological interventions focused on stress management have demonstrated effectiveness in women prior to IVF. Mindfulness-based programs have also been explored as a means to reduce stress and improve psychological well-being in infertile women. Modifying coping mechanisms of infertile spouses through interventions could potentially increase well-being and decrease distress.

8.4.1 Definition and Types of Coping

Coping refers to the behavioral and emotional efforts that individuals implement to manage unexpected stressors and changes or to regulate a situation to their desired state. In the context of infertility, coping mechanisms are the various ways in which individuals and couples confront and attempt to manage the significant stress associated with the inability to conceive and often the arduous process of infertility treatment. Coping is considered an important determinant of psychological adjustment during this challenging experience.

Various coping strategies are employed by individuals facing infertility stress. Dyadic coping refers to the ways in which couples cope together with infertility, viewing it as a shared problem and working to support each other. The effectiveness of these coping strategies can vary depending on individual personalities, the stage of infertility or treatment, and the support systems available. Health professionals can play a crucial role in helping individuals and couples identify and utilize adaptive coping mechanisms to improve their well-being throughout their infertility journey. Emotional approach coping involves processing and expressing emotions related to infertility. For instance, one study found that men's high use of emotional approach coping was associated with decreased depressive symptoms in women after a negative pregnancy result [14]. Problem-focused coping centers on actively trying to solve the problems associated with infertility. A husband's use of problem-focused coping has been linked to decreased depressive symptoms in their partner after a failed insemination [14]. Similar results were obtained when resorting to positive reinterpretation, positive reappraisal, and growth, which involves finding positive meaning in the experience of infertility. A number of individuals turn to their faith or self-controlling coping as a way to cope with the stress of infertility.

Evasive coping or avoidance involves trying to avoid thinking about or dealing with the stressors of infertility. Low use of avoidance coping by women was linked to decreased depressive symptoms in men after a negative pregnancy result. Conversely, high use of evasive coping by women was associated with a higher sense of life purpose in men during treatment [40]. Weak social support seeking by women was also associated with a higher sense of life purpose in men.

Distancing involves trying to create emotional distance from the problem. Men's increased distancing was associated with women's elevated depressive symptoms before treatment. Planful problem-solving is a more active form of problem-focused coping, involving making plans to address the infertility. Mindfulness involves focusing on the present moment without judgment and has shown effectiveness in improving psychological health in women undergoing infertility treatment [26]. Mindfulness-based interventions, such as mobile applications, can improve psychological health in women undergoing infertility treatment. Mindfulness practices help individuals focus on the present moment without judgment, potentially reducing anxiety and stress. Mindful Self-Compassion (MSC) therapy has shown promise in reducing psychological distress, psychopathological symptoms, and hopelessness in infertile women undergoing IVF by improving self-compassion and compassion for others. Self-compassion by being kind and understanding toward oneself in the face of infertility-related suffering has been shown to be relevant in managing the emotional burden. Self-compassion can buffer against hostility and reduce self-criticism, blame, and censure. Acceptance and commitment focus on enhancing an individual's emotional bond with their thoughts and feelings, promoting cognitive flexibility. Cultivating hope can help individuals adapt and cope positively with the challenges of infertility. Relaxation techniques such as meditation, deep breathing, guided imagery, and yoga have been shown to reduce negative emotions and anxiety scores in women undergoing infertility treatment. Yoga intervention specifically increased the quality of life and decreased negative feelings and thoughts associated with infertility [41].

8.4.2 Active Versus Avoidant Coping

Individuals employ various coping styles to manage the stress of infertility, which involves behavioral and emotional efforts to deal with stressors. Two contrasting styles are active problem-solving and seeking information versus avoidance and denial.

Active problem-solving and seeking information can manifest in several ways. Some individuals actively gather information about IVF procedures from medical professionals and experienced individuals as a form of psychological preparation and to predict what awaits them. Seeking health information is considered very important for psychological adjustment to illness. This information seeking can be an active way of coping and lowering anxiety. Furthermore, planful problem-solving is a specific subscale of coping that involves making plans to address the infertility. Research has shown that when men use problem-focused coping, it can be associated with decreased depressive symptoms in women after a negative pregnancy result. This may be because it signals the man's investment in the process.

Conversely, avoidance and denial are also utilized as coping mechanisms. Some individuals avoid seeking information about IVF, stating they feel more comfortable with less information as a form of psychological defense to not feel bad or cope poorly. Avoidance is also identified as a subscale in coping assessments. In one study, men with male factor infertility were found to avoid thinking about their infertility problem and disclosing their situation. Similarly, men who had failed ICSI distanced themselves from families with children. Evasive coping or avoidance by women has been linked to a higher sense of life purpose in men during treatment in one study. This suggests that sometimes avoiding difficult topics or emotions might make the spouse feel unburdened. However, men's increased distancing has also been associated with women's elevated depressive symptoms before treatment, possibly because women feel unsupported [41].

It is important to note that both active information seeking and avoidance can be ways to cope and lower anxiety for different individuals. The effectiveness of a particular coping style can depend on individual personalities and the specific stage of infertility or treatment. Health professionals can assist couples in identifying and using adaptive coping mechanisms. Interventions can also be designed to modify coping mechanisms to improve well-being and decrease distress in infertile spouses.

Psychological interventions, including positive thinking counseling and cognitive reconstruction, can effectively reduce mental health disorders, depression, and anxiety in women undergoing infertility treatments. Cognitive reconstruction aims to modify irrational thoughts that contribute to negative behaviors. Psychotherapy can provide a safe space for couples to express emotions, improve communication, and develop coping mechanisms. Addressing psychological problems like depression, anxiety, and stress may also help increase the chance of conception.

Open communication between partners about infertility can be a direct way of addressing the problem as a couple and seeking solutions together. Considering lifestyle modifications might be a direct approach in some cases of infertility, as modifiable lifestyle factors like smoking and psychological stress can affect semen quality in men. Health-promoting lifestyle programs are considered essential in ART to potentially improve pregnancy results. Actively seeking information about IVF (problem-focused coping strategy) can help reduce anxiety (emotion-focused coping strategy). Furthermore, the effectiveness of different coping styles can vary among individuals and across different stages of the infertility journey. Addressing the psychological needs of couples is considered a crucial aspect of successful infertility treatment alongside physical interventions [40].

Individuals seek information about infertility and its treatment through various sources, and this behavior can serve as a significant coping mechanism. Gathering information can be a form of much-needed psychological preparation, helping individuals predict what awaits them in procedures like IVF. Consultations with doctors are frequently chosen as the most acceptable source of information on IVF. Nurses also serve as information sources and play a crucial role in supporting the treatment process by helping patients understand their situation. They can offer counseling and enhance emotional resilience. While the internet is a significant source for some infertile couples seeking additional information, emotional and social support, and self-help, others actively avoid online information, feeling it can increase stress and questioning its reliability. Individuals often seek information from other women with more experience with IVF. Others choose to get a smaller amount of information or actively avoid it as a form of psychological defense to not feel bad or cope poorly. This can also be a way of coping and lowering anxiety for some individuals. The potential impact of information-seeking behavior on anxiety can vary. For some, gathering information provides a sense of control and preparedness, thereby lowering anxiety. However, for others, the sheer volume of clinical information can be overwhelming, and exposure to varied or potentially negative information, especially online, can increase stress and anxiety. This highlights the importance of reliable and accessible information from healthcare professionals. Healthcare teams should communicate clearly and offer counseling as an option to aid in coping with infertility and its treatment [41].

8.4.3 The Role of Social Support as a Coping Mechanism

Social support plays a crucial role in buffering the stress associated with infertility from partners, family, friends, and support groups. The support from a partner is particularly significant. Studies reveal that mutual support and enhanced communication between partners can strengthen their bond throughout the infertility journey. When men provide emotional approach coping or problem-focused coping, it is associated with decreased depressive symptoms in women after a negative pregnancy result. Conversely, a husband's increased distancing can lead to elevated depressive symptoms in women. Furthermore, partner emotional support has been directly linked to lower perceived stress in women undergoing ART. Marital status itself has been associated with greater social well-being, highlighting the importance of spousal support during fertility challenges. In IVF-ET couples, fertility stress and marital quality often affect each other, indicating the interdependence of these factors. A wife's increased communication and ability to cope with infertility stress can improve her husband's marital quality [40].

While family and friends can provide social support, their support may sometimes be limited if they have not personally experienced IVF. They might also offer unwanted advice or struggle to understand the complexities of infertility, potentially adding to the stress. Infertility is often described as something not widely discussed in social circles, leading to feelings of isolation and being misunderstood. Despite these challenges, social support from family and community members, especially those with prior IVF experiences, is appreciated.

Many individuals seek support from others who understand their situation. Support groups, peer members, online forums, and information resources are sought after to resolve stress, address relationship issues, share experiences with others, and obtain practical information. These platforms provide a space to connect with individuals facing similar challenges, offering a sense of community and shared understanding that can be lacking in broader social circles.

Research indicates that social support is a crucial factor in helping couples develop infertility-related coping strategies and decrease stress. Infertile women may develop resilience through various ways of confronting infertility stress with the support of friends, family, and healthcare professionals. Conversely, a lack of social support has been associated with higher postpartum depressive symptoms. The perception of adequate social support can act as a buffer against the negative emotional impact of infertility [42].

In conclusion, while support from family and friends can be valuable, the consistent and understanding support from a partner is paramount in managing infertility stress. Additionally, connecting with others through support groups and online communities can provide a unique form of validation and shared experience. Healthcare professionals should recognize the importance of social support and encourage couples to seek and utilize these resources throughout their infertility journey. Maladaptive coping strategies such as self-blame and substance abuse can unfortunately worsen their psychological distress. Health professionals could design interventions based on modifying the coping mechanisms of infertile spouses to increase levels of well-being and decrease levels of distress. Systemic and dyadic approaches in counseling could help couples adjust to the demands of infertility. Coping strategies during infertility treatment are multifaceted and have significant implications for psychological well-being. Problem-focused and emotional approach coping by partners can be beneficial, while avoidant and emotion-oriented coping may sometimes be detrimental. Interventions that foster adaptive coping mechanisms like self-compassion, mindfulness, and dyadic coping can potentially mitigate the psychological distress associated with infertility.

8.5 The Dyadic Experience: Infertility as a Shared Stressor

Infertility is not merely an individual issue but significantly impacts both partners within a relationship, making it a dyadic stressor. Both women and men experience considerable psychological distress due to infertility. Women may face stress, grief, inability to focus, shock, insomnia, anxiety, withdrawing from others, a sense of hopelessness, guilt, and shame. Similarly, men also report psychological, social, and sexual challenges. The diagnosis of infertility itself can be a nerve-racking experience for couples, leading to feelings like anger, guilt, sadness, depression, anxiety, and loss of self-confidence and self-esteem in both partners.

The infertility journey and its treatments can strain the intimate relationship between partners due to long treatments, stressful appointments, and changes in mood and libido caused by trauma, medications, and treatments. Studies reveal that the fertility stress level of wives undergoing IVF-ET is often significantly higher than that of their husbands. However, this does not diminish the stress experienced by men, and the emotional well-being of one partner can significantly affect the other. Some research indicates that men might suppress their emotional needs to support their partners, whom they perceive as suffering more.

Infertility can either cause conflicts in relationships or, with support, help couples grow stronger. Couples express a desire for counseling to be able to talk through the infertility experience and grow stronger through it. The mutual influence of spouses should not be overlooked, and psychological support for both partners is essential. Dyadic coping, which refers to how couples cope with stress together, is particularly relevant in the context of infertility. Infertility is rooted in the couple's relationship. Stronger dyadic coping can decrease partnership conflict and improve the ability to cope with stressful events, leading to improved relationship satisfaction and marital adjustment. Studies have found that dyadic coping mediates the relationship between fertility stress and marital quality in IVF-ET couples. The fertility stress of both wives and husbands can impact their marital quality through their dyadic coping efforts [6, 40].

Therefore, healthcare professionals should recognize infertility as a shared stressor and consider interventions that target both individuals within the couple and their dyadic coping mechanisms to reduce fertility stress and improve marital quality. Counseling and emotional support offered to both partners can help them develop infertility-related coping strategies and decrease stress.

8.5.1 Impact on Marital Quality and Intimacy

Infertility significantly impacts marital satisfaction, communication, and intimacy within a couple, often creating substantial challenges but also offering opportunities for growth.

Infertility can be a major source of stress that negatively affects marital quality. Couples may experience a range of difficult emotions, including anger, guilt, sadness, depression, anxiety, and a loss of self-confidence and self-esteem, which can strain their relationship. The financial burden of infertility treatment also adds to the stress. Research indicates that the fertility stress level of wives undergoing IVF-ET can be significantly higher than their husbands', though both partners experience distress. This stress can lead to decreased marital quality compared to fertile couples. However, mutual support and enhanced communication throughout the infertility journey can strengthen the bond between partners. Stronger dyadic coping, the ability of couples to cope with stress together, has been shown to decrease partnership conflict and improve the ability to handle stressful events, ultimately influencing marital quality positively. Conversely, a lack of support can contribute to spousal relationship strain. Marital quality is even considered the most important source of support during infertility treatment.

8.5.2 Communication

The infertility journey can either cause conflicts within a relationship or help couples grow stronger through the experience. Open and effective communication is crucial for navigating the emotional challenges. Studies have revealed that partners provide mutual support through enhanced communication. Therapists can play a vital role by providing a safe space for couples to express their emotions, which they may find difficult to discuss with each other, especially men in some societies [7]. Addressing psychological problems through therapy can also aid in developing better communication among partners. However, differences in how each partner copes with infertility can sometimes lead to misunderstandings or feelings of being unsupported. For instance, increased distancing by men during the pretreatment period has been associated with women's elevated depressive symptoms, potentially because women feel their partners do not share their worries. Conversely, wives' increased communication and ability to cope with infertility stress can be conducive to maintaining harmonious relationships, positively impacting their husbands' marital quality. Couples are encouraged to view infertility as a shared problem and work together by sharing information and discussing worries.

8.5.3 Intimacy

Infertility and its treatments often have a negative impact on a couple's sexual intimacy. The pressure of "sex on demand," scheduled around ovulation cycles rather than being a spontaneous expression of intimacy, can lead to a decrease in libido and pleasure for women. Some women may experience physical discomfort such as vaginal dryness and sensitive breasts. The long treatments, stressful appointments, and mood changes and decreased libido resulting from the trauma of infertility and medication can strain the intimate relationship. Women have reported less pleasure and a decrease in sexual activity, with some even experiencing a cessation of sexual activity for years due to their infertility journey. Furthermore, the primary goal of sexual intercourse can shift from pleasure to conception, impacting the emotional connection associated with intimacy. Even drugs used in infertility treatment, like clomiphene citrate, can cause side effects such as anxiety and irritability, further affecting intimacy. Research also suggests that women with infertility may experience fewer or diminished orgasms compared to fertile counterparts. Treatment outcomes can also affect men's sexual functioning and relationship quality, often driven more by psychological factors than hormonal ones.

Overall, infertility presents significant challenges to marital satisfaction, communication, and intimacy. However, with open communication, mutual support, dyadic coping, and professional psychological support when needed, couples can navigate these difficulties and potentially strengthen their relationship. Recognizing infertility as a shared stressor is crucial for fostering resilience within the couple.

8.5.4 Dyadic Coping

Dyadic coping refers to how couples manage stress together, recognizing that stress experienced by one partner can become shared (dyadic stress) due to their interdependence. It encompasses not only an individual's coping efforts but also the communication between partners about the stressor and the joint coping responses they undertake as a couple. The goal of dyadic coping is to restore or maintain the well-being of both individuals while promoting a healthy relationship characterized by reciprocal trust, mutual closeness, and intimacy [40].

Men's increased distancing during the pretreatment period was linked to elevated depressive symptoms in women. Conversely, men's high use of emotional approach coping, problem-focused coping, or positive reinterpretation before treatment was associated with decreased depressive symptoms in women after a negative pregnancy result.

Women's high use of emotion-oriented coping was related to increased distress in men during different stages of infertility treatment. Similarly, women's high use of self-controlling coping prior to treatment was associated with increased depressive symptoms or distress in men. In contrast, women's low use of avoidance or religious coping before treatment was linked to decreased depressive symptoms in men after a negative pregnancy result.

Stronger dyadic coping is associated with decreased partnership conflict, improved ability to cope with stressful events, and greater relationship satisfaction and marital adjustment. Specifically in couples undergoing IVF-ET, dyadic coping mediates the relationship between fertility stress and marital quality. This means that how well couples cope together significantly affects how their fertility-related stress impacts their marital relationship.

Given the interconnectedness of coping within a couple, healthcare professionals should consider dyadic approaches when designing interventions for infertility. Understanding how one partner's coping strategies can protect or harm the other's well-being can inform the development of more effective support for both individuals within the relationship. The mutual influence of spouses should not be overlooked in clinical practice, and encouraging open communication and collaborative coping efforts may be crucial for improving psychological outcomes for couples facing infertility. Support from a partner has also been shown to be associated with significantly lower perceived stress.

Research has identified several ways in which one partner's coping strategies during infertility treatment can influence the other partner's psychological well-being. A systematic review by Moutzouri et al. specifically examined this interpersonal level of coping, revealing significant associations between the coping mechanisms of one partner and the emotional adjustment of the other [40]. The review found that men's increased distancing and undermining as a way to cope with fertility problems during the pretreatment period was associated with elevated depressive symptoms in women. This may occur because women might perceive their partners as not sharing their worries or being equally committed to having children, leading to feelings of being unsupported. Conversely, men's high use of emotional approach coping, problem-focused coping, or positive reinterpretation before treatment was linked to decreased depressive symptoms in women after a negative pregnancy result. This suggests that when men actively engage with their emotions, focus on solutions, or find positive meaning in the situation, it can buffer their partners from emotional distress following unsuccessful treatment. Additionally, men's low use of substances was associated with an increased sense of life purpose in women during the treatment/IVF period. In the case of women, their high use of emotion-oriented coping was related to increased distress in men during different stages of infertility treatment. This might be because when both partners are primarily focused on emotional responses rather than problem-solving, men may experience greater distress, especially given the demanding nature of infertility treatment. Furthermore, women's high use of self-controlling coping during the pretreatment period was associated with increased depressive symptoms or distress in men. This could reflect a traditional behavior where men are less likely to share their difficulties, and when women also adopt a highly self-controlled approach, men might feel less opportunity for mutual support. When women do not rely on avoidance or solely on religious coping, it might positively impact their partners' emotional state after treatment failure. Interestingly, women's high use of evasive coping or low use of substances or weak social support seeking was associated with men's high sense of life purpose during the treatment period. One possible explanation is that women might be hiding their worries to protect their spouse, leading the men to feel less burdened and experience a higher sense of purpose. The findings from this systematic review highlight that the impact of a partner's coping strategy is not universal but depends on the specific coping mechanism employed and the stage of the infertility journey [40].

These insights suggest that healthcare professionals should consider these dyadic influences when designing psychological interventions for infertile couples. Interventions that aim to modify maladaptive coping mechanisms and promote supportive coping strategies within the couple have the potential to improve the psychological well-being of both partners. The mutual influence of spouses and the importance of dyadic coping, where couples cope with stress together, is crucial for navigating the challenges of infertility.

The Actor-Partner Interdependence Model (APIM) is a statistical framework used to analyze dyadic data, such as data from couples, by simultaneously examining the influence of each partner on their own outcomes (actor effects) and on their partner's outcomes (partner effects). In the context of couples undergoing in vitro fertilization (IVF), APIM can be applied to understand the reciprocal influences of stress and coping [6]. Traditional approaches often examine the impact of an individual's stress or coping on their own well-being. However, APIM acknowledges the interdependence between partners in a close relationship. During the stressful IVF journey, one partner's experience of stress and their coping mechanisms can directly affect the other partner's stress levels and coping responses.

8.6 Exploring Gendered Experiences of Infertility Treatment

Research suggests several potential differences in how men and women experience and express emotions related to infertility [8]. Women often report higher levels of stress, anxiety, and depression compared to men during infertility and IVF treatment. This may be partly due to the significant importance placed on motherhood and parenthood for women in many societies, leading to greater social and psychological pressure. Infertility can be viewed as a failure to achieve a normative identity for women. Furthermore, women are often perceived as primarily responsible for reproduction, which can contribute to their increased stress. The diagnostic and treatment processes for infertility are also typically more invasive and demanding for women.

The study by Ye et al. found that while the level of hope in women undergoing IVF-ET for the first time did not differ significantly from men, women reported significantly lower fertility quality of life and greater negative emotions such as stress, anxiety, and depression [10]. This aligns with other research indicating that women experience higher levels of depression, cognitive dysfunction, anxiety, and general psychological problems, along with lower self-esteem, compared to men facing infertility.

8.6.1 Men's Experiences

Historically, research and clinical attention have predominantly focused on the female experience of infertility. However, men also experience significant psychological distress related to infertility and its treatment. Men may grapple with feelings of inadequacy, emasculation, and a loss of their masculine identity. They may also experience stress related to diagnostic procedures, such as semen analysis, and the pressure to perform sexually on demand.

Men's coping styles and their ways of expressing emotional distress may differ from women's, which can sometimes lead to their experiences being overlooked. However, studies have highlighted the psychological, social, marital, and sexual implications of male infertility treatment. Men also have specific needs in the clinical setting that require attention and support. It is crucial to acknowledge and address the gender differences in how men and women cope with infertility stress during physical interventions and counseling [7].

Men may experience great difficulty expressing their emotions due to societal norms. However, social research has increasingly focused on the male perspective, revealing that childless men are equally invested in experiencing parenthood and suffer elevated anxiety due to infertility. Men with male factor infertility are a particularly vulnerable group, displaying a higher risk for sexual, emotional, and psychological strain. Studies have also shown that men undergoing treatment for male infertility may have an avoidant coping mechanism, and their self-esteem, relationship quality, and sexual functions can be tied to treatment outcomes [7]. Psychological evaluations indicate that urological surgery can have a lasting impact on infertility-specific stress. Treatment failure can lead to feelings of depression, grief, and inadequacy. Men tend to have an avoidant coping mechanism throughout fertility treatment, and their self-esteem can be tied to treatment outcomes. For instance, successful testicular sperm extraction (TESE) can improve overall and family-related self-esteem, while failed TESE can significantly lower self-esteem across various domains. Feelings of being stressed, emasculated, and depressed have also been reported. Surgical treatments can affect the sexual functioning of infertile men. The impact of TESE outcomes on sexual function appears to be psychologically driven, whereas improvements after microsurgical varicocelectomy are primarily evident in hypogonadal men [43]. Men with failed TESE may experience a significant decrease in erectile function, intercourse satisfaction, and orgasmic function. This negative impact can be independent of changes in testosterone levels. Microsurgical varicocelectomy seems to improve erectile function in infertile men with preoperative hypogonadism, likely due to the normalization of testosterone levels. However, this improvement in sexual function is not always associated with successful treatment of subfertility. Similar to women, the pressure of timed intercourse for conception can also affect spontaneity and satisfaction in men [13]. Psychological strain experienced by men undergoing infertility treatment can also negatively affect their sexual function. Couples may also experience a loss of satisfying sexual life, with sex becoming a scheduled task rather than a spontaneous event once infertility treatments begin. Some research indicates that men might experience psychosomatic distress and stress more often than women, which correlates with lower quality of life, although they might report higher relationship satisfaction [40].

Interestingly, a study using the Actor-Partner Interdependence Model (APIM) found that wives' fertility stress can significantly affect their husbands' marital quality, highlighting the interconnectedness of their emotional experiences [6]. This suggests that even if men do not express their emotions in the same way as women, they are still affected by their partner's stress. The study also found that wives generally had higher fertility stress and lower levels of dyadic coping and marital quality compared to their husbands. This gender disparity might make it challenging for men to fully empathize with their spouses.

There is a need for better inclusion, communication, education, and resource provision to address reported issues of marginalization and uncertainty in men. Clinicians should strive to provide patients with a comprehensive understanding of their condition, treatment processes, expected outcomes, and alternative options. The need for emotional support and better communication from medical staff has been emphasized. Men feel more involved when clinicians discuss their concerns, provide information on the general experiences of infertile men, and offer opportunities to talk about their wishes for fatherhood. Routine psychosocial screening in cases of severe male infertility and follow-up after surgical treatment failure are likely beneficial [44]. Healthcare professionals should also provide comprehensive education and written resources from both medical and psychosocial standpoints. Continued communication with and inclusion of the male partner throughout the whole management process will benefit the overall patient experience. Online support groups have also been suggested as a complementary resource.

In conclusion, while both men and women experience significant emotional distress due to infertility, there appear to be differences in the intensity of certain emotions and how they are expressed. Women often report higher negative emotional states and face greater societal pressures, while men might struggle with emotional expression and adopt different coping mechanisms yet are still significantly impacted by the challenges of infertility and their partner's experience. Understanding these gender-specific experiences is crucial for providing effective psychological support to couples undergoing infertility treatment.

8.7 Psychological Interventions and Support Programs for Infertility

Given the significant psychological impact of infertility, providing adequate support and interventions is crucial. Healthcare professionals should be aware of the mental health needs of individuals and couples undergoing fertility treatment and offer appropriate resources and referrals. This includes open and empathetic communication, psychological counseling and therapy, psychoeducational interventions, and support groups. It is important to address the potential for postpartum mental illness in individuals who have undergone infertility treatment. Studies suggest a possible link between infertility treatment and an increased risk of postpartum depression. Therefore, ongoing support and monitoring of mental health during and after pregnancy are essential [45].

8.7.1 Need for Psychological Support

It is crucial to integrate psychological support into infertility care due to the significant mental health challenges faced by individuals and couples undergoing diagnosis and treatment, particularly in IVF. Infertility is more than just a medical problem; it profoundly affects mental health, leading to stress, guilt, emptiness, anxiety, and depression. As already discussed, studies indicate that infertile couples experience greater stress and have an increased risk of developing psychological disorders compared with healthy couples. This psychological distress can, in turn, negatively impact fertility.

Psychological interventions have demonstrated effectiveness in reducing mental health disorders, depression, and anxiety among individuals with infertility. Stress management is a focal point in counseling interventions, aiming to boost coping mechanisms. Techniques such as positive thinking and cognitive reconstruction can significantly reduce perceived stress. Mindfulness-based interventions, including mobile applications, have also shown promise in reducing depression and anxiety and increasing mindfulness and self-efficacy. Mindful Self-Compassion (MSC) therapy can improve life satisfaction and mental well-being by reducing psychological distress, psychopathological symptoms, and hopelessness in infertile women and couples undergoing IVF [40].

Healthcare professionals provide comprehensive psychological support alongside medical treatment. Relying solely on physical treatments for infertility may not be enough; addressing psychological needs is crucial for successful treatment. The American Society for Reproductive Medicine (ASRM) regards a fertility/mental health counselor as a recommended component in ART clinics [46].

Making mental health professionals mandatory in ART facilities could provide a beneficial source of support. Healthcare professionals should be able to provide compassionate and empathetic care, give adequate information and time, and empower patients throughout the process. Counseling, provided individually, as a couple, or in a group, can address the extraordinary situation-specific needs of patients. It focuses on the emotional crisis associated with unfulfilled wishes and the stress of repeated interventions with narrow success rates. Psychotherapy can provide a safe space to express emotions, aid in developing coping mechanisms and decision-making, and improve communication between partners. Starting counseling before medical intervention is ideal.

Integrating psychological support into infertility care is essential for addressing the significant emotional distress experienced by patients, potentially improving treatment outcomes, and enhancing overall well-being. This support should be comprehensive, encompassing clear explanations, empathetic care, and access to various psychological interventions throughout the infertility journey.

8.7.2 Mindfulness-Based Interventions

Mindfulness-Based Stress Reduction (MBSR) and Mindful Self-Compassion (MSC) programs are valuable psychological interventions for managing the significant stress, anxiety, and depression experienced by infertile women undergoing IVF. These programs aim to improve well-being and coping mechanisms.

MBSR, grounded in Kabat-Zinn's work, focuses on cultivating awareness of the present moment without judgment [47]. It typically involves practices like mindfulness meditation and mindful movement over several weeks. Studies have shown that MBSR and other mindfulness-based interventions (MBIs) can effectively reduce stress, anxiety, and depression in infertile women. For example, the experimental group using a mindfulness-based mobile application showed significant reductions in depression and anxiety, alongside increases in mindfulness, self-efficacy, and adjustment levels [48]. Meta-analyses have also confirmed the efficacy of psychological interventions, including mindfulness, in improving mental health outcomes for women undergoing infertility treatments [49].

MSC, a program that builds upon mindfulness, aims to cultivate a compassionate and understanding connection with oneself, particularly when facing difficulties. It involves practices designed to increase self-compassion, compassion for others, mindfulness, and life satisfaction. Research indicates that MSC therapy can reduce psychological distress, psychopathological symptoms, and hopelessness in infertile women undergoing IVF. It can also enhance emotional resilience and reduce self-criticism [50].

Both MBSR and MSC can be adapted to address the unique challenges of infertility. For instance, mindfulness practices can be customized to the stages of IVF treatment. A mobile application developed for infertility included audio recordings tailored to specific stages like oocyte retrieval and embryo transfer. These tailored exercises included body scans focusing on the uterus and ovaries and visualizations of the uterine lining. The mindfulness content can also incorporate themes related to drug administration, ovarian awareness, and pre-/post-embryo transfer awareness [51].

Nurses play a crucial role in supporting these interventions by creating a supportive environment, offering emotional support, and teaching stress management strategies like mindfulness. They can guide patients in applying these techniques throughout the IVF process [26].

Both MBSR and MSC are valuable non-pharmacological approaches that can be effectively applied and adapted to help infertile women manage stress, anxiety, and depression associated with IVF treatment, ultimately contributing to their overall well-being. Integrating such psychological support into standard infertility care is increasingly recognized as essential.

8.7.3 Cognitive Restructuring and Cognitive Behavioral Therapy (CBT)

Cognitive restructuring techniques are valuable tools in helping individuals undergoing infertility treatment, particularly IVF, identify and modify negative thought pattern. This approach is based on the premise that irrational thoughts can lead to negative emotions and behaviors, and by changing these underlying thoughts, individuals can experience improved well-being.

In the context of infertility, women often experience significant psychological distress, including stress, anxiety, and depression. Cognitive restructuring interventions aim to address this by teaching individuals to become aware of their negative thoughts related to infertility. These thoughts might include feelings of failure, guilt, hopelessness about conceiving, or unfairness.

The process of cognitive restructuring typically involves several steps. Individuals learn to recognize the automatic, often negative thoughts that arise in response to infertility-related situations, such as a failed treatment cycle or seeing a pregnant woman. Once identified, these thoughts are critically examined. Individuals are encouraged to question the evidence supporting these thoughts and to consider alternative, more balanced perspectives. For example, a thought like "I will never get pregnant" might be challenged by considering the possibility of future treatment options or the fact that many people do eventually conceive. The core of cognitive restructuring involves replacing irrational or negative thoughts with more realistic and positive ones. This does not necessarily mean forcing oneself to think positively all the time but rather developing a more balanced and rational outlook. By modifying negative thought patterns, individuals can develop more effective coping mechanisms for dealing with the stressors of infertility treatment.

Several studies highlight the effectiveness of cognitive restructuring in reducing stress and improving mental health in infertile women. A randomized controlled trial involving women with recurrent failed IVF cycles demonstrated that positive thinking counseling and cognitive reconstruction significantly reduced perceived stress [52]. This intervention involved individual face-to-face counseling sessions focused on teaching these skills. The findings align with other research showing that cognitive behavioral programs can reduce psychosocial problems associated with infertility by increasing awareness of stress-triggering thoughts and enhancing the ability to communicate emotions [53].

Cognitive restructuring techniques empower infertile individuals to identify their negative thought patterns, challenge their validity, and replace them with more balanced perspectives. This process can lead to reduced stress, anxiety, and depression, ultimately contributing to improved psychological well-being throughout their infertility journey. Therapists and counselors in infertility centers are recommended to utilize these therapeutic approaches to address the psychological issues faced by infertile women.

8.7.4 Counseling and Therapy

Individual and couples counseling plays a vital role in addressing the emotional challenges associated with infertility, which is more than just a medical condition and significantly impacts mental health. Infertility can lead to stress, guilt, anxiety, and depression. Healthcare systems should recognize the importance of providing comprehensive psychological support alongside medical treatment [54].

Individual counseling offers a safe space for individuals to express their emotions related to unfulfilled wishes and the stress of repeated interventions with uncertain outcomes. It can help individuals navigate feelings of failure, guilt, and hopelessness. Psychotherapy can aid in developing coping mechanisms and decision-making throughout the treatment process. For individuals struggling to accept their infertility, therapy can provide support in exploring available options.

Couples counseling is equally crucial as infertility is often a shared experience that can strain intimate relationships due to long treatments, stressful appointments, and changes in mood and libido. Counseling provides a platform for couples to talk through their infertility experience and grow stronger together. It can improve communication between partners, helping them navigate the individual stages of denial, anger, blame, shame, and despair that they may experience differently. Addressing psychological problems within the couple's dynamic may even help increase the chance of conception. Studies indicate that couples desire counseling to resolve stress and relationship issues [27, 41, 55].

Tailoring counseling sessions to specific needs is paramount. Infertility counseling differs from routine gynecological consultations by focusing on the emotional crisis arising from an unfulfilled life goal [56]. Counseling should ideally begin before any medical intervention to provide initial support. It addresses situation-specific needs, such as high distress periods, pregnancy after infertility, facing the end of treatment, or considering third-party donor programs. The type of counseling (individual, couple, or group) should be matched to the patient's preferences and the nature of their challenges. For instance, dyadic coping, the way couples manage stress together, is significantly associated with marital quality in IVF-ET couples, suggesting that interventions can be tailored to enhance these coping mechanisms. Furthermore, understanding the different stages of infertility treatment is essential for tailoring support effectively. Healthcare professionals, including nurses, midwives, and mental health professionals, should be knowledgeable about psychosocial factors to provide empathetic care, adequate information, and empower patients throughout their journey. Integrating mental health professionals into ART facilities is a recommended and potentially beneficial source of tailored support.

8.7.5 Practical Challenges in Implementing Interventions

Several potential barriers can hinder participation in psychological support programs for individuals and couples undergoing infertility treatment, including time commitment and initial emotional discomfort.

Psychological interventions, such as counseling sessions, require a significant time investment. The need for regular attendance and engagement in homework assignments can be challenging for individuals already managing demanding IVF treatment schedules involving numerous appointments and potential travel. The very thought of failure after such a high cost, including time, can lead to distress. Furthermore, maintaining a regular mindfulness practice, even with a mobile application, can be difficult for participants due to the demands of their daily lives [50]. On the other hand, short counseling sessions or interventions that do not adequately address the intense grief and emotional challenges of infertility may not be effective in encouraging continued participation.

In addition, engaging with psychological support often requires individuals to confront and explore difficult emotions such as sadness, anger, frustration, loss of self-esteem, and hopelessness associated with infertility Some individuals might be hesitant to delve into these feelings due to the potential for increased emotional discomfort, as one participant described avoiding online information to prevent feeling bad. Mindfulness practices, while beneficial in the long run, can initially elicit unpleasant or upsetting emotions as individuals become more aware of their thoughts and feelings. This initial uneasiness can be a barrier to starting or continuing therapy if not handled appropriately. The alternation between hope and despair during IVF treatment can also make individuals wary of engaging in processes that might bring difficult emotions to the surface, especially after treatment failures.

Beyond these primary barriers, other factors can also play a role. Some individuals may be hesitant to participate in couples counseling due to privacy concerns or cultural stereotypes. Shame surrounding infertility can also be a significant stressor, potentially making individuals avoid seeking support. In addition, there may be a perceived lack of benefit or misunderstanding about the value of psychological support or may believe it will not significantly impact their chances of conceiving. Financial constraints can also be a barrier to accessing psychological services. Furthermore, the logistical demands of ART, including time to navigate insurance and attend appointments, can make additional commitments like therapy seem overwhelming.

Addressing these barriers through clear communication about the benefits of psychological support, flexible scheduling options, ensuring privacy and confidentiality, and providing culturally sensitive and effective interventions is crucial to improve participation and ultimately the psychological well-being of individuals and couples undergoing infertility treatment.

8.8 The Influence of Lifestyle Factors on Reproductive Health

Modifiable lifestyle factors such as diet, physical activity, stress management, and weight play an important role in influencing reproductive health in both men and women [57].

Diet plays a crucial role in fertility. For women, a proper diet before pregnancy is essential. Anti-inflammatory diets and the Mediterranean diet, rich in antioxidants, flavonoid resources, and unsaturated fatty acids while low in processed and red meats, are highlighted as beneficial for fertility. Adequate folate and selenium intake, along with low cholesterol consumption, can positively impact sperm parameters in men. Conversely, high saturated fat and calcium intake may negatively affect sperm quality. Excessive caffeine consumption may have detrimental effects, while moderate caffeine intake shows a positive association with sperm motility. Alcoholic has been linked to decreased semen quality [58].

Physical activity is another vital factor. Regular, moderate physical activity can improve fertility outcomes, particularly in obese women undergoing IVF. Exercise may reduce oxidative stress and chronic inflammation in the testes for men. However, excessive exercise might negatively impact the hypothalamic-pituitary-adrenal axis. A sedentary lifestyle is associated with lower health-related quality of life in infertile individuals.

Weight, as indicated by body mass index (BMI), significantly affects reproductive health in both sexes [59]. In women, obesity is linked to infertility. In men, elevated BMI is negatively correlated with sperm concentration and testosterone levels. Adiposity can lead to reduced testosterone and increased estradiol, disrupting spermatogenesis. Weight reduction through lifestyle changes can improve hormonal profiles and semen quality. Being overweight or obese in men is associated with reduced fertility [60, 61].

Stress management is critical due to the significant psychological distress associated with infertility. Infertility and ART treatments can lead to high levels of anxiety and stress. Psychological support and stress management training can improve the quality of life and potentially increase the chances of achieving pregnancy. Psychological stress in men is associated with reduced sperm motility and concentration. Lifestyle interventions should integrate stress management techniques. Dyadic coping, how couples manage stress together, significantly impacts marital quality during IVF-ET.

Modifiable lifestyle factors such as diet, physical activity, stress management, and maintaining a healthy weight are crucial determinants of reproductive health in both men and women. Addressing these factors through lifestyle interventions and psychological support programs can potentially improve fertility outcomes and overall well-being [62, 63].

8.8.1 Lifestyle Interventions in Infertility Treatment

Lifestyle interventions encompassing nutrition, physical activity, and stress management are increasingly recognized for their potential benefits for infertile couples undergoing ART. The development of these programs often involves a multistep approach, starting with a thorough understanding of the lifestyle factors of infertile couples.

Health-promoting lifestyle programs are considered essential in ART to enhance pregnancy results and live births. These programs, when combined with IVF, can influence the outcome of fertilization. Lifestyle interventions can modify dietary patterns, with diets rich in antioxidants, flavonoid resources, and unsaturated fatty acids being beneficial for fertility. Adequate intake of folate and selenium, and low cholesterol consumption, can positively impact sperm parameters in men. Regular, moderate physical activity can improve fertility outcomes, especially in obese women undergoing IVF. Exercise may reduce oxidative stress and chronic inflammation in the testes for men. Lifestyle interventions increase individuals' life satisfaction and promote health and lifespan.

Addressing psychological needs alongside physical treatments is crucial for successful infertility treatment. Proper methods within lifestyle programs can help reduce anxiety and stress. Stress management becomes a focal point in counseling interventions for infertility. Tailored literature-based programs including stress reduction alongside nutrition and physical activity are being developed for IVF/ ICSI interventions [57].

8.9 Conclusion and Future Directions

Infertility and its treatment are significant life events that extend far beyond the physical realm, profoundly impacting the psychological well-being of individuals and couples. Undergoing IVF introduces various stressors. The emotional distress, relational strain, and the challenges associated with ART can impact the outcome of the treatment itself, and there is evidence that it may affect the offspring. This highlights the need for a holistic approach to infertility care that integrates psychological support with medical interventions. Coping strategies and dyadic support play a crucial role in managing the psychological impact of infertility and IVF. Psychological interventions, such as counseling and psychotherapy, are vital in addressing the mental health challenges associated with infertility treatment. This support should be tailored to address the specific stressors and emotional needs at different stages of treatment. Providing comprehensive information, empathetic care, and adequate time for patients to express their concerns is also vital. Integrating mental health professionals into fertility clinics can provide a beneficial source of support and improve the overall patient experience. Addressing the psychological well-being of infertile individuals and couples is crucial for improving their quality of life and potentially their reproductive outcomes. Healthcare professionals must be sensitive to the emotional needs of their patients, providing open communication and resources for psychological counseling and fostering supportive environments. Recognizing and addressing the unique experiences of both men and women is essential for promoting better psychological adjustment and overall well-being throughout the infertility journey [7, 12, 50].

Future research should continue to explore effective interventions and strategies to mitigate the psychosocial burden of infertility and enhance the quality of life for those striving to build a family. Longitudinal studies are essential to understand the long-term psychological impact of infertility treatment. Additional research is needed to understand whether ART-related stress is associated with negative physical health outcomes in mothers and their offspring over the long term. Further research is warranted on the effectiveness of different psychological interventions. There is also a recognized need for specific psychological interventions for all infertile women due to the negative effects of unsuccessful IVF cycles. The exploration of personalized approaches to psychological support is also suggested. Future research should consider context-specific factors in fertility care. Further research can use comparative analyses in diverse populations to elucidate whether infertility involves specific moderating effects or amplifies general trends. More comprehensive assessment of psychological distress is needed.

Finally, further research on male experiences is warranted. Future studies should explore the emotional well-being of relationships during infertility treatment, especially for more vulnerable patient groups, and verify the need to support not only the patient but also the couple confronting the issue together. More research is needed to clarify the relationship between personality traits and infertility treatments in both men and women. Single mothers, same sex couples and surrogates also need to be included in future studies.

References

1. Sun H, Gong TT, Jiang YT, Zhang S, Zhao YH, Wu QJ. Global, regional, and national prevalence and disability-adjusted life-years for infertility in 195 countries and territories, 1990-2017: results from a global burden of disease study, 2017. Aging (Albany NY). 2019;11(23):10952–91. https://doi.org/10.18632/aging.102497.
2. WHO. Infertility prevalence estimates, 1990–2021. Geneva: World Health Organization; 2023. Licence: CC BY-NC-SA 3.0 IGO
3. Baker VL, Dyer S, Chambers GM, Keller E, Banker M, de Mouzon J, Elgindy E, Bai FM, Ishihara O, Jwa SC, Kupka MS, Zegers-Hochschild F, Adamson GD. International Committee for Monitoring Assisted Reproductive Technologies (ICMART): world report for cycles conducted in 2017-2018. Hum Reprod. 2025:deaf049. https://doi.org/10.1093/humrep/deaf049. Epub ahead of print. PMID: 40239109.
4. European IVF Monitoring Consortium (EIM) for the European Society of Human Reproduction and Embryology (ESHRE), Smeenk J, Wyns C, De Geyter C, Kupka M, Bergh C, Saiz CI, De Neubourg D, Rezabek K, Tandler-Schneider A, Rugescu I, Goossens V. ART in Europe, 2019: results generated from European registries by ESHRE†. Hum Reprod. 2023;38(12):2321–38. https://doi.org/10.1093/humrep/dead197. PMID: 37847771; PMCID: PMC10694409.
5. Sharma A, Shrivastava D. Psychological problems related to infertility. Cureus. 2022;14(10):e30320. https://doi.org/10.7759/cureus.30320. PMID: 36407201; PMCID: PMC9661871.
6. Song X, Zhao J, Xiao Z, Ye H, Dong S, Hu L, Cai Z. The actor-partner interdependence model of fertility stress and marital quality among couples undergoing in vitro fertilization and embryo transfer: The mediating role of dyadic coping. Stress Health. 2024;40(6):e3483. https://doi.org/10.1002/smi.3483. Epub 2024 Oct 22. PMID: 39435725; PMCID: PMC11636441.
7. Wu W, La J, Schubach KM, Lantsberg D, Katz DJ. Psychological, social, and sexual challenges affecting men receiving male infertility treatment: a systematic review and implications for clinical care. Asian J Androl. 2023;25(4):448–53. https://doi.org/10.4103/aja202282. PMID: 36412462; PMCID: PMC10411259.
8. Peterson SK, Jennings Mayo-Wilson L, Spigel L, Morgan I, Parker A. Health care experiences of individuals accessing or undergoing in vitro fertilization (IVF) in the U.S.: a narrative review of qualitative studies. Front. Reprod Health. 2025;7:1490917. https://doi.org/10.3389/frph.2025.1490917.
9. Pfeiffer A, Schweizer-Arau A, Popovici RM, Vogel A, von Hasselbach Y, Beissner F, Meissner K. Nurturing hope: reproductive outcomes with Sinosomatics following unsuccessful in vitro fertilization attempts. Complement Med Res. 2024;31(4):367–75. https://doi.org/10.1159/000539408. Epub 2024 May 20. PMID: 38768578; PMCID: PMC11343086.
10. Ye H, Zhao J, Zou Y, Song X, Xu M, Zhang Y, Zhang L, Wang G. Correlations among hope, fertility quality of life and negative emotions for couples undergoing their first in vitro fertilization-embryo transfer: a cross-sectional analysis. Reprod Health. 2025;22(1):10. https://doi.org/10.1186/s12978-025-01954-x. PMID: 39876018; PMCID: PMC11776239.

11. Li CC, Hwang JL, Ko YL, Chen HH, Chien LY. Factors associated with postpartum depressive symptoms among women who conceived with infertility treatment. Acta Psychol. 2023;238:103987. https://doi.org/10.1016/j.actpsy.2023.103987. Epub 2023 Jul 17. PMID: 37467654.
12. Lu Q, Cheng Y, Zhou Z, Fan J, Chen J, Yan C, Zeng X, Yang J, Wang X. Effects of emotions on IVF/ICSI outcomes in infertile women: a systematic review and meta-analysis. J Assist Reprod Genet. 2025; https://doi.org/10.1007/s10815-025-03388-7. Epub ahead of print. PMID: 39875719.
13. Park JC. Assessment of anxiety, depression, and sexual dysfunction in women undergoing fertility treatment. Clin Exp Reprod Med. 2025;52(1):38–43. https://doi.org/10.5653/cerm.2024.07465. Epub 2025 Feb 28
14. Ďurašková G, Hampl R, Dostál D. Infertility stress and coping strategies in women and men undergoing in vitro fertilization treatment. Ceska Gynekol. 2025;90(1):14–21. https://doi.org/10.48095/cccg202514. PMID: 40117254.
15. Ozturk A, Aba YA, Sik BA. The relationship between stigma, perceived social support and depression in infertile Turkish women undergoing in vitro fertilization-embryo transfer. Arch Psychiatr Nurs. 2021;35(5):434–40. https://doi.org/10.1016/j.apnu.2021.05.009. Epub 2021 Jun 15. PMID: 34561056.
16. Morgan I, Tucker C, Palmquist AEL, Baker S, Mayo-Wilson LJ, Martin CL, Hernandez N, Clarke L. Mapping fertility trajectories: an endarkened narrative inquiry of Black women's fertility experiences and pathways through infertility treatment. Soc Sci Med. 2025;376:118082. https://doi.org/10.1016/j.socscimed.2025.118082.
17. Zhou Y, Sun Z, Song J. Research progress on the impact of anxiety and depression on embryo transfer outcomes of in vitro fertilization. Zhejiang Da Xue Xue Bao Yi Xue Ban. 2023;52(1):61–7. https://doi.org/10.3724/zdxbyxb-2022-0473. PMID: 37283119; PMCID: PMC10293778.
18. Ražić Pavičić A, Jakšić N, Jakovina T, Skočić Hanžek M, Miškulin I, Gregurek R. The role of psychological factors in the outcome of in vitro fertilization in women with primary infertility. Psychiatr Danub. 2022;34(Suppl 10):104–14. PMID: 36752249.
19. Roberts L, Renati S, Solomon S, Montgomery S. Women and infertility in a Pronatalist culture: mental health in the slums of Mumbai. Int J Womens Health. 2020;12:993–1003. https://doi.org/10.2147/IJWH.S273149. PMID: 33192102; PMCID: PMC7654515.
20. Koert E, Daniluk JC. When time runs out: reconciling permanent childlessness after delayed childbearing. J Reprod Infant Psychol. 2017;35(4):342–52. https://doi.org/10.1080/02646838.2017.1320363. Epub 2017 May 9. PMID: 29517370.
21. Kruglova K, O'Connell SBL, Dawadi S, Gelgoot EN, Miner SA, Robins S, Schinazi J, Zelkowitz P. An mHealth app to support fertility patients navigating the world of infertility (Infotility): development and usability study. JMIR Form Res. 2021;5(10):e28136. https://doi.org/10.2196/28136. PMID: 34636741; PMCID: PMC8548975.
22. Leigh L, Skuthan A. The effect of IVF treatments for infertility on occupational balance. OTJR (Thorofare N J). 2025;45(1):12–20. https://doi.org/10.1177/15394492241267255. Epub 2024 Aug 1. PMID: 39087238.
23. Sousa-Leite M, Costa R, Figueiredo B, Gameiro S. Discussing the possibility of fertility treatment being unsuccessful as part of routine care offered at clinics: patients' experiences, willingness, and preferences. Hum Reprod. 2023;38(7):1332–44. https://doi.org/10.1093/humrep/dead096. PMID: 37196325; PMCID: PMC10320487.
24. Moutzouroulia A, Asimakopoulou Z, Tzavara C, Asimakopoulos K, Adonakis G, Kaponis A. The impact of infertility on the mental health of women undergoing in vitro fertilization treatment. Sex Reprod Healthc. 2025;43:101072. https://doi.org/10.1016/j.srhc.2025.101072. Epub 2025 Jan 27. PMID: 39884254.
25. Shah JS, Dodge LE, Vaughan DA, Rooney KL, Penzias AS, Domar AD. Impact of empathic physician contact on patient anxiety and distress during the waiting period after embryo transfer: a randomized controlled trial. Reprod Biomed Online. 2022;45(3):425–31. https://doi.org/10.1016/j.rbmo.2022.04.021. Epub 2022 May 5. PMID: 35750588.

26. İnam Ö, Satılmış İG. The effect of mindfulness-based nursing support on the psychosocial status of women receiving infertility treatment: a randomized controlled trial. BMC Womens Health. 2025;25(1):127. https://doi.org/10.1186/s12905-025-03659-6. PMID: 40114156; PMCID: PMC11924654.
27. Soleimani R, Ansari F, Hamzehgardeshi Z, Elyasi F, Moosazadeh M, Yazdani F, Shahidi M, Shiraghaei N, Karimi M, Hemati T, Pejmanmanesh M. Perceived stress reduction through an infertility coaching program: a randomized controlled clinical trial. Sci Rep. 2023;13(1):14511. https://doi.org/10.1038/s41598-023-41845-4. PMID: 37666933; PMCID: PMC10477300.
28. Chai Y, Li Q, Wang Y, Niu B, Chen H, Fan T, Ke X, Zou H. Cortisol dysregulation in anxiety infertile women and the influence on IVF treatment outcome. Front Endocrinol (Lausanne). 2023;14:1107765. https://doi.org/10.3389/fendo.2023.1107765. PMID: 37383394; PMCID: PMC10299854.
29. Mínguez-Alarcón L, Chagnon O, Tanaka A, Williams PL, James-Todd T, Ford JB, Souter I, Rexrode KM, Hauser R, Chavarro JE. Preconception stress and pregnancy serum glucose levels among women attending a fertility center. J Endocr Soc. 2024;8(1):bvad152. https://doi.org/10.1210/jendso/bvad152. PMID: 38178907; PMCID: PMC10766068.
30. Ni Y, Huang L, Tong C, Qian W, Fang Q. Analysis of the levels of hope and influencing factors in infertile women with first-time and repeated IVF-ET cycles. Reprod Health. 2021;18(1):200. https://doi.org/10.1186/s12978-021-01248-y. PMID: 34627302; PMCID: PMC8502316.
31. Calhaz-Jorge C, De Geyter CH, Kupka MS, Wyns C, Mocanu E, Motrenko T, Scaravelli G, Smeenk J, Vidakovic S, Goossens V. Survey on ART and IUI: legislation, regulation, funding and registries in European countries: the European IVF-monitoring Consortium (EIM) for the European Society of Human Reproduction and Embryology (ESHRE). Hum Reprod Open. 2020;2020(1):hoz044. https://doi.org/10.1093/hropen/hoz044. PMID: 32042927; PMCID: PMC7002185.
32. Ombelet W, Van Blerkom J, Boshoff G, Huyser C, Lopes F, Nargund G, Sallam H, Vanmechelen K, Campo R. Now is the time to introduce new innovative assisted reproduction methods to implement accessible, affordable, and demonstrably successful advanced infertility services in resource-poor countries. Hum Reprod Open. 2025;2025(1):hoaf001. https://doi.org/10.1093/hropen/hoaf001. PMID: 39935763; PMCID: PMC11810638.
33. Nachtigall RD, MacDougall K, Davis AC, Beyene Y. Expensive but worth it: older parents' attitudes and opinions about the costs and insurance coverage for in vitro fertilization. Fertil Steril. 2012;97(1):82–7. https://doi.org/10.1016/j.fertnstert.2011.10.019.
34. Vu M, Stuehling D, Li D, Alur-Gupta S. Fertility care for all: impact of New York State's medicaid expansion on infertility care. J Assist Reprod Genet. 2024;41(2):423–8. https://doi.org/10.1007/s10815-023-02979-6.
35. Blakely B, Williams J, Mayes C, Kerridge I, Lipworth W. Conflicts of interest in Australia's IVF industry: an empirical analysis and call for action. Hum Fertil. 2019;22:230–7. https://doi.org/10.1080/14647273.2017.1390266.
36. https://dier.gov.mt/en/Employment-Conditions/Leave/Pages/IVF-leave.aspx. Accessed on 20 April 2025.
37. Yan Y, Ma Y, Xu L, Lv Y. Impact of perceived social support on anxiety and depression in women undergoing in vitro fertilization-embryo transfer: the role of psychological resilience. J Assist Reprod Genet. 2025;42(1):231–42. https://doi.org/10.1007/s10815-024-03308-1. Epub 2024 Nov 6. PMID: 39505778; PMCID: PMC11805728.
38. Mirzaasgari H, Momeni F, Pourshahbaz A, Keshavarzi F, Hatami M. The role of psychological distress in the relationship between personality dimensions and pregnancy outcome of women undergoing assisted reproductive treatment (IVF/ICSI). Iran J Psychiatry. 2023;18(2):153–64. https://doi.org/10.18502/ijps.v18i2.12366. PMID: 37383963; PMCID: PMC10293695.
39. Gupta A, Lu E, Thayer Z. The influence of assisted reproductive technologies-related stressors and social support on perceived stress and depression. BMC Womens Health. 2024;24(1):431. https://doi.org/10.1186/s12905-024-03262-1. PMID: 39068405; PMCID: PMC11282751.
40. Moutzouri M, Sarantaki A, Koulierakis G, Gourounti K. Coping strategies associated with emotional adjustment during the dyadic experience of infertility and its treat-

ment: a systematic review. J Mother Child. 2024;28(1):61–9. https://doi.org/10.34763/jmotherandchild.20242801.d-24-00013. PMID: 39043203; PMCID: PMC11265839.
41. Mitrović M, Ćirović N, Janković I, Spasić Šnele M, Opsenica Kostić J, Guberinić M, Trenkić M. Representations of in vitro fertilization in the first cycle of IVF in women. Health Psychol Behav Med. 2024;13(1):2444245. https://doi.org/10.1080/21642850.2024.2444245. PMID: 39777053; PMCID: PMC11702993.
42. Assaysh-Öberg S, Borneskog C, Ternström E. Women's experience of infertility & treatment - a silent grief and failed care and support. Sex Reprod Healthc. 2023;37:100879. https://doi.org/10.1016/j.srhc.2023.100879. Epub 2023 Jun 20. PMID: 37356208.
43. Arya ST, Dibb B. The experience of infertility treatment: the male perspective. Hum Fertil. 2016;19:242–8.
44. Mikkelsen AT, Madsen SA, Humaidan P. Psychological aspects of male fertility treatment. J Adv Nurs. 2013;69:1977–86.
45. Ali ZE, Liperis G, Mincheva M, Serdarogullari M, Uraji J, Ammar OF, Fraire-Zamora JJ. From stress to success: exploring methods addressing psychosocial stress in couples trying to conceive. Hum Reprod. 2023;38(11):2277–9. https://doi.org/10.1093/humrep/dead159. PMID: 37558266.
46. https://www.asrm.org/globalassets/_asrm/practice-guidance/practice-guidelines/pdf/fertility-evaluation-of-infertile-women-a-committee-opinion.pdf. Accessed 2 April 2025.
47. Ludwig DS, Kabat-Zinn J. Mindfulness in medicine. JAMA. 2008;300(11):1350–2. https://doi.org/10.1001/jama.300.11.1350. PMID: 18799450.
48. Carolino N, Cunha M, Pinto-Gouveia J, Gameiro S, Galhardo A. KindMap: an e-mental health tool to promote the well-being and mental health of people facing infertility-study protocol for a feasibility randomised control trial. BMJ Open. 2024;14(12):e087447. https://doi.org/10.1136/bmjopen-2024-087447. PMID: 39653558; PMCID: PMC11628952.
49. Wen Y, Li X, Shu W, Zhang H, Shen Z, Huang Z. The effects of mindfulness therapy on infertile female patients: a meta-analysis. Technol Health Care. 2024;32(6):4983–97. https://doi.org/10.3233/THC-240174. PMID: 38943413; PMCID: PMC11612955.
50. Sahraian K, Abdollahpour Ranjbar H, Namavar Jahromi B, Cheung HN, Ciarrochi J, Habibi AM. Effectiveness of mindful self-compassion therapy on psychopathology symptoms, psychological distress and life expectancy in infertile women treated with in vitro fertilization: a two-arm double-blind parallel randomized controlled trial. BMC Psychiatry. 2024;24(1):174. https://doi.org/10.1186/s12888-023-05411-6. PMID: 38429659; PMCID: PMC10908010.
51. Bai CF, Cui NX, Xu X, Mi GL, Sun JW, Shao D, Li J, Jiang YZ, Yang QQ, Zhang X, Cao FL. Effectiveness of two guided self-administered interventions for psychological distress among women with infertility: a three-armed, randomized controlled trial. Hum Reprod. 2019;34(7):1235–48. https://doi.org/10.1093/humrep/dez066. PMID: 31242506.
52. Bal Z, Uçar T. The effect of cognitive behavioural therapy and eye movement desensitization and reprocessing techniques on infertile women: a randomized controlled trial. Reprod Biomed Online. 2024;48(2):103612. https://doi.org/10.1016/j.rbmo.2023.103612. Epub 2023 Oct 13. PMID: 38199076.
53. Koochaksaraei FY, Simbar M, Khoshnoodifar M, Faramarzi M, Nasiri M. Interventions promoting mental health dimensions in infertile women: a systematic review. BMC Psychol. 2023;11(1):254. https://doi.org/10.1186/s40359-023-01285-1. PMID: 37653562; PMCID: PMC10472670.
54. Soltani M, Shairi MR, Roshan R, Rahimi CR. The impact of emotionally focused therapy on emotional distress in infertile couples. Int J Fertil Steril. 2014;7(4):337.
55. Masoumi SZ, Abdoli S, Kazemi F, Pilehvari S, Ahmadpanah M, Khodakarami B, Fazli F. Stress management through cognitive reconstruction and positive thinking in women with recurrent failed in vitro fertilization: a randomized controlled trial. BMC Psychiatry. 2025;25(1):119. https://doi.org/10.1186/s12888-025-06533-9.
56. Yazdani F, et al. Counseling-supportive interventions to decrease infertile women's perceived stress: a systematic review. Electron Phys. 2017;9(6):4694.

57. Malekpour P, Hasanzadeh R, Javedani Masroor M, Chaman R, Motaghi Z. Effectiveness of a mixed lifestyle program in couples undergoing assisted reproductive technology: a study protocol. Reprod Health. 2023;20(1):112. https://doi.org/10.1186/s12978-023-01652-6. PMID: 37528465; PMCID: PMC10394976.
58. Sharma R, Biedenharn KR, Fedor JM, Agarwal A. Lifestyle factors and reproductive health: taking control of your fertility. Reprod Biol Endocrinol. 2013;11:66. https://doi.org/10.1186/1477-7827-11-66.
59. Service CA, Puri D, Al Azzawi S, Hsieh TC, Patel DP. The impact of obesity and metabolic health on male fertility: a systematic review. Fertil Steril. 2023;120(6):1098–111. https://doi.org/10.1016/j.fertnstert.2023.10.017.
60. Amoah BY, Yao Bayamina S, Gborsong C, Owusu H, Asare GA, Yeboah EK, Ablakwa J, Hammond G. Modifiable lifestyle factors and male reproductive health: a cross-sectional study in IVF clinic attendees in Ghana. Front Reprod Health. 2025;7:1520938. https://doi.org/10.3389/frph.2025.1520938. PMID: 40008399; PMCID: PMC11850308.
61. Bocu K, Boeri L, Mahmutoglu AM, Vogiatzi P. Can lifestyle changes significantly improve male fertility: a narrative review? Arab. J Urol. 2024:1–11. https://doi.org/10.1080/2090598.2024.2421626.
62. Alfaraj S, Alfagih A, Al-Zahrani EF, Aljahdali GL, Alrabieaa H, Alsalman F, Gill R, Albadah B. Prevalence of psychological stress among women attending the Assisted Reproductive Technology (ART) unit at King Abdulaziz Medical City: a COVID-19 pandemic experience. Cureus. 2023;15(10):e47145. https://doi.org/10.7759/cureus.47145. PMID: 37859679; PMCID: PMC10582646.
63. Bogović A, Potkonjak AM, Djaković I, Vraneš HS. Depression, anxiety, and stress in infertile couples during the COVID-19 pandemic: the consequences we face. JBRA Assist Reprod. 2024;28(1):9–12. https://doi.org/10.5935/1518-0557.20230018. PMID: 37962946; PMCID: PMC10936920.

9 Assessment of Biomarkers Involved in the Transmission of Maternal Psychological Stress Through the Placenta to the Fetus

Isotta Triulzi, Sergio Martinez-Vazquez, Almudena Escudero, and Rafael A. Caparros-Gonzalez

Abstract

Maternal psychological stress during pregnancy can lead to neurological disorders in offspring, such as anxiety, depression, attention-deficit/hyperactivity disorder, and autism, as well as child's immune system alteration and preterm birth.

This chapter reviews current evidence on how maternal psychological stress crosses the placenta and reaches the fetus. Maternal stress activates multiple placental pathways that influence fetal development, negatively impacting its prenatal and postnatal development. This occurs primarily through activation of the hypothalamic-pituitary-adrenal axis, alteration of placental blood flow, release of proinflammatory cytokines, and oxidative stress, with cortisol as the main mediator. Alteration of the mother gut microbiota composition, catecholamines, serotonin, and tryptophan production compromised fetal microbiome, immune system, and neurodevelopment.

I. Triulzi (✉)
Institute of Management, Scuola Superiore Sant'Anna, Pisa, Italy
e-mail: Isotta.Triulzi@santannapisa.it

S. Martinez-Vazquez
Department of Nursing, University of Jaen, Jaen, Spain

Consortium for Biomedical Research in Epidemiology and Public Health CIBERESP, Madrid, Spain

A. Escudero
Faculty of Health Sciences, Department of Nursing, University of Granada, Granada, Spain

R. A. Caparros-Gonzalez
Faculty of Health Sciences, Department of Nursing, University of Granada, Granada, Spain

Instituto de Investigacion Biosanitaria ibs.GRANADA, Granada, Spain

R. A. Caparros-Gonzalez (ed.), *Maternal Stress during Pregnancy and Postpartum*, https://doi.org/10.1007/978-3-032-09245-8_9

The chapter advocates integrative preventive strategies—psychosocial support, antioxidant-rich nutrition, and nutritional interventions—to mitigate maternal stress and safeguard long-term offspring health.

Keywords

Maternal stress · Biomarker · Placenta · Cortisol · Immune system · Reactive oxygen species, Microbiota · Catecholamines; Serotonin and tryptophan

9.1 Introduction

During pregnancy, maternal psychological stress can cross the placenta and reach the developing fetus. The vulnerability experienced by pregnant women can have a significant influence on the maternal experience and on the development of the fetus, a phenomenon known as fetal programming [1] .

It is a complex phenomenon that can be categorized according to different dimensions, such as the intensity, duration, and variability of stress. Its expression varies depending on both present and past experiences, which represent a common pathway through which diverse environmental and individual factors can influence the fetus development.

It is known that the transfer of maternal stress from mother to fetus is the result of the interaction of several transfer mechanisms that operate synergistically [2].

Excessive maternal cortisol can penetrate the placenta due to its lipophilic nature and affect the activity of the fetal hypothalamic-pituitary-adrenal (HPAA) axis , thus producing long-lasting and even permanent behavioral and cognitive changes in the offspring [3]. In response to psychological stress, brain structures activate maternal HPAA, resulting in the release of cortisol into the maternal circulation. Although the placental enzyme 11beta-hydroxysteroid dehydrogenase type 2 (11ß-HSD-2) inactivates most of the maternal cortisol, psychosocial stress can compromise this barrier, as it reduces the activity of 11ß-HSD-2, exposing the fetus to elevated levels of cortisol. Fetal exposure to elevated cortisol levels is associated with a variety of detrimental consequences in the offspring [4, 2].

Furthermore, during the course of pregnancy, the placenta shows an increased demand for oxygen to support fetal growth, which raises mitochondrial activity and makes it more susceptible to oxidative stress. This phenomenon involves an imbalance in the body's oxidation-reduction processes, caused by the excessive production of reactive oxygen species (ROS; also called oxygen free radicals) that exceed the capacity of cellular homeostasis to neutralize them [5]. Such oxidative stress can affect the placenta and fetal membranes, having both positive and negative repercussions depending on its intensity and duration. A moderate and well-regulated level of physiological oxidative stress is required to ensure the proper development and function of the placenta, including processes such as trophoblast cell migration and invasion, placental remodeling, vascular development, and organogenesis during the early stages of gestation. In addition, oxidative stress contributes to signaling pathways that promote the onset of full-term labor [6].

However, when the balance is compromised by prolonged or intense stress and free radical levels reach high concentrations, oxidative stress can cause severe damage to biological molecules, resulting in a number of pathophysiological and pathological changes, including cellular apoptosis. Therefore, when oxidative stress exceeds the antioxidant capacity of the placenta, tissue damage occurs [5].

The aim of this chapter is to describe the main mechanisms of maternal stress transmission to the fetus through the placenta, as well as the direct effects that maternal stress can have on both the fetus and the postnatal period.

9.2 Biomarkers

Cortisol is by far the most well-known stress hormone. If stress were the highest-grossing film in the history of cinema, cortisol would be the star. But a good film is not only made with a star, it also requires a strong supporting cast and skilled professionals to make it shine. The same happens with maternal stress: several biomarkers are involved in the process and can reach the fetus. A good example of those biomarkers can be found in a systematic review published by Rakers et al. in 2020 [1]. In this chapter, we present broader information on some of the main l biomarkers involved in the transmission of maternal psychological stress from the mother to the fetus including proinfiammatory cytokines, ROSs, gut microbiota composition, catecholamines, serotonin and tryptophan.

9.2.1 Cortisol

Cortisol is known as the primary stress hormone, as its release reflects the activation of the hypothalamic-pituitary-adrenal (HPA) axis [7].

To better understand how cortisol works, I invite you, the reader, to take part in an on an imaginative task. Imagine you are peacefully walking down the street; it is a sunny day, spring has arrived, and you are thinking of your favorite song. Suddenly, you hear a noise which reminds of the sound of a heavy object falling to the ground, followed by a terrifying scream. You have just witnessed a car run over someone.

This experience might produce a certain level of discomfort and lead to the release s of cortisol. Experiencing a stressful situation triggers the activation of the HPA axis. During this process, you receive information through your senses (you might hear a noise witness an accident, or smell a particular odor), which stimulates your amygdala and hippocampus - two regions of the brain involved in emotion processing and memory, respectively.

After your brain has started processing this information, the hypothalamus sends a signal to the hypophysis (or pituitary gland, located in the brain) which stimulates the release of cortisol from the adrenal glands (situated on top of the kidneys) [8]. During pregnancy, maternal cortisol crosses the placenta and may alter foetal nervous system development, especially if elevated in early pregnancy. Research indicates that high cortisol levels in early gestation are associated with slower cognitive development and lower mental scores in the first year of life. Conversely, high levels towards the end of pregnancy may promote brain maturation and cognitive development. Thus, the impact of high cortisol appears to depend on the stage of pregnancy during which the mother experiences significant stress.

Assessment of cortisol, a key biomarker in the transmission of maternal psychological stress through the placenta to the fetus, can be performed using a variety of biological matrices [9]. Previous studies among pregnant women have measured cortisol levels in saliva, urine, blood, amniotic fluid, breast milk, earwax, and hair. Some matrices offer advantages, while others present certain limitations. Measuring cortisol levels in saliva, urine, blood, amniotic fluid, or breast milk provides information on acute stress responses and requires a trained professional for sample collection and storage. However, in most cases, these procedures can be invasive. For example, I, obtaining a blood sample or amniotic fluid sample may itself may induce psychological stress and consequently elevate cortisol levels [10]. Moreover, cortisol assessment in these matrices can be affected by environmental variables, including time of day, sampling procedures rand food intake.

To overcome the limitations of the previous matrices, researchers often need to collect repeated samples over 24 hours and across several days to estimate chronic cortisol concentrations. This procedure is usually expensive, inconvenient for pregnant women, and associated with a greater likelihood of incomplete sample collection or participant dropout. Given these limitations, researchers have explored alternative matrices to allow for more reliable and less invasive measurements of chronic cortisol concentrations, which are less influenced by environmental factors. The most innovative and noninvasive method is the measurement of cortisol in hair samples.

According to previous studies, free cortisol becomes incorporated into the hair shaft during its growth. The main source of free cortisol is passive diffusion, although there is evidence that it can also be deposited through sebum secretions, with minor local production of cortisol occurring in the hair follicle [11]. Hair grows an average of 1 cm per month; hair cortisol reflects the cortisol available in other matrices and are linked to chronic stress exposure rather than acute stress responses.

Hair cortisol has been reported to be less affected by confounding variables and covariates than cortisol measured from other matrices. Nevertheless, it is recommended to wash hair samples with isopropanol to remove any residual cortisol from sebum or sweat.

9.2.2 Cytokines and Immune System

Previous studies suggest that the release of maternal cytokines is involved in the transmission of maternal psychological stress to the developing fetus. Cytokines are a group of soluble polypeptides that can act as mediators of signaling between cells with endocrine effects and associated with immunomodulation. Cytokines have a protein nature and can suppress or stimulate inflammation processes through a variety of mechanisms such as alteration of T-cell differentiation, vascular permeability, or liberation of proteins (acute phase). It has been suggested that an excess of cytokines may modify the development of the fetal brain by a direct modification of glial cells in the fetus [12].

Certain cytokines (e.g., TNF-α, IL-6) may stimulate the hypothalamic-pituitary-adrenal axis and therefore promotes the release of cortisol. In respect to levels of cytokines during pregnancy, a previous study found a certain increase in maternal cytokines during low-risk pregnancies (in humans). Nevertheless, an additional study has informed on stable circulating cytokines levels during normal human pregnancies [13].

Some epidemiological studies have associated maternal immune activation related to antenatal infections with later neuropsychiatric (and also immunological and metabolic) diseases. Nevertheless, this finding usually comes from animal studies and not from human's data. Recent findings on small cohorts in humans reflect a lack of association between maternal cytokine levels and the development of psychosis in the offspring later in life. Besides, although certain positive associations have been found between certain maternal cytokines and a higher risk of neuropsychiatric illnesses in the offspring, these findings could not be replicated in future studies [14].

Maternal cytokines can be transferred to the fetus through the placenta. The placenta itself can produce cytokines that are released into the fetal blood circulation after exposure to maternal stress. Nevertheless, it is still unknown whether maternal psychological stress can directly produce the release of placental cytokines.

Besides, certain gestational diseases, such as preeclampsia, according to the article by [8], are linked to a series of issues related with the placenta and blood flow, such as abnormal placentation, ischemia, placental reperfusion, syncytiotrophoblast detachment, among others. These alterations cause oxidative stress, increased inflammatory cytokines (proinflammatory IL-6), and an abnormal inflammatory response, which aggravates the function of endothelial cells and results in adverse complications for the fetus. The research of Graham et al. (2022) [15] on the effect of maternal stress on children's brain development is increasingly being considered to understand the biological pathways related to inflammation.

9.2.3 Reactive Oxygen Species

Reactive oxygen species (ROS) are highly reactive molecules derived from oxygen (including superoxide anion radicals, hydrogen peroxide, singlet oxygen, and hydroxyl radicals) [16, 17] that are produced during normal metabolic processes, mainly in the mitochondrial matrix. While they serve as important regulatory signals for various cellular functions [18], excessive levels of ROS can lead to oxidative stress, resulting in damage to cellular components when they surpass the protective capabilities of antioxidants [16, 17]. This damage can affect particularly to DNA and proteins. In addition, mitochondria are especially vulnerable to oxidative stress, which can disrupt mitochondrial membrane potential and trigger apoptosis [16]. Additionally, oxidative stress can cause sterol auto-oxidation [16, 19]. Interestingly, ROS can have dual roles in cancer cells, where they may induce autophagic cell death or act as a cytoprotective mechanism through the induction of autophagy [17, 19].

The generation of ROS is an unavoidable consequence of oxygen metabolism. When ROS levels exceed the body's antioxidant defenses, oxidative stress (OS) occurs, leading to significant physiological repercussions [20, 21]. Psychosocial stress is among various factors that can contribute to oxidative stress [1]. Research has shown that oxidative stress during gestation can adversely affect fetal development, resulting in outcomes ranging from miscarriage to metabolic disorders, which may play a role in fetal programming for later life [22–24]. Heightened oxidative stress, coupled with insufficient antioxidant protection, may contribute to recurrent pregnancy loss, although many aspects of how oxidative stress impacts pregnancy outcomes remain unclear [25]. Oxidative stress has been found to induce modifications in the fetal epigenome, providing potential mechanistic insights into fetal programming, including implications for the hypothalamic-pituitary-adrenal (HPA) axis [26–28].

Due to their high reactivity and short half-life, ROS are not likely to be directly transferred from the mother to the fetus [29]. However, studies indicate that there may be interactions between the oxidative stress systems of the mother and fetus, although the precise mechanisms remain poorly understood. Evidence suggests that prenatal stress may indirectly induce oxidative stress by negatively affecting utero-placental perfusion (UPP), which can have detrimental effects on brain organization and function [30–32]. It is emphasized that the biological responses that safeguard against cellular stress, including oxidative stress responses and heat shock systems, are integral to understanding and preventing disruptions in prenatal brain development [18]. Mechanisms such as heat shock proteins (HSPs) and antioxidants are promising targets for developing treatments for brain diseases and other disorders. Dysregulation of these protective systems may contribute to neuropsychiatric disorders but is also essential for safeguarding the brain under pathological conditions [18].

Additionally, maternal catecholamines such as norepinephrine (NE) and epinephrine (E) may contribute to this indirect transfer of stress, adversely impacting fetal growth and development through their effects on UPP [33, 34].

The main role of the placenta is to facilitate the exchange of nutrients and oxygen between the mother and the fetus. Any disruption in these processes can lead to hypoxia, which is often caused by oxidative stress. Various factors can interfere with placental function, resulting in complications during pregnancy [35, 36]. OS is crucial for normal placental function during pregnancy [23]; however, an excess of oxidative stress can lead to placental dysfunction and serious complications [21, 37]. Moderate oxidative stress is necessary for appropriate placental development, while excessive levels can result in premature aging of the placenta and complications such as preeclampsia, fetal death, and preterm delivery [23, 24, 35]. Identifying biomarkers for oxidative stress and placental aging may be critical in preventing and managing these complications, thereby mitigating their negative impact on families and healthcare systems. Furthermore, exists a significant association between reduced antioxidant activity and pregnancy-related issues, such as spontaneous abortions linked to oxidative stress [38]. This imbalance adversely affects maternal health and fetal development by impairing placental function and the delivery of oxygen and nutrients to the fetus.

In summary, imbalances in oxidative stress during pregnancy can lead to complications and health issues in adulthood. It is evident that oxidative stress, associated with the production of reactive oxygen species, plays both beneficial [39–41] and detrimental [33–36] roles in placental function and fetal development. Disruptors of this balance, such as nutritional imbalances, inflammation, and lipotoxicity, can negatively affect fetal growth. A balanced diet, such as the Mediterranean diet rich in antioxidants [42–44], has been shown to reduce oxidative stress biomarkers and inflammation, thereby enhancing maternal health and fetal development.

9.2.4 Microbiota

Researchers have recently hypnotized that maternal microbiota plays a role in the maternal-fetal stress transfer. Stress influences gut microbial composition, and the gut modulates the body's response [45]. Gut microbiota modulates hosts' physiology, immune response, central nervous function, neurocognition, behavior, and neuroendocrine system. Its alteration has an impact on fetal development during pregnancy [46].

Pregnancy is characterized by a state of mild inflammation, along with significant metabolic and microbiota alterations. The maternal hormonal cascades facilitate fetal development, and the gut microbiota, along with the maternal vaginal and oral microbiota, undergoes significant compositional changes [47, 48]. Numerous differences have been observed in microbiota between women at the end of pregnancy and those in early pregnancy or nonpregnant women: Some studies have identified an increase in proteobacteria, bifidobacteria, and lactic acid-producing bacteria (including specific Lactobacillus strains), accompanied by a reduction in the abundance of butyrate-producing bacteria from the second trimester onward [47], while another study have reported an increase in Bacteroidetes, with a decrease in Verrucomicrobia and Tenericutes [49]. Although researchers have observed changes in microbiota during pregnancy, there is no consensus on how they change. There remains no clear consensus on the nature of these changes, as different techniques have been adopted for the microbiota analysis. Moreover, a multitude of factors influence the microbiota during pregnancy, including individual-specific factors (diet, age, body mass index, weight gain, and comorbidities) as well as population-level factors (ethnicity, geography, and environmental influences). Distinguishing the effects of these factors—such as diet [50]—from those of pregnancy on gut microbiota changes is a complex challenge. These modifications may either be a response to the physiological changes occurring during pregnancy or play a role in driving these physiological adaptations in the mother or supporting fetal development [51].

Several studies suggest that the neonatal microbiome is inherited from the maternal microbiome during parturition, as the fetus passes through the birth canal and comes into contact with the vaginal microbiota that colonize the previously sterile fetal gut. In the case of cesarean section, the neonatal microbiome may instead be influenced by the maternal skin microbiome [47]. However, in recent years, the assumption that the placenta is a sterile organ and gain mother microbiome during parturition has been challenged by various scientists and a consensus has not been reached yet. Human research moves slowly due to ethical concerns and difficulties in accessing samples, remaining a highly contentious topic. Several studies have proposed that the placenta may harbor bacteria and potentially even its own microbiome [52]. A study of Park et al. 2023 [53] found "evidence of microbial colonization in traditionally considered sterile intrauterine environments and in the fetal gastrointestinal tract. The distinct bacterial composition in meconium, the first stool passed by newborns, supports the hypothesis that microbial colonization occurs during normal pregnancy." However, this hypothesis was not accepted by some scientists [54]. A recent study indicated that the microbial signals detected are likely due to contamination during the collection of fetal samples or during DNA extraction and sequencing [55].

Since the maternal microbiome is key for developing and maintaining the immune system in adults and the immune system can affect the microbiota, a similar interaction can exist between maternal gut microbiome and fetal immune responses [51]. Although it's unlikely that placenta and fetus contain bacteria, the maternal microbiome may still be able to affect the fetal immune system through an indirect way with bacterial products or microbiota-derived metabolites, such as short-chain fatty acids (SCFAs), secondary bile acids and tryptophan derivatives, and small pieces of bacteria (lipopolysaccharides and flagellin), that can be found in the fetus and/or placenta [47, 51].

Bacterial metabolites such as short-chain fatty acids (SCFAs) can affect the immune response of the mother and the fetus and can cross the placenta. SCFAs have been detected in higher concentration in the maternal gut or blood [56] and in cord blood [57] in pregnant women compared to nonpregnant individuals. This may be due to change in microbiome compositions as the SCFA-producing bacteria increases during pregnancy. Moreover, SCFAs influence brain activity through several pathways: modulate concentrations of neurotransmitters (e.g., GABA, serotonin, glutamate) and neurotropic factors, involved in the emotional processes; protect against neuroinflammation; attenuate the response to stress induced by the HPA axis [58].

Secondary bile acids and tryptophan derivatives (i.e., indoles) are able to affect the immune response and have been detected in the fetus. As for the SCFAs, secondary bile acids and tryptophan derivatives production increases during pregnancy due to modification in the gut microbiome compositions. Small pieces of bacteria (lipopolysaccharides (LPS) and flagellin) from the mother's gut may reach the baby, helping the baby's immune system learn to recognize friendly versus harmful bacteria [47, 59].

These metabolites have an effect in fetal immune response in mice and adult individuals as have been described in the review of Faas et al. [51]. Further research is needed to shed light on the role and actions of these metabolites in pregnant women.

Prenatal stress has widespread effects on offspring through abnormal immune development and behavioral deficits. The microbiome can play a crucial role in mediating the effects of stress on offspring through its influence on the immune system and the production of metabolites. The microbiota-derived metabolites cross the fetus and can affect immune and neurodevelopment.

Maternal stress-induced dysbiosis affects immune development and increases the risk of inflammatory disorders and deficit in infant neurodevelopment in offspring. Sun et al. (2021) [60] reported that prenatal stress impairs intestinal barrier function in the mother and in the offspring and predisposes offspring to *colitis* in adulthood through persistent gut dysbiosis. Balla et al. (2024) [61] showed that *allergic* predisposition in offspring can be derived from early life triggers such as maternal influence in shaping perinatal immunity (immature fetal immune system and mucosal barriers undergo periods of plasticity), mothers' epigenetics, metabolic, diet, and microbioma. Gur et al. (2017) [62] linked maternal stress to alteration of composition of gut microbial communities (through alteration of cytokine levels in the intrauterine environment) and birth outcomes, such as prematurity and neurodevelopment. Also, Vuong et al. (2020) [63] have emphasized the role of maternal gut microbiota in *fetal brain development*. Dysbiosis caused by maternal stress interferes with the production of critical metabolites that regulate neurogenesis and neural circuit formation. The study highlighted how impaired axonogenesis and reduced thalamocortical axon growth in the fetal brain can result from disrupted microbial signals, with downstream effects on behavior and cognition in offspring. Complementing these findings, a 2024 study in *Nature Molecular Psychiatry* [64] further supports the connection between maternal stress, gut dysbiosis, and neurodevelopment. It underscores the lasting effects of maternal stress on the offspring's hypothalamic-pituitary-adrenal (HPA) axis and immune regulation, which collectively influence vulnerability to psychiatric and neurological disorders later in life.

These findings suggest a complex interaction between maternal microbioma, immune system, endocrine system, inflammation, and behavioral abnormalities in maternal stress.

9.2.5 Catecholamines

Catecholamines, specifically norepinephrine (NE) and epinephrine (EPI), play a crucial role in the body's rapid response to stress. These catecholamines function as the body's immediate response system to stress, as it activated within seconds of exposure. Upon release, they enter the bloodstream, providing a fast and immediate physiological reaction to stress, in contrast to the activation of the hypothalamic-pituitary-adrenal axis (HPAA), which takes tens of minutes to release its effector hormone, cortisol, and reach peak serum concentration. The sympathoadrenal medullary system (SAMS) serves as the body's first-line of defense against stress, initiating a rapid response within seconds after stress exposure [65]. Plasma catecholamine levels largely reflect sympathetic nervous system activity during acute stress situations [46, 66].

Despite the importance of catecholamines in maternal stress response, their direct impact on fetal development remains debated since maternal catecholamines do not easily cross the placenta in significant amounts due to their hydrophilic nature [67, 68]. They can indirectly affect the fetus by altering uteroplacental perfusion (UPP). NE is a potent vasoconstrictor that can increase vascular tone in the uterus and placenta, reducing blood flow and oxygen supply to the fetus. This effect is mediated by α-adrenergic receptors, which are highly responsive in uterine arteries, making them particularly susceptible to stress-induced vasoconstriction [69, 70].

Human studies have reported inconsistent findings regarding the association between maternal psychological stress and fetal circulation. Some studies have found a correlation between high maternal stress and reduced umbilical blood flow [71], whereas others have not observed significant changes [72]. This variability is attributed to the transient nature of stress-induced uterine blood flow changes, which are not always captured in resting-state Doppler ultrasound measurements.

In animal models, acute maternal stress has been shown to cause significant reductions in uterine blood flow, leading to fetal metabolic adaptations. Studies in sheep indicate that stress-induced vasoconstriction can trigger a shift to anaerobic metabolism in the fetus, accompanied by an increase in fetal catecholamine levels. Such metabolic shifts suggest that the fetus can detect and respond to reduced oxygen availability, possibly leading to long-term developmental consequences [34, 73].

Moreover, chronic stress exposure during pregnancy has been linked to impairments in placental catecholamine metabolism. The placenta normally plays a crucial role in clearing catecholamines from the fetal circulation, maintaining fetal homeostasis. However, stress-induced disturbances in placental catecholamine clearance mechanisms can lead to elevated fetal catecholamine levels, which have been associated with adverse pregnancy outcomes such as intrauterine growth restriction (IUGR) and preterm birth [74].

In summary, while maternal catecholamines may not directly cross the placenta in significant amounts, their influence on uteroplacental perfusion and fetal stress responses should be taken in consideration. The assessment of catecholamines in maternal and fetal compartments serves as a valuable biomarker for evaluating the impact of maternal stress on fetal health outcomes. Future research should focus on the potential therapeutic strategies to mitigate these stress-related adverse outcomes [46, 70].

9.2.6 Serotonin and Tryptophan

During pregnancy, the placenta is formed as a temporary organ and is vital to the preservation of pregnancy and fetal development. During embryonic brain development, placenta is an important source of hormones and neurotransmitters [75, 76].

Tryptophan, as the sole precursor of serotonin, mainly derived from diets, is essential for neurodevelopment and immunomodulation [77]. Gestational tryptophan fluctuation may account for the maternal-fetal transmission in determining neuroembryogenesis with long-lasting effects on psychological development. Personality disorders and social exclusion are related to psychosocial problems, leading to impaired social functioning. However, it is not clear how the fluctuation in mother-child transmission regulates the neuroendocrine development and gut microbiota composition in progeny due to that tryptophan metabolism in pregnant women is affected by multiple factors, such as diets (tryptophan-enriched or tryptophan-depleted diet), emotional mental states (anxiety, depression), health status (hypertension, diabetes), and social support as well as stresses and management skills [77].

Gestational experiences may reprogram fetal brain development and increase vulnerability to bullying. Thus, the adverse maternal-fetal transmission is maternal distress [78]. Tryptophan (Trp), an essential amino acid primarily obtained from dietary sources in the small intestine, plays a crucial role during pregnancy. Tryptophan (Trp), an essential amino acid, can be only obtained through the diet. Adults need 3.5 mg of L-Trp/kg body weight/day to maintain nitrogen balance [79]. It serves as the exclusive precursor for serotonin (5-hydroxytryptophan, 5-HT) and is vital for fetal brain development through both direct and indirect pathways involving 5-HT. Trp is transported to the fetal brain where it is converted into 5-HT by the enzyme tryptophan hydroxylase (TPH) 2. Additionally, TPH1 in the placenta also synthesizes 5-HT, which is then delivered to the fetal brain [80]. Disturbances in serotonergic (5-HTergic) function are linked to various psychopathological conditions. Changes in Trp metabolism are a key biological indicator of prenatal maternal stress; for instance, lower plasma levels of both Trp and KYN have been observed in cases of severe gestational anxiety and depression [78]. Trp is essential for fetal brain development and programming [81]. Since the metabolites of both pathways are involved in fetal development and programming, any perturbations in their homeostasis can have serious developmental and functional consequences [82, 83]. The rate-limiting enzyme for the synthesis of tryptophan to kynurenine in the placenta is activated by proinflammatory cytokines and stress hormones, respectively, during maternal stress [84].

Antenatal stress negatively impacts neuroembryogenesis by altering the placental Trp-KYN metabolism, which produces various neuroactive metabolites, such as kynurenic acid (KYNA), 3-hydroxykynurenine (3-HK), and quinolinic acid (QUIN). This alteration sets the stage for neuropathological conditions and associated psychiatric disorders [85]. Additionally, individuals with gestational diabetes mellitus frequently exhibit elevated levels of urinary Trp and purine metabolites [86]. An excessive increase in Trp levels can compromise pregnancy by impairing T-cell suppression, a phenomenon observed in conditions like preeclampsia [87] which is notably a significant obstetric risk factor for schizophrenia [88]. Elevated cortisol levels resulting from maternal stress can cross the placenta, impacting neuroembryonic development and neuroendocrine function, leading to enduring changes in cognitive and behavioral outcomes throughout life [89]. Moreover, antenatal stress can reduce the diversity of gut microbes that metabolize Trp in both the mother and offspring, thereby altering fetal exposure to Trp and its metabolites. This disruption can mediate atypical fetal neurogenesis and subsequently affect the microbial development of the progeny [90].

Beyond its function in neurotransmission, embryonic serotonin or 5-HT has been recognized for its involvement in regulating neurodevelopmental processes. As a neurotransmitter, 5-HT plays an important role in regulating emotions, learning, and memory [80, 91]. A specific group of 5-HT1-receptors found in the developing fetal forebrain plays a role in how serotonergic signaling influences the response of thalamocortical axons to guidance cues, as demonstrated in both laboratory and live models. This effect of 5-HT on the wiring of the fetal brain raises significant questions about the origins of this neurotransmitter during pregnancy [80]. Traditionally, it was believed that the sources of 5-HT affecting brain development were either maternal transport to the fetus or production by raphe neurons in the fetal brainstem. Recent findings, however, highlight a novel function for placental metabolic pathways in influencing fetal brain development, underscoring the crucial interactions between the mother, placenta, and fetus, as well as the role of 5-HT in the fetal programming of mental health disorders in adulthood [80].

Maternal stress during pregnancy is associated with an increased risk of psychiatric disorders in offspring, such as anxiety, depression, schizophrenia, and autism [76, 92]. Maternal stress leads to behavioral changes and alterations in tryptophan metabolism in the offspring, with effects that vary by sex. Disruptions in both the 5-HT and KYN pathways may contribute to the emotional disturbances seen in individuals who were exposed to stress in utero [92]. Other studies found evidence in that PAE may inhibit SERT expression while simultaneously promoting increased TPH1 protein expression in human placenta. This may result in increased 5-HT in fetal circulation known to affect neurodevelopment [93]. Placental serotonin is recognized as a key component of fetoplacental physiology and can be influenced by environmental factors such as maternal diet, drugs, stress, and immune activation. Disturbances in placental serotonin signaling during critical developmental periods may have long-lasting consequences for the health and behavior of the offspring [94]. Therefore, the ability to prevent environmental modulation of placental serotonin, and hence negative effects on the developing fetus, is of great importance [91]. Consequently, variations in maternal diet or medication use during pregnancy can influence placental Trp levels, which in turn can modify placental 5-HT synthesis, the maternal-fetal supply of Trp and 5-HT, fetal concentrations of 5-HT, gut microbiota composition, and both endocrine and neuroendocrine development. Ultimately, these changes can affect the psychosocial development of the offspring.

In conclusion, the intricate interplay between maternal health, dietary factors, and psychosocial influences during pregnancy significantly shapes fetal neurodevelopment and long-term psychological outcomes. The role of tryptophan as a precursor for serotonin underscores its importance in maintaining healthy maternal-fetal communication and ensuring optimal brain development in the offspring. Disturbances in tryptophan metabolism and serotonergic signaling, driven by maternal stress, diet, and health conditions, can lead to adverse neurodevelopmental consequences, increasing the risk of psychiatric disorders in later life. It becomes increasingly clear that addressing maternal well-being and environmental factors is crucial for fostering healthy neurodevelopment and mitigating the risk of psychological issues in children. Therefore, strategies aimed at optimizing maternal nutrition, reducing stress, and enhancing social support during pregnancy are essential for promoting healthier outcomes for future generations.

9.3 Conclusion

This chapter shows that maternal psychological stress during pregnancy can be transmitted to the fetus through several biological mechanisms, affecting negatively both their prenatal and postnatal development.

The main mechanisms of transmission of maternal stress to the fetus through the placenta include the activation of the hypothalamus-pituitary-adrenal (HPA) axis, where stress activates the HPA axis in the mother, increasing the production of cortisol, which can cross the placenta. Cortisol is the main mediator of the transfer of stress from the mother to the fetus. Although the placenta inactivates part of this cortisol, high levels of maternal stress can overcome this protective barrier. The direct effects of maternal stress on the fetus and in the postnatal stage include an increase of the risk of neurological disorders such as anxiety, depression, ADHD, and autism, as well as an increased risk of premature birth, low birth weight, and growth restriction intrauterine.

In addition, maternal stress can alter blood flow to the placenta, compromising the supply of oxygen and nutrients to the fetus. Stress induces the release of proinflammatory cytokines that can cross the placenta and affect the intrauterine environment. Also, excess oxidative stress can damage placental function and contribute to complications such as preeclampsia. Alterations in the mother microbiome can affect placenta and, consequently, the fetus microbiome, immune system, and neurodevelopment. Finally, changes are observed in the supply of energy to the tissues fetoplacental due to elevated levels of glucocorticoids, which affects adaptability metabolic rate of the fetus.

Strategies that can reduce maternal stress and enhance environmental factors (social support), maternal nutrition, and maternal well-being are essential for promoting healthier outcomes for future generations.

References

1. Rakers F, Rupprecht S, Dreiling M, Bergmeier C, Witte OW, Schwab M. Transfer of maternal psychosocial stress to the fetus. Neurosci Biobehav Rev. Elsevier Ltd. 2020;117:185–97.
2. Dowell J, Elser BA, Schroeder RE, Stevens HE. Cellular stress mechanisms of prenatal maternal stress: heat shock factors and oxidative stress. Neurosci Lett [Internet]. 2019;709:134368. Available from: https://doi.org/10.1016/j.neulet.2019.134368.
3. Caparros-Gonzalez R, Torre-Luque A, Romero-Gonzalez B, Quesada-Soto J, Alderdice F, Peralta-Ramírez M. Stress during pregnancy and the development of diseases in the offspring: a systematic-review and meta-analysis. Midwifery. 2021;97:192939.

4. Delagneau G, Twilhaar ES, Testa R, van Veen S, Anderson P. Association between prenatal maternal anxiety and/or stress and offspring's cognitive functioning: a meta-analysis. Child Dev. 2023;94(3):779–801.
5. Jovandaric MZ, Dugalic S, Babic S, Babovic IR, Milicevic S, Mihajlovic D, et al. Programming factors of Neonatal intestinal Dysbiosis as a cause of disease. Int J Mol Sci. 2023;24(6):5723.
6. Sultana Z, Qiao Y, Maiti K, Smith R. Involvement of oxidative stress in placental dysfunction, the pathophysiology of fetal death and pregnancy disorders. Reproduction [Internet]. 2023;166(2):25–38. Available from: https://doi.org/10.1530/REP-22-0278.
7. Caparros-Gonzalez R, Romero-Gonzalez B, Strivens-Vilchez H, Gonzalez-Perez R, Martinez-Augustin O, Peralta-Ramirez MI. Hair cortisol levels, psychological stress and psychopathological symptoms as predictors of postpartum depression. PLoS One. 2017;12(8):1–17.
8. Chiarello D, Abad C, Rojas D, Toledo F, Vázquez C, Mate A, et al. Oxidative stress: Normal pregnancy versus preeclampsia. Acta Mol Basis Dis. 2020;1866(2):165354.
9. Meyer JS, Novak MA. Assessment of prenatal stress-related cortisol exposure: focus on cortisol accumulation in hair and nails. Dev Psychobiol. 2021;63(3):409–36.
10. Wosu AC, Valdimarsdóttir U, Shields AE, Williams DR, Williams MA. Correlates of cortisol in human hair: implications for epidemiologic studies on health effects of chronic stress. Ann Epidemiol [Internet]. 2013;23(12):797–811.e2. Available from: https://pubmed.ncbi.nlm.nih.gov/24184029
11. Marceau K, Wang W, Robertson O, Shirtcliff EA. A systematic review of hair cortisol during pregnancy: reference ranges and methodological considerations. Psychoneuroendocrinology. 2020;122:104904.
12. Ratnayake U, Quinn T, Walker DW, Dickinson H. Cytokines and the neurodevelopmental basis of mental illness. Front Neurosci. 2013;7:180.
13. Makhseed M, Raghupathy R, Azizieh F, Farhat R, Hassan N, Bandar A. Circulating cytokines and CD30 in normal human pregnancy and recurrent spontaneous abortions. Hum Reprod. 2000;15(9):2011–7.
14. Allswede DM, Buka SL, Yolken RH, Torrey EF, Cannon TD. Elevated maternal cytokine levels at birth and risk for psychosis in adult offspring. Schizophr Res. 2016;172(1–3):41–5.
15. Graham AM, Doyle O, Tilden EL, Sullivan EL, Gustafsson HC, Marr M, et al. Effects of maternal psychological stress during pregnancy on offspring brain development: considering the role of inflammation and potential for preventive intervention. Biol Psychiatry Cogn Neurosci Neuroimaging. 2022;7(5):461–70.
16. Dunlop C, Whyte P. 8 - Is Oxygen Toxic?. Editor(s): Clifford S. Deutschman, Patrick J. Neligan. Evidence-Based Practice of Critical Care, W.B. Saunders. 2010;45–50 ISBN 9781416054764, https://doi.org/10.1016/B978-1-4160-5476-4.00008-0. (https://www.sciencedirect.com/science/article/pii/B9781416054764000080).
17. Kanabur P, Ramasamy R. Nutraceutical Therapy in Male Infertility, Editor(s): Michael K. Skinner, Encyclopedia of Reproduction (Second Edition), Academic Press, 2018;333–339. ISBN 9780128151457, https://doi.org/10.1016/B978-0-12-801238-3.64787-6. (https://www.sciencedirect.com/science/article/pii/B9780128012383647876).
18. Dowell J, Elser BA, Schroeder RE, Stevens HE. Cellular stress mechanisms of prenatal maternal stress: heat shock factors and oxidative stress. Neurosci Lett. 2019;709:134368.
19. Hayat MA. Chapter 1 - Introduction to Autophagy: Cancer, Other Pathologies, Inflammation, Immunity, Infection, and Aging, Volume 7, Editor(s): M.A. Hayat, Autophagy: Cancer, Other Pathologies, Inflammation, Immunity, Infection, and Aging, Academic Press, 2015;1–53. ISBN 9780128010433, https://doi.org/10.1016/B978-0-12-801043-3.00001-7. (https://www.sciencedirect.com/science/article/pii/B9780128010433000017).
20. Rakers F, Rupprecht S, Dreiling M, Bergmeier C, Witte OW, Schwab M. Transfer of maternal psychosocial stress to the fetus. Neurosci Biobehav Rev. 2020;117:185–97.
21. Thompson LP, Al-Hasan Y. Impact of oxidative stress in Fetal programming. J Pregnancy. 2012;2012:1–8.
22. Jansson T, Powell TL. Role of the placenta in fetal programming: underlying mechanisms and potential interventional approaches. Clin Sci. 2007;113(1):1–13.

23. Myatt L. Review: reactive oxygen and nitrogen species and functional adaptation of the placenta. Placenta. 2010;31:S66–9.
24. Burton GJ, Yung HW, Cindrova-Davies T, Charnock-Jones DS. Placental endoplasmic reticulum stress and oxidative stress in the pathophysiology of unexplained intrauterine growth restriction and early onset Preeclampsia. Placenta. 2009;30:43–8.
25. Zejnullahu VA, Zejnullahu VA, Kosumi E. The role of oxidative stress in patients with recurrent pregnancy loss: a review. Reprod Health. 2021;18(1):207.
26. Godfrey KM, Lillycrop KA, Burdge GC, Gluckman PD, Hanson MA. Epigenetic mechanisms and the mismatch concept of the developmental origins of health and disease. Pediatr Res. 2007;61(5 Part 2):5R–10R.
27. Niu Y, DesMarais TL, Tong Z, Yao Y, Costa M. Oxidative stress alters global histone modification and DNA methylation. Free Radic Biol Med. 2015;82:22–8.
28. Szumiel I. Ionizing radiation-induced oxidative stress, epigenetic changes and genomic instability: the pivotal role of mitochondria. Int J Radiat Biol. 2015;91(1):1–12.
29. Reth M. Hydrogen peroxide as second messenger in lymphocyte activation. Nat Immunol. 2002;3(12):1129–34.
30. Burton GJ, Hung TH. Hypoxia-reoxygenation; a potential source of placental oxidative stress in normal pregnancy and Preeclampsia. Fetal Matern Med Rev. 2003;14(2):97–117.
31. Dreiling M, Bischoff S, Schiffner R, Rupprecht S, Kiehntopf M, Schubert H, et al. Stress-induced decrease of uterine blood flow in sheep is mediated by alpha 1-adrenergic receptors. Stress. 2016;19(5):547–51.
32. Thakor AS, Herrera EA, Serón-Ferré M, Giussani DA. Melatonin and vitamin C increase umbilical blood flow via nitric oxide-dependent mechanisms. J Pineal Res. 2010;49(4):399–406.
33. Levine TA, Alderdice FA, Grunau RE, McAuliffe FM. Prenatal stress and hemodynamics in pregnancy: a systematic review. Arch Womens Ment Health. 2016;19(5):721–39.
34. Rakers F, Bischoff S, Schiffner R, Haase M, Rupprecht S, Kiehntopf M, et al. Role of catecholamines in maternal-fetal stress transfer in sheep. Am J Obstet Gynecol. 2015;213(5):684.e1–9.
35. Schoots MH, Gordijn SJ, Scherjon SA, van Goor H, Hillebrands JL. Oxidative stress in placental pathology. Placenta. 2018;69:153–61.
36. Sultana Z, Qiao Y, Maiti K, Smith R. Involvement of oxidative stress in placental dysfunction, the pathophysiology of fetal death and pregnancy disorders. Reproduction. 2023;166(2):R25–38.
37. Turpin CA, Sakyi SA, Owiredu WK, Ephraim RKD, Anto EO. Association between adverse pregnancy outcome and imbalance in angiogenic regulators and oxidative stress biomarkers in gestational hypertension and preeclampsia. BMC Pregnancy Childbirth. 2015;15(1):189.
38. Grzeszczak K, Łanocha-Arendarczyk N, Malinowski W, Ziętek P, Kosik-Bogacka D. Oxidative stress in pregnancy. Biomolecules. 2023;13(12):1768.
39. Qanungo S, Mukherjea M. Ontogenic profile of some antioxidants and lipid peroxidation in human placental and fetal tissues. Mol Cell Biochem. 2000;215(1–2):11–9.
40. Jauniaux E, Gulbis B, Burton GJ. The human first trimester gestational Sac limits rather than facilitates oxygen transfer to the Foetus—a review. Placenta. 2003;24:S86–93.
41. Hussain T, Murtaza G, Metwally E, Kalhoro DH, Kalhoro MS, Rahu BA, et al. The role of oxidative stress and antioxidant balance in pregnancy. Mediat Inflamm. 2021;2021:9962860.
42. Casas I, Nakaki A, Pascal R, Castro-Barquero S, Youssef L, Genero M, et al. Effects of a Mediterranean diet intervention on maternal stress, well-being, and sleep quality throughout gestation-the IMPACT-BCN trial. Nutrients. 2023;15(10):2362.
43. Tuttolomondo A, Simonetta I, Daidone M, Mogavero A, Ortello A, Pinto A. Metabolic and vascular effect of the Mediterranean diet. Int J Mol Sci. 2019;20(19):4716.
44. Visioli F, Grande S, Bogani P, Galli C. The role of antioxidants in the Mediterranean diets: focus on cancer. Eur J Cancer Prev. 2004;13(4):337–43.
45. Cryan JF, O'riordan KJ, Cowan CSM, Sandhu KV, Bastiaanssen TFS, Boehme M, et al. The microbiota-gut-brain axis. Physiol Rev. 2019;99(4):1877–2013.
46. Collins JM, Keane JM, Deady C, Khashan AS, McCarthy FP, O'Keeffe GW, et al. Prenatal stress impacts foetal neurodevelopment: temporal windows of gestational vulnerability.

Neurosci Biobehav Rev [Internet]. 2024;164(June):105793. Available from: https://doi.org/10.1016/j.neubiorev.2024.105793.
47. Miko E, Csaszar A, Bodis J, Kovacs K. The Maternal–Fetal gut microbiota axis: physiological changes, dietary influence, and modulation possibilities. Life MDPI. 2022;12:424.
48. Nuriel-Ohayon M, Neuman H, Koren O. Microbial changes during pregnancy, birth, and infancy. Front Microbiol. Frontiers Media SA. 2016;7:1031.
49. Liu J, Yang H, Yin Z, Jiang X, Zhong H, Qiu D, et al. Remodeling of the gut microbiota and structural shifts in Preeclampsia patients in South China. Eur J Clin Microbiol Infect Dis. 2017;36(4):713–9.
50. Al Rubaye H, Adamson CC, Jadavji NM. The role of maternal diet on offspring gut microbiota development: a review. J Neurosci Res [Internet]. 2021 [cited 2025 Feb 20];99(1):284–93. Available from: https://onlinelibrary.wiley.com/doi/full/10.1002/jnr.24605.
51. Faas MM, Smink AM. Shaping immunity: the influence of the maternal gut bacteria on fetal immune development. Semin Immunopathol [Internet]. 2025;47(1) Available from: https://doi.org/10.1007/s00281-025-01039-8.
52. Aagaard K, Ma J, Anton K. The placenta Harbors a unique microbiome. Sci Transl Med. 2015;6(237):229–62.
53. Park JY, Yun H, Lee S, Been KHJ, Jung YH, Choi CW, et al. Comprehensive characterization of maternal, fetal, and neonatal microbiomes supports prenatal colonization of the gastrointestinal tract. Sci Rep. 2023;13(1):4652.
54. Perez-Muñoz ME, Arrieta MC, Ramer-Tait AE, Walter J. A critical assessment of the "sterile womb" and "in utero colonization" hypotheses: implications for research on the pioneer infant microbiome. Microbiome. 2017;5(1):1–19.
55. Kennedy KM, de Goffau MC, Perez-Muñoz ME, Arrieta MC, Bäckhed F, Bork P, et al. Questioning the fetal microbiome illustrates pitfalls of low-biomass microbial studies. Nature. 2023;613(7945):639–49.
56. Zubcevic J, Watkins J, Lin C, Bautista B, Hatch HM, Tevosian SG, et al. Nicotine exposure during Rodent pregnancy alters the composition of maternal gut microbiota and abundance of maternal and amniotic short chain fatty acids. Metabolites. 2022;12(8):735.
57. Ilyés T, Pop M, Surcel M, Pop DM, Rusu R, Silaghi CN, et al. First comparative evaluation of short-chain fatty acids and vitamin-K-dependent proteins levels in mother–newborn pairs at birth. Life. 2023;13(3):847.
58. Moianu A, Şerban G, Andone S. The role of short-chain fatty acids in microbiota–gut–brain cross-talk with a focus on amyotrophic lateral sclerosis: a systematic review. Int J Mol Sci [Internet]. 2023 [cited 2025 Feb 21];24(20):15094. Available from: https://pmc.ncbi.nlm.nih.gov/articles/PMC10606032/.
59. Pessa-Morikawa T, Husso A, Kärkkäinen O, Koistinen V, Hanhineva K, Iivanainen A, et al. Maternal microbiota-derived metabolic profile in fetal murine intestine, brain and placenta. BMC Microbiol [Internet]. 2022;22(1):1–16. Available from: https://doi.org/10.1186/s12866-022-02457-6.
60. Sun Y, Xie R, Li L, Jin G, Zhou B, Huang H, et al. Prenatal maternal stress exacerbates experimental Colitis of offspring in adulthood. Front Immunol. 2021;12(November):1–17.
61. Balla J, Rathore AP, St. John AL. Mechanisms and risk factors for perinatal allergic disease. Curr Opin Immunol [Internet]. 2024;91:102505. Available from: https://doi.org/10.1016/j.coi.2024.102505.
62. Gur TL, Worly BL, Bailey MT. Stress and the commensal microbiota: importance in parturition and infant neurodevelopment. Front Psychiatry. Frontiers Media SA. 2015;6:5.
63. Vuong HE, Pronovost GN, Williams DW, Coley EJL, Siegler EL, Qiu A, et al. The maternal microbiome modulates fetal neurodevelopment in mice. Nature [Internet]. 2020;586(7828):281–6. Available from: https://doi.org/10.1038/s41586-020-2745-3.
64. Hudobenko J, Di Gesù CM, Mooz PR, Petrosino J, Putluri N, Ganesh BP, et al. Maternal dysbiosis produces long-lasting behavioral changes in offspring. Mol Psychiatry [Internet]. 2024;(February):1–12. Available from: https://doi.org/10.1038/s41380-024-02794-0.

65. Ulrich-Lai YM, Herman JP. Neural regulation of endocrine and autonomic stress responses. Nat Rev Neurosci [Internet]. 2009 [cited 2025 Feb 21];10(6):397–409. Available from: https://www.nature.com/articles/nrn2647.
66. Kvetnansky R, Sabban EL, Palkovits M. Catecholaminergic systems in stress: structural and molecular genetic approaches. Physiol Rev [Internet]. 2009 [cited 2025 Feb 21];89(2):535–606. Available from: https://journals.physiology.org/doi/10.1152/physrev.00042.2006.
67. Saarikoski S. Development of noradrenaline uptake in the human foetal heart. Experientia. 1977;33(2):251–3.
68. Sodha RJ, Proegler M, Schneider H. Transfer and metabolism of norepinephrine studied from maternal-to-fetal and fetal-to-maternal sides in the in vitro perfused human placental lobe. Am J Obstet Gynecol. 1984;148(4):474–81.
69. Civantos Calzada B, Aleixandre De Artiñano A. Alpha-adrenoceptor subtypes. Pharmacol Res. 2001;44(3):195–208.
70. Dreiling M, Bischoff S, Schiffner R, Rupprecht S, Kiehntopf M, Schubert H, et al. Stress-induced decrease of uterine blood flow in sheep is mediated by alpha 1-adrenergic receptors. Stress [Internet]. 2016 [cited 2025 Feb 21];19(5):547–51. Available from: https://www.tandfonline.com/doi/abs/10.1080/10253890.2016.1203417.
71. Helbig A, Kaasen A, Malt UF, Haugen G. Does antenatal maternal psychological distress affect placental circulation in the third trimester?. PLoS One [Internet]. 2013 [cited 2025 Feb 21];8(2):e57071. Available from: https://journals.plos.org/plosone/article?id=10.1371/journal.pone.0057071.
72. Monk C, Feng T, Lee S, Krupska I, Champagne FA, Tycko B. Distress during pregnancy: epigenetic regulation of placenta glucocorticoid-related genes and fetal neurobehavior. Am J Psychiatry [Internet]. 2016 [cited 2025 Feb 21];173(7):705–13. Available from: https://psychiatryonline.org/doi/10.1176/appi.ajp.2015.15091171.
73. Gu W, Jones CT. The effect of elevation of maternal plasma catecholamines on the fetus and placenta of the pregnant sheep. J Dev Physiol. 1986;8(3):173–86.
74. Bzoskie L, Yen J, Tseng YT, Blount L, Kashiwai KPJ. Human placental norepinephrine transporter mRNA: expression and correlation with fetal condition at birth. Placenta. 1997;18(2–3):205–10.
75. Rosenfeld CS. The placenta-brain-axis. J Neurosci Res. 2021;99(1):271–83.
76. Rosenfeld CS. Placental serotonin signaling, pregnancy outcomes, and regulation of fetal brain development†. Biol Reprod. 2020;102(3):532–8.
77. Huang X, Feng Z, Cheng HW. Perspective: gestational Tryptophan fluctuation altering Neuroembryogenesis and psychosocial development. Cells. 2022;11(8):1270.
78. Keane JM, Khashan AS, McCarthy FP, Kenny LC, Collins JM, O'Donovan S, et al. Identifying a biological signature of prenatal maternal stress. JCI Insight. 2021;6(2):e143007.
79. Sainio EL, Pulkki K, Young SN. L-Tryptophan: biochemical, nutritional and pharmacological aspects. Amino Acids. 1996;10(1):21–47.
80. Bonnin A, Levitt P. Fetal, maternal, and placental sources of serotonin and new implications for developmental programming of the brain. Neuroscience. 2011;197:1–7.
81. Staud F, Karahoda R. Trophoblast: the central unit of fetal growth, protection and programming. Int J Biochem Cell Biol. 2018;105:35–40.
82. Hadden C, Fahmi T, Cooper A, Savenka AV, Lupashin VV, Roberts DJ, et al. Serotonin transporter protects the placental cells against apoptosis in caspase 3-independent pathway. J Cell Physiol. 2017;232(12):3520–9.
83. Bonnin A, Levitt P. Placental Source for 5-HT that Tunes Fetal brain development. Neuropsychopharmacology. 2012;37(1):299–300.
84. Hong J, Lu X, Wang J, Jiang M, Liu Q, Lin J, et al. Triphenyl phosphate disturbs placental tryptophan metabolism and induces neurobehavior abnormal in male offspring. Ecotoxicol Environ Saf. 2022;243:113978.
85. Notarangelo FM, Schwarcz R. Restraint stress during pregnancy rapidly raises Kynurenic acid levels in mouse placenta and Fetal brain. Dev Neurosci. 2016;38(6):458–68.

86. Law KP, Han TL, Mao X, Zhang H. Tryptophan and purine metabolites are consistently upregulated in the urinary metabolome of patients diagnosed with gestational diabetes mellitus throughout pregnancy: a longitudinal metabolomics study of Chinese pregnant women part 2. Clin Chim Acta. 2017;468:126–39.
87. Badawy AAB. The tryptophan utilization concept in pregnancy. Obstet Gynecol Sci. 2014;57(4):249.
88. Jones P, Cannon M. The new epidemiology of Schizophrenia. Psychiatr Clin N Am. 1998;21(1):1–25.
89. Glover V, O'Connor TG, O'Donnell K. Prenatal stress and the programming of the HPA axis. Neurosci Biobehav Rev. 2010;35(1):17–22.
90. Galley JD, Chen HJ, Antonson AM, Gur TL. Prenatal stress-induced disruptions in microbial and host tryptophan metabolism and transport. Behav Brain Res. 2021;414:113471.
91. Bondarenko N, Lifantseva N, Voronova S, Melnikova V. The placenta as the main source of serotonin in ontogenetic dynamics: inflammation-induced modulation of placental serotonin can be prevented by immunoglobulin administration. Int J Mol Sci. 2024;25(24):13532.
92. Moura CA, Cagni FC, Costa LRF, Tiago PRF, Croyal M, Aguesse A, et al. Maternal stress during pregnancy in mice induces sex-dependent behavioral alterations in offspring along with impaired Serotonin and Kynurenine pathways of Tryptophan metabolism. Dev Neurosci. 2022;44(6):603–14.
93. Ruyak SL, Noor S, DiDomenico J, Sun MS, Fernandez Oropeza AK, Rodriguez DE, et al. Effects of prenatal opioid and alcohol exposures on immune and serotonin factors in human placenta. Exp Neurol. 2022;353:114057.
94. Vachalova V, Kumnova F, Synova T, Anandam KY, Abad C, Karahoda R, et al. Metformin inhibits OCT3-mediated serotonin transport in the placenta. Biomed Pharmacother. 2024;179:117399.

The Role of the Brain–Gut Axis in Maternal Stress and Its Detrimental Consequences

10

Alena Lochmannová and Colin R. Martin

Abstract

Maternal psychological stress is increasingly recognised as a critical environmental factor that influences fetal development and programming through the brain–gut axis. This bidirectional network, comprising neural, endocrine, immune and microbial pathways, plays a central role in how maternal stress is communicated to both the mother and fetus. During pregnancy, heightened psychosocial stress activates the HPA axis, which disrupts gut microbiota, increases intestinal permeability and promotes systemic inflammation, which can cross the placental barrier, impacting fetal neurodevelopment. This chapter explores the mechanisms through which maternal stress alters the brain–gut axis during pregnancy, focusing on microbial shifts, immune responses and neuroendocrine disruptions. It highlights the role of the maternal gut microbiota in fetal health and underscores the importance of interventions such as dietary fibre, probiotics and stress-reduction techniques to preserve gut-brain homeostasis and optimise maternal and fetal health outcomes.

Keywords

Maternal stress · Brain–gut axis · Fetal neurodevelopment · HPA axis · Gut microbiota · Pregnancy · Immune signalling · Microbial diversity · Prenatal stress · Neuroinflammation · Maternal health · Intervention strategies

A. Lochmannová (✉)
Department of Infectious Diseases and Travel Medicine, Faculty of Medicine in Pilsen, Charles University, Prague, Czech Republic
e-mail: Alena.Lochmannova@lfp.cuni.cz

C. R. Martin
Institute for Health and Wellbeing, University of Suffolk, Ipswich, UK
e-mail: colinmartin.bssr@proton.me

R. A. Caparros-Gonzalez (ed.), *Maternal Stress during Pregnancy and Postpartum*, https://doi.org/10.1007/978-3-032-09245-8_10

10.1 Introduction

Maternal psychological stress is increasingly recognised as a bona fide developmental teratogen—an environmental influence capable of disrupting fetal growth and programming. Large observational cohorts show that stress exposure during gestation, whether indexed by a formal psychiatric diagnosis or by self-reported worries about finances, work, social relationships or pregnancy itself, remains an independent predictor of lower birth weight and more than doubles the adjusted odds of pre-term birth after biomedical and sociodemographic covariates are controlled [1–3]. These associations are thought to be transmitted through tightly coupled autonomic, neuroendocrine and immune pathways linking the mother to the fetus.

Perinatal epidemiology therefore adopts pragmatic, clinically grounded criteria to flag pregnancies in which psychosocial load is likely to shape biology. Antenatal care teams generally consider any documented mood- or anxiety-related diagnosis, together with charted concerns such as previous traumatic births, inadequate social support, financial insecurity or work strain, as indicators of heightened stress liability [2]. Across studies that apply similarly broad definitions, psychosocial burden consistently retains predictive power for pre-term delivery [3] and related complications [4, 5] after classical obstetric risk factors are accounted for. This clinical framing legitimises routine psychosocial screening in obstetrics and provides the conceptual bridge to mechanistic work on stress-responsive pathways—including the neuroendocrine and immune loops that constitute the brain–gut axis—through which maternal experience is conveyed to the developing fetus [6].

A second window of vulnerability opens once the infant is born. Abrupt hormonal withdrawal, sleep fragmentation and the relentless demands of caregiving generate a distinct pattern of maternal post-partum stress that reaches well beyond the transient "baby blues." Cross-sectional data from 486 Czech mothers show that women who perceive little emotional or instrumental support report markedly poorer post-partum well-being and receive less partner assistance than their better-supported peers [7]. Complementary evidence from a Croatian cohort underscores both the breadth and the clinical salience of this burden: Everyday hassles—fatigue, worries about infant nurturing, body changes and strained couple relationships—accumulate across the entire first post-partum year, and roughly one in three first-time mothers manifests clinically significant symptoms of depression, anxiety or stress, two-thirds of which would be missed by depression-only screening [8]. Taken together, these findings reveal the social contingency and diagnostic under-recognition of maternal post-partum stress and underscore the need for comprehensive psychosocial assessment and targeted support during this second critical window.

Building on this clinical framing, current mechanistic work converges on the brain–gut axis as a circular, bidirectional network that links the central nervous system, the enteric nervous system, hypothalamic–pituitary–adrenal (HPA) stress circuitry, systemic immunity and the intestinal microbiome [9]. Three partially overlapping signalling channels support this dialogue—neural, endocrine and immune—and each can be modulated by, and in turn remodel, the resident microbiota. Neural traffic is routed primarily through the vagus nerve and the enteric nervous system. Afferent fibres arising from mucosal endings convey mechanical and chemical information to the nucleus tractus solitarius and dorsal motor nucleus, while efferent parasympathetic and sympathetic fibres regulate motility, secretion and epithelial permeability in a top-down direction. Enteroendocrine cells situated at the mucosal interface translate luminal signals into neural messages by releasing serotonin, cholecystokinin, glucagon-like peptide-1 and peptide YY, all of which activate vagal afferents [10]; the vagus nerve is therefore often described as the "gut–brain super-highway" [9, 11]. Endocrine dialogue centres on glucocorticoids, catecholamines and gut-derived peptides. Activation of the maternal HPA axis releases cortisol and adrenaline, molecules that diffuse across the epithelium and alter microbial gene expression, whereas gut hormones such as glucagon-like peptide-1 and peptide YY, liberated in response to nutrient and microbial stimuli, feed back to hypothalamic centres that govern appetite and autonomic tone [10]. Clinical data likewise confirm that stress-driven elevations in circulating cortisol markedly promote gut dysbiosis [12]. In parallel, immune signalling conveys microbiota- and damage-associated molecular patterns as well as cytokines (e.g., IL-6, TNF-α) into the bloodstream, synchronising peripheral inflammatory status with central stress-processing networks [10] and influencing mood, cognition and pain thresholds [9]. Microbial metabolites constitute a potent fourth messenger set. Fermentation of dietary fibre yields the short-chain fatty acids acetate, propionate and butyrate in an approximate 60:25:15 ratio [13]. These SCFAs reinforce epithelial tight junctions, temper mucosal and systemic inflammation; stimulate the release of anorexigenic peptides; and—after transport across the blood–brain barrier via monocarboxylate transporters—modulate neuroinflammation and behaviour [10, 13]. The microbiota and enteroendocrine cells also synthesise classical neurotransmitters such as serotonin, dopamine and γ-aminobutyric acid, which act locally on gut function and remotely on mood and cognition [9]. Because these neural, endocrine, immune and microbial circuits are embedded in closed feedback loops, perturbations at any node—such as the sustained HPA activation, dysbiosis and low-grade inflammation that accompany maternal psychological stress—can propagate throughout the system. This systems-level plasticity provides a plausible biological bridge by which maternal experience is transduced into endocrine, immune and metabolic cues that influence placental function, fetal programming and, in the postpartum period, maternal mental health [14].

Pregnancy superimposes profound hormonal and immunological remodelling on the brain–gut axis [15]. Rising concentrations of oestrogens, progesterone and placenta-derived corticotropin-releasing hormone shift maternal microbial community structure, loosen epithelial tight junctions and recalibrate HPA axis feedback sensitivity—changes that safeguard nutrient flow to the fetus and immunotolerance at the maternal–fetal interface yet leave the system highly vulnerable to psychosocial challenge [16]. When maternal stress activates this sensitised HPA axis, surges of cortisol and catecholamines disturb gut ecology, exacerbate barrier permeability and amplify systemic pro-inflammatory signalling capable of reaching the placenta [10]. Animal and human data demonstrate that such neuroendocrine–microbial feedback feeds forward: Gestational stress alters maternal gut diversity and composition during late pregnancy, is mirrored in the neonatal colon, and associates with changes in hippocampal plasticity and microglial density in both dam and offspring [16]. Complementing these mechanistic findings, a prospective cohort of 95 pregnant individuals showed that lower α-diversity early in gestation predicted greater bowel symptoms, heightened perceived helplessness and poorer coping capacity postpartum [6]. A broader translational review concludes that psychological stress consistently reshapes microbiota across diverse paradigms and that microbiota-targeted interventions—pro- and prebiotics or dietary fibre—can attenuate HPA hyper-reactivity and stress-related behaviours, although rigorous human trials remain limited [17]. Collectively, these observations position pregnancy as a period in which physiological endocrine adjustments both harness and expose the brain–gut circuitry, making maternal microbiome–neuroendocrine crosstalk a principal conduit through which psychological stress is translated into obstetric risk and fetal programming signals.

From a translational perspective, probing stress-driven alterations in the pregnancy-adapted brain–gut circuit offers three strategic dividends. First, early-gestation microbial diversity already stratifies psychological resilience, providing a pragmatic biomarker for directing antenatal resources [6]. Second, experimental evidence shows that gestational stress remodels maternal and neonatal microbiota in parallel with changes in hippocampal plasticity, indicating modifiable causal leverage [16]. Third, an integrative review confirms that stress-related microbial shifts can be attenuated by gut-directed approaches—probiotics, prebiotics, fermentable fibre—thereby moderating stress phenotypes, although rigorous obstetric trials remain scarce [17]. Taken together, these findings underscore that the brain–gut axis is both measurable and malleable, positioning it as an ideal platform for biomarker discovery, psychobiotic therapeutics and precision stress-reduction protocols aimed at averting downstream obstetric and neurodevelopmental morbidity.

This chapter first delineates the neurobiological architecture of the brain–gut axis and the physiological adaptations that occur during pregnancy; it then dissects molecular and cellular mechanisms by which maternal stress compromises this network, summarises clinical consequences for mother and child and discusses current and emerging intervention strategies. By integrating animal and human evidence, the chapter aims to refine conceptual models of prenatal programming and inform multidisciplinary approaches to safeguarding maternal and fetal health.

10.2 Neurobiology of the Brain–Gut Axis

The neural "high command" of the brain–gut network is the HPA axis, which translates psychological challenge into the endocrine language of corticotropin-releasing hormone, adrenocorticotropic hormone and circulating glucocorticoids. These hormones reach the intestinal wall within minutes and can modify motility, epithelial permeability and even microbial gene expression [18]. Running in parallel is the enteric nervous system—an intrinsic network of myenteric and submucosal neurons embedded in the gut wall that generates autonomous reflexes for secretion, blood flow and peristalsis yet remains tightly coupled to central autonomic nuclei through dense vagal and sympathetic projections [19]. The third node, the gut microbiome, contributes an extensive additional gene repertoire and a pharmacopoeia of bioactive molecules—short-chain fatty acids (SCFAs), indole derivatives and microbially synthesised neurotransmitters—that interact with immune and neuronal sensors in the mucosa [18].

Communication among these three nodes proceeds along four intertwined conduits. Neural traffic dominates the fast lane: Viscerosensory information encoded by vagal and sympathetic afferents ascends to the nucleus tractus solitarius, while descending parasympathetic and sympathetic fibres fine-tune motility, secretion and barrier integrity, continually reshaping the microbial habitat. Endocrine signalling forms a slower chemical loop; HPA-derived cortisol and catecholamines feed forward to the gut, whereas gut hormones such as glucagon-like peptide-1 and peptide YY enter the circulation and act on hypothalamic and brain stem nuclei. Immune dialogue adds a third layer: Cytokines released from lamina propria cells in response to stress or microbial cues circulate systemically or activate vagal chemoreceptors, synchronising peripheral inflammatory tone with central stress circuitry. Finally, microbial mediators—notably the SCFAs acetate, propionate and butyrate, together with indole metabolites and bacterially derived serotonin or γ-aminobutyric acid—reach the brain via the circulation or through afferent-neuron activation, closing a dense web of feedback loops that allows the gut to act simultaneously as both sensor and effector of central states [18, 19].

10.3 Changes in the Brain–Gut Axis During Pregnancy

Pregnancy constitutes an extraordinary biological state characterised by profound systemic remodelling. While the endocrine and metabolic recalibrations of gestation have long been recognised, only recently has the maternal gut microbiota been identified as a key driver and modulator of these adaptations, with consequences that extend to both maternal and offspring health [20].

Gestation initiates a tightly orchestrated endocrine immune programme that reshapes gastrointestinal physiology. Escalating concentrations of oestrogen and progesterone progressively slow gastric emptying and intestinal transit, augment mucin production and remodel bile acid pools, together widening the absorptive window for calories and micronutrients needed to sustain fetal growth and maternal adipose accretion. Concomitantly, pregnancy is accompanied by a controlled, low-grade pro-inflammatory milieu that recalibrates gut-associated immune signalling and remodels epithelial permeability—changes regarded as preparatory for the immunological challenges of parturition [21].

Beyond their influence on motility, ovarian steroids exert barrier protective actions. In females, hormones such as oestrogen and progesterone play crucial roles in modulating both the gut microbiome and brain function [22]. Oestrogen upregulates tight junction proteins and mucus secretion, whereas progesterone relaxes smooth muscle layers, jointly altering epithelial permeability and luminal flow [21]. In parallel, placental corticotrophin-releasing hormone escapes negative feedback control, driving a trimester-dependent rise in circulating cortisol. Hypercortisolism increases gut permeability and amplifies gut-derived inflammatory signalling—hallmarks of stress-related dysregulation of the brain–gut axis [23–25].

Diet can modulate this response. Fermentation of soluble dietary fibre yields SCFAs—acetate, propionate and butyrate—that reinforce epithelial tight junctions, stimulate enteroendocrine release of glucagon-like peptide 1 and peptide YY and dampen hypothalamic–pituitary–adrenal activity, collectively lowering maternal cortisol concentrations [26].

Dynamic fluctuations in circulating oestrogen appear to influence microbiome diversity; lower oestrogen phases have been linked to decreases in α-diversity and an enrichment of opportunistic Proteobacteria, whereas oestrogen peaks tend to preserve saccharolytic communities. Peripartum dysbiosis in concert with abrupt steroid withdrawal postpartum has been implicated in approximately 10–15% of cases of postpartum depression, underscoring the enduring impact of gestational brain–gut reprogramming on maternal mental health [22].

Metagenomic profiling reveals a trimester-specific succession from a diverse, butyrate-rich community in early pregnancy to a Proteobacteria-enriched, low-diversity profile at term—an ecological shift that parallels the metabolic pivot toward fat storage and heightened inflammatory vigilance [20, 21, 27]. Low dietary fibre intake accelerates this transition, curtailing SCFA production and favouring pathogenic overgrowth, whereas fibre-rich diets maintain saccharolytic taxa and buffer cortisol-mediated stress responses [26].

Total bacterial load rises while α-diversity declines between the first and third trimesters because of an expansion of Actinobacteria (notably Bifidobacterium) and Proteobacteria alongside a depletion of the butyrate producer Faecalibacterium. Between-subject (β) diversity increases in tandem with weight gain, insulin resistance and elevated faecal cytokines—physiological changes reminiscent of metabolic syndrome yet adaptive in pregnancy [20].

Landmark germ-free mouse experiments demonstrated that third trimester microbiota induce adiposity, insulin resistance and low-grade mucosal inflammation in otherwise healthy hosts—definitively proving a causal role for late gestation communities in orchestrating pregnancy-specific metabolic adaptation [20, 27]. Consistent with this, calorimetric analyses recorded an ≈10% rise in faecal energy density between the first and third trimesters, suggesting altered nutrient extraction dynamics that favour maternal fetal energy availability [27]. Maternal gut profiles remain distinct from pre-pregnancy baselines for at least 1 month postpartum, with sustained β-diversity; this period coincides with a steep decline in ovarian steroids and persistent low-grade inflammation, both proposed contributors to the delayed microbiome restitution [20, 27].

Population-specific evidence underscores that microbiome trajectories are not uniform across ethnic groups. In a prospective cohort of 55 Chinese women, both α- and β-diversity increased across gestation, accompanied by a decline in Bacteroidetes and an expansion of Proteobacteria. Gestational diabetes mellitus

(GDM) emerged as the main determinant of between-subject variation: GDM pregnancies displayed higher late gestation diversity but reduced dispersion, with enrichment of Ruminococcus gnavus and Bacteroides vulgatus—species positively correlated with insulin signalling and lipopolysaccharide biosynthesis pathways. In contrast, non-GDM pregnancies were characterised by higher abundances of Bacteroides coprocola and Prevotella copri, taxa inversely linked to these pro-inflammatory routes [28].

Pregnancy-driven surges in oestrogen, progesterone and cortisol orchestrate a systemic shift in gastrointestinal motility, barrier integrity and immune tone while simultaneously sculpting a trimester-specific microbial ecology that favours energy harvest and immune priming. These adaptations are largely beneficial, ensuring optimal substrate supply for fetal growth and preparing the mother for the metabolic demands of late gestation and lactation. Yet the same hormone-dependent circuitry and microbiome plasticity render the maternal brain–gut axis exquisitely sensitive to exogenous modifiers—nutritional quality, psychosocial stress and metabolic disorders such as gestational diabetes—whose downstream effects on maternal and infant health remain incompletely understood.

10.4 The Impact of Stress on the Brain–Gut Axis in Pregnant Women

Prenatal stress is increasingly recognised as a critical factor capable of disrupting the delicate communication along the microbiota–gut–brain axis, with consequences that extend beyond the maternal organism to fetal neurodevelopment. This bidirectional axis comprises neural, immune and endocrine components that communicate through neuroactive metabolites, cytokines and microbial products. During pregnancy, maternal exposure to psychological stress—manifested as anxiety, depression or exposure to interpersonal violence—activates the HPA axis, leading to increased secretion of corticotropin-releasing hormone, cortisol and pro-inflammatory cytokines, which in turn impact gut microbiota composition and barrier function [29, 30].

Alterations in maternal gut microbiota in response to prenatal stress include increased representation of potentially pro-inflammatory genera such as Staphylococcus and Rothia [30] together with a concomitant depletion of beneficial butyrate producers such as Eubacterium and Oscillospira [31]. These shifts do not necessarily reduce alpha diversity but indicate a dysbiotic profile that may compromise mucosal immunity and increase intestinal permeability. The downstream effects may involve microbial translocation and systemic inflammation, which together with elevated maternal cortisol levels may allow cytokines such as interleukin-6 (IL-6) or chemokines like CCL2 to cross the placental barrier, thereby affecting fetal brain development [29].

Beyond psychosocial stressors, environmental pollutants represent an additional dimension of prenatal stress capable of altering the gut–brain axis. Exposure to toxicants such as heavy metals, phthalates, Bisphenol A (BPA) and particulate matter has been linked to gut dysbiosis, impaired intestinal barrier function and dysregulation of SCFA production—mechanisms closely tied to both maternal mental health and fetal neurodevelopment. These pollutants may further modulate neurotransmitter synthesis (e.g., serotonin, GABA), impact microbial metabolite availability and potentiate neuroinflammation, thereby exacerbating HPA axis dysregulation and fetal vulnerability to neurodevelopmental disorders [32].

Maternal microbial dysregulation thus emerges as a central pathway by which various forms of prenatal stress—psychological or environmental—can program long-term consequences in offspring via the gut–brain axis. The transmission of altered microbial profiles to the neonate during birth and early life further compounds these risks, underscoring the need for an integrated understanding of microbial, neuroendocrine and inflammatory pathways during pregnancy [29, 30, 32].

In line with this, a landmark longitudinal study demonstrated that higher levels of maternal prenatal stress—measured through both psychological distress and elevated salivary cortisol—were significantly associated with alterations in the infant gut microbiota. Specifically, increased maternal stress was linked to greater relative abundance of pro-inflammatory genera such as Escherichia, Serratia and Enterobacter, and a reduction in beneficial taxa including Lactobacillus and Bifidobacterium [33]. These microbial signatures were also associated with increased gastrointestinal and allergic symptoms in infants, indicating early-life health implications of prenatal stress-mediated dysbiosis. The findings further suggest that maternal stress may create a selective intrauterine and perinatal environment through HPA axis activation, altered immune signalling and changes in maternal gut ecology, all of which contribute to the colonisation patterns observed in neonates.

Adding a further layer of complexity, hormonal regulation—particularly via oestrogen—appears to modulate stress responses along the brain–gut axis. Oestrogen is known to influence gut epithelial integrity, immune activation and microbial community structure. During pregnancy, fluctuating oestrogen levels interact with stress pathways and can either buffer or exacerbate GBA dysfunction depending on the hormonal context. Chronic stress is capable of altering oestrogen receptor signalling and impairing the protective roles of oestrogens within the gastrointestinal tract. In particular, reduced oestrogen-mediated anti-inflammatory effects and compromised mucosal protection may heighten susceptibility to gut permeability and systemic inflammation, further amplifying brain–gut dysregulation during gestation [34].

Recent advances focusing explicitly on the inflammatory dimension of the gut–brain axis refine this picture further. A comprehensive review by Morys, Małecki and Nowacka Chmielewska [35] underscores that stress-elicited inflammatory cascades simultaneously erode the intestinal barrier and the blood–brain barrier (BBB) through downregulation of tight junction proteins such as claudin 5, occludin and ZO 1. Compromised barriers permit systemic translocation of lipopolysaccharide and pro-inflammatory cytokines—including IL 1β, IL 6, TNF α and the chemokines CCL2/CCL5—which can reach the maternal–fetal interface and potentiate neuroinflammatory signalling. Central to this process is activation of pattern recognition receptors (e.g., TLR4, NOD-like receptors) and the NLRP3 inflammasome in enteric immune cells and microglia; pharmacological or probiotic strategies that dampen NLRP3 activity restore BBB integrity and ameliorate stress-induced behavioural phenotypes in preclinical models. The review further delineates three complementary immune-mediated conduits—systemic, cellular and neuronal—through which gut dysbiosis communicates with the brain; all are modulated by HPA axis hormones and are therefore particularly pertinent during pregnancy, when glucocorticoid surges can skew Th17/Treg balance and prime microglial reactivity. Conversely, microbiota-derived SCFAs—notably butyrate, propionate and acetate—have been shown to fortify epithelial and endothelial tight junctions, inhibit TLR-mediated neuroinflammation and support microglial metabolic fitness, suggesting therapeutic avenues via dietary fibre enrichment, targeted probiotics or faecal microbiota transplantation [35]. These insights reinforce the proposition that nutritional and microbial interventions aimed at preserving gut and neurovascular barrier integrity may buffer the impact of prenatal stress on fetal neurodevelopment.

Building on these mechanistic insights, an integrative scoping review by Ryan, O'Mahony, Leahy Warren, Philpott and Mulcahy [31] systematically mapped seven human studies that concurrently examined perinatal maternal stress and the maternal gut, infant gut and/or human milk microbiomes. Across five of the seven studies, higher subjective or physiological stress exposures were associated with increased abundance of potentially pathogenic genera—including Erwinia, Serratia, Haemophilus and Bacteroides—and with a relative depletion of health-promoting taxa such as Lactococcus, Lactobacillus and Akkermansia. Although one study presented a contrasting pattern, the aggregate evidence converges on a stress-related shift toward a more pro-inflammatory microbial milieu. The review further noted that maternal stress altered microbial α- and β-diversity in both mothers and infants, with the strongest divergence in infant community structure emerging after the first postnatal month. Methodological heterogeneity—particularly in stress metrics and covariate control—was highlighted as a key driver of between-study inconsistencies, underscoring the value of integrating subjective questionnaires with objective biomarkers such as cortisol or cytokine panels.

Of particular relevance to vertical transmission pathways, Ryan et al. emphasised the human milk microbiome as an under-investigated yet potentially critical conduit linking maternal stress to infant gut colonisation. Human milk—described as "mother nature's prototypical probiotic food" [36]—supplies both commensal microbes and bioactive metabolites that seed and nourish the neonatal microbiota; stress-related perturbations of this ecosystem could therefore propagate dysbiosis across generations [31]. Nevertheless, none of the reviewed studies simultaneously profiled maternal stress, milk microbiota and infant gut outcomes, representing a prominent knowledge gap that future longitudinal cohorts should address.

Collectively, the scoping review positions perinatal stress as a modifiable determinant of the maternal gut–milk–infant gut continuum and reinforces the strategic importance of the first 1000 days of life in preventive interventions aimed at preserving microbial diversity and limiting the early expansion of Proteobacteria-dominated, inflammation-prone communities [31].

Complementing these empirical findings, emerging conceptual work reframes the microbiota–gut–brain axis as a non-transplacental conduit through which prenatal stress can shape early neurodevelopment. Rotem Kohavi and colleagues [37] argue that maternal anxiety and depression—ranging from daily hassles to traumatic events—can perturb the gestational microbiome in ways that are transmitted to the offspring, thereby supplementing classic transplacental pathways such as cortisol transfer or psychotropic medication exposure. They synthesise human and animal evidence demonstrating that prenatal stress-induced dysbiosis interfaces with multiple stress-responsive systems: heightened HPA axis activity, altered serotonergic signalling, changes in placental function and immune dysregulation. Each of these mechanisms can be consolidated—or, conversely, mitigated—by the maternal gut microbiome [37].

The authors highlight that disturbances in microbial composition are a hallmark of numerous neurodevelopmental disorders and that gestational dysbiosis linked to maternal stress is already documented. They advocate for longitudinal tracking of molecular and microbial biomarkers throughout gestation to identify critical windows of vulnerability and to inform precision interventions. In particular, dietary fibre enrichment, probiotic supplementation and other microbiome-targeted strategies are proposed as promising avenues to confer resilience against the neurodevelopmental impacts of prenatal stress [37].

Prenatal stress reshapes the maternal microbiota–gut–brain axis by altering microbial communities, weakening epithelial and neurovascular barriers and heightening inflammatory and neuroendocrine signalling that can extend to the fetus. Yet these same pathways reveal actionable leverage points—dietary fibre, probiotics and targeted anti-inflammatory measures—that hold promise for restoring gut–brain homeostasis and supporting healthy neurodevelopment. Clarifying these mechanisms sets the stage for evaluating how such microbiota-driven perturbations manifest in maternal health and fetal outcomes.

10.5 Consequences for the Mother and the Fetus

Prenatal psychological distress—manifesting chiefly as depressive and anxious symptoms—reshapes the maternal gut microbiota and amplifies systemic inflammation, leaving the mother more vulnerable to infection-related morbidities during gestation [38, 39].

Through the microbiota–immune–brain axis, stress-linked dysbiosis allows pro-inflammatory cytokines and microbially derived metabolites to reach the fetal milieu. These signals can activate fetal microglia, weaken the blood–brain barrier and interfere with synaptogenesis and myelination, thereby compromising early brain development [39]. Pregnancy appears especially sensitive: Microbial metabolites produced in the maternal gut—rather than live bacteria—may traverse the blood–placental barrier and tune fetal immune responses [40].

Longitudinal human evidence indicates that distinctive microbiome profiles associated with high maternal distress partly mediate the link between antenatal mood symptoms and poorer infant cognitive and motor outcomes, underscoring the microbiome as a conduit through which psychological stress is biologically embedded in the offspring [38]. Complementary mechanistic work highlights three interconnected pathways—reduced short-chain-fatty-acid production, exaggerated T-helper-17 activity and altered tryptophan–serotonin metabolism—that collectively foster neuroinflammation and perturb fetal brain maturation [41]. Critical windows spanning preconception, gestation, birth and early postnatal life appear to determine how microbiome perturbations translate into later neurodevelopmental vulnerability [40].

A large prospective cohort further shows that the maternal prenatal microbiome—not the infant's own microbiota—explains the greatest variance in neurodevelopment across the first year of life; taxa such as Fusobacteria support fine-motor outcomes when present prenatally yet predict poorer performance when dominant postnatally [42]. In keeping with this susceptibility, a review documents that prenatal stress reduces maternal and offspring pools of short-chain fatty acids—central modulators of serotonergic signalling and anti-inflammatory tone—thereby amplifying stress reactivity and impairing cognition later in life [43].

Integrative work also emphasises that perinatal stress can imprint lasting epigenetic changes in hippocampal and prefrontal circuits, predisposing the child to long-term cognitive deficits and heightened stress sensitivity [29]. Extending evidence to the very first stage of colonisation, a prospective cohort that enrolled 465 pregnant women (with meconium available for 348 neonates) showed that mothers in the high-negative-emotion stress profile bore neonates with reduced meconium α-diversity and lower abundances of several potentially beneficial genera compared with low-stress and resilience (high-ACEs–low-negative emotion) profiles [44].

Although early research focused on direct transplacental cortisol or medication transfer, emerging models now position the maternal gut microbiome as an additional non-transplacental route by which stress signals reach the fetus. These models suggest that microbial, neuroendocrine, immune and autonomic pathways converge to influence neurodevelopment and highlight the promise of dietary or probiotic interventions to bolster resilience during critical windows [37].

These perturbations extend beyond the brain. Stress-induced immune activation is associated with impaired placental transport, growth restriction and earlier labour, thereby increasing the likelihood of low birth weight, pre-term delivery and later neurodevelopmental disorders in the child [39, 41].

Prenatal psychological distress initiates an inflammatory cascade that compromises placental transport, restricts fetal growth and predisposes the neonate to preterm birth and later neurodevelopmental difficulties. Mounting evidence identifies the maternal gut microbiome as the pivotal relay in this pathway—and, importantly, as an adaptable biological system. Dietary modification, pre- and probiotics and other microbiota-directed strategies therefore present realistic opportunities to dampen inflammatory signalling, stabilise placental function and support optimal brain maturation from the earliest stages of life.

10.6 Clinical and Research Implications

The clinical and research implications of these insights span screening, intervention and investigation. Routine prenatal care should move beyond depression checklists to incorporate brief, validated stress inventories alongside emerging biological indices—salivary cortisol patterns, serum zonulin or claudin concentrations, faecal short-chain fatty acid profiles and microbial diversity metrics—to create composite risk scores that flag pregnancies at greatest neurodevelopmental risk [44, 45]. Such multimodal screening could be deployed in obstetric clinics or via home-based kits, enabling dynamic monitoring of maternal stress–microbiome signals across gestation.

Interventions must be equally multifaceted and evidence driven. Nutritional strategies that optimise macronutrient balance and micronutrient sufficiency—particularly fibre intake to sustain butyrate-producing taxa—and support exclusive breastfeeding can shape microbial succession and barrier function in both mother and infant [46, 47]. Probiotic and prebiotic supplements selected for their psychobiotic potential may attenuate HPA-axis hyper-reactivity and systemic inflammation, while structured stress management programmes (mindfulness, cognitive-behavioural skills) address the psychosocial drivers of dysbiosis [43]. Embedding these modalities within a coordinated care model—where obstetricians, mental health specialists, dietitians and paediatricians collaborate—ensures that biological screening translates into targeted support rather than mere risk labelling.

From a public health perspective, antenatal classes and community programmes should integrate nutrition education, microbiome-friendly recipes and stress-reduction workshops, coupled with subsidised access to fibre-rich foods and quality probiotics. Such low-cost, scalable initiatives can shift population risk curves and foster resilience long before birth.

Research must now advance to deliver precision perinatal care. Large, longitudinal mother–infant cohorts with strain-resolved metagenomic and metabolomic profiling will be critical to identify the microbial taxa and metabolites that mediate stress effects and to define the gestational windows most amenable to intervention [48]. Randomised trials combining dietary, microbial and psychosocial strategies should extend follow-up into childhood to determine whether early manipulation of the microbiota–gut–brain axis yields sustained cognitive, behavioural and metabolic benefits. Finally, guideline development—grounded in robust cost-effectiveness analyses—will be essential to translate this emerging science into routine obstetric practice, with the goal of safeguarding both maternal well-being and optimal neurodevelopment from life's very beginning.

10.7 Conclusions

This chapter has demonstrated that maternal psychological stress operates as a bona fide developmental teratogen by engaging the brain–gut axis—a complex, bidirectional network of neural, endocrine, immune and microbial pathways.

Epidemiological evidence links heightened psychosocial burden in pregnancy and the postpartum period to obstetric complications, suboptimal fetal growth and enduring neurodevelopmental vulnerability. Mechanistic studies clarify how stress-induced HPA axis activation alters gut ecology, compromises barrier integrity and amplifies systemic inflammation, thereby transmitting adverse signals across the placenta and, during parturition and breastfeeding, seeding neonatal microbial communities with dysbiotic profiles. These disturbances not only jeopardise early synaptogenesis, myelination and microglial programming but also perpetuate a feedback loop that sustains maternal stress phenotypes and heightens risk for postnatal mental health disorders.

Critically, the gut microbiome emerges as both a sentinel and a steward of maternal–fetal health. Its remarkable plasticity underlies opportunities for intervention: Dietary modification, targeted psychobiotics and structured stress management programmes can recalibrate microbial composition, reinforce epithelial and neurovascular barriers and temper inflammatory signalling. Integrating these approaches within a multidisciplinary perinatal care framework—linking obstetricians, mental health specialists, dietitians and paediatricians—will be essential to translate biomarker-driven screening into tailored prevention and therapy. Looking forward, precision research that combines longitudinal, strain-resolved microbiome profiling with rigorous clinical trials must define causal windows, validate microbial and metabolite mediators and document long-term benefits for both mother and child. By reframing prenatal distress as a modifiable biological exposure, this work paves the way for interventions capable of safeguarding placental function and optimising neurodevelopment from life's very beginning.

References

1. DiPietro JA. Maternal stress in pregnancy: considerations for Fetal development. J Adolesc Health. 2012;51(2, Supplement):S3–8.
2. Lilliecreutz C, Larén J, Sydsjö G, Josefsson A. Effect of maternal stress during pregnancy on the risk for preterm birth. BMC Pregnancy Childbirth. 2016;16(1):5.
3. Copper RL, Goldenberg RL, Das A, Elder N, Swain M, Norman G, et al. The preterm prediction study: maternal stress is associated with spontaneous preterm birth at less than thirty-five weeks' gestation. Am J Obstet Gynecol. 1996;175(5):1286–92.
4. Rondó PHC, Ferreira RF, Nogueira F, Ribeiro MCN, Lobert H, Artes R. Maternal psychological stress and distress as predictors of low birth weight, prematurity and intrauterine growth retardation. Eur J Clin Nutr. 2003;57(2):266–72.
5. van den Heuvel MI, Hect JL, Smarr BL, Qawasmeh T, Kriegsfeld LJ, Barcelona J, et al. Maternal stress during pregnancy alters fetal cortico-cerebellar connectivity in utero and increases child sleep problems after birth. Sci Rep. 2021;11(1):2228.
6. Long ES, Penalver Bernabe B, Xia K, Azcarate-Peril MA, Carroll IM, Rackers HS, et al. The microbiota-gut-brain axis and perceived stress in the perinatal period. Arch Womens Ment Health. 2023;26(2):227–34.
7. Lochmannová A, Martin CR. Exploring the role of social support in postpartum well-being with a psychometric approach. Bratisl Med J [Internet]. 2025.; Available at https://doi.org/10.1007/s44411-025-00060-5.

8. Nakić Radoš S, Brekalo M, Matijaš M. Measuring stress after childbirth: development and validation of the Maternal Postpartum Stress Scale. J Reprod Infant Psychol. 2023;41(1):65–77.
9. Petrut SM, Bragaru AM, Munteanu AE, Moldovan AD, Moldovan CA, Rusu E. Gut over mind: exploring the powerful gut–brain axis. Nutrients. 2025;17(5):842.
10. Kasarello K, Cudnoch-Jedrzejewska A, Czarzasta K. Communication of gut microbiota and brain via immune and neuroendocrine signaling. Front Microbiol. 2023;14:1118529.
11. Furness JB, Callaghan BP, Rivera LR, Cho HJ. The enteric nervous system and gastrointestinal innervation: integrated local and central control. Adv Exp Med Biol. 2014;817:39–71.
12. Misiak B, Łoniewski I, Marlicz W, Frydecka D, Szulc A, Rudzki L, et al. The HPA axis dysregulation in severe mental illness: can we shift the blame to gut microbiota? Prog Neuro-Psychopharmacol Biol Psychiatry. 2020;102:109951.
13. Mansuy-Aubert V, Ravussin Y. Short chain fatty acids: the messengers from down below. Front Neurosci [Internet]. 2023:17. Available at: https://www.frontiersin.org. https://www.frontiersin.org/journals/neuroscience/articles/10.3389/fnins.2023.1197759/full.
14. Sarkar A, Lehto SM, Harty S, Dinan TG, Cryan JF, Burnet PWJ. Psychobiotics and the manipulation of bacteria–gut–brain signals. Trends Neurosci. 2016;39(11):763–81.
15. Gupta PD. ClinicSearch. 2025 [citován 3. květen 2025]. Importance of changes in the Gut Microbiota Milieu during pregnancy and beyond. Available at: https://clinicsearchonline.org/article/importance-of-changes-in-the-gut-microbiota-milieu-during-pregnancy-and-beyond.
16. Pawluski JL, Murail P, Grudet F, Bys L, Golubeva AV, Bastiaanssen T, et al. Gestational stress and perinatal SSRIs differentially impact the maternal and neonatal microbiome-gut-brain axis. J Neuroendocrinol. 2023;35(7):e13261.
17. Molina-Torres G, Rodriguez-Arrastia M, Roman P, Sanchez-Labraca N, Cardona D. Stress and the gut microbiota-brain axis. Behav Pharmacol. 2019;30(2 and 3-Spec Issue):187–200.
18. Mayer EA, Nance K, Chen S. The gut–brain axis. Annu Rev Med. 2022;73:439–53.
19. Bercik P, Collins SM, Verdu EF. Microbes and the gut-brain axis. Neurogastroenterol Motilit. 2012;24(5):405–13.
20. Nuriel-Ohayon M, Neuman H, Koren O. Microbial changes during pregnancy, birth, and infancy. Front Microbiol [Internet]. 2016:7. Available at: https://www.frontiersin.org. https://www.frontiersin.org/journals/microbiology/articles/10.3389/fmicb.2016.01031/full.
21. Edwards SM, Cunningham SA, Dunlop AL, Corwin EJ. The maternal gut microbiome during pregnancy. MCN Am J Matern Child Nurs. 2017;42(6):310.
22. Kour H, Andola S. The crucial link between gut health, mental well-being, and hormonal fluctuations in females. Indian J Health Sci Biomed Res kleu. 2024;17(3):311.
23. Zheng G, Victor Fon G, Meixner W, Creekmore A, Zong Y, Dame KM, et al. Chronic stress and intestinal barrier dysfunction: glucocorticoid receptor and transcription repressor HES1 regulate tight junction protein Claudin-1 promoter. Sci Rep. 2017;7(1):4502.
24. Gangestad SW, Caldwell Hooper AE, Eaton MA. On the function of placental corticotropin-releasing hormone: a role in maternal-fetal conflicts over blood glucose concentrations. Biol Rev Camb Philos Soc. 2012;87(4):856–73.
25. La Torre D, Van Oudenhove L, Vanuytsel T, Verbeke K. Psychosocial stress-induced intestinal permeability in healthy humans: what is the evidence? Neurobiol Stress. 2023;27:100579.
26. Fabiani H, Tan HT. The importance of dietary fiber on stress hormone in pregnancy: a literature review. J Midwifery. 2020;5(1):13–9.
27. Koren O, Goodrich JK, Cullender TC, Spor A, Laitinen K, Bäckhed HK, et al. Host Remodeling of the gut microbiome and metabolic changes during pregnancy. Cell. 2012;150(3):470–80.
28. Li M, Zhang G, Cui L, Zhang L, Zhou Q, Mu C, et al. Dynamic changes in gut microbiota during pregnancy among Chinese women and influencing factors: a prospective cohort study. Front Microbiol [Internet]. 2023:14. Available at: https://www.frontiersin.org. https://www.frontiersin.org/journals/microbiology/articles/10.3389/fmicb.2023.1114228/full.
29. Rubinstein MR, Burgueño AL, Quiroga S, Wald MR, Genaro AM. Current understanding of the roles of gut–brain axis in the cognitive deficits caused by perinatal stress exposure. Cells. 2023;12(13):1735.

30. Mepham J, Nelles-McGee T, Andrews K, Gonzalez A. Exploring the effect of prenatal maternal stress on the microbiomes of mothers and infants: a systematic review. Dev Psychobiol. 2023;65(7):e22424.
31. Ryan N, O'Mahony S, Leahy-Warren P, Philpott L, Mulcahy H. The impact of perinatal maternal stress on the maternal and infant gut and human milk microbiomes: a scoping review. PLoS One. 2025;20(2):e0318237.
32. Singh S, Sharma P, Pal N, Kumawat M, Shubham S, Sarma DK, et al. Impact of environmental pollutants on gut microbiome and mental health via the gut–brain axis. Microorganisms. 2022;10(7):1457.
33. Zijlmans MAC, Korpela K, Riksen-Walraven JM, de Vos WM, de Weerth C. Maternal prenatal stress is associated with the infant intestinal microbiota. Psychoneuroendocrinology. 2015;1(53):233–45.
34. Jiang Y, Greenwood-Van Meerveld B, Johnson AC, Travagli RA. Role of estrogen and stress on the brain-gut axis. Am J Physiol Gastrointest Liver Physiol. 2019;317(2):G203–9.
35. Morys J, Małecki A, Nowacka-Chmielewska M. Stress and the gut-brain axis: an inflammatory perspective. Front Mol Neurosci. 2024;17:1415567.
36. McGuire MK, McGuire MA. Human Milk: mother nature's prototypical probiotic food? Adv Nutr. 2015;6(1):112–23.
37. Rotem-Kohavi N, Keane J, Clarke G, Dinan TG, Cryan JF, McCarthy FP, et al. The microbiome-gut-brain axis: a new window to view the impact of prenatal stress on early neurodevelopment. In: Wazana A, Székely E, Oberlander TF, editors. Prenatal stress and child development [Internet]. Cham: Springer International Publishing; 2021. p. 165–91. Available at: https://doi.org/10.1007/978-3-030-60159-1_8.
38. Fan X, Zang T, Wu N, Liu J, Sun Y, Slack J, et al. The mediating effect of maternal gut microbiota between prenatal psychological distress and neurodevelopment of infants. J Affect Disord. 2024;362:893–902.
39. Park JC, Im SH. The gut-immune-brain axis in neurodevelopment and neurological disorders. Microbiome Res Rep. 2022;1(4):23.
40. Nuzum ND, Deady C, Kittel-Schneider S, Cryan JF, O'Mahony SM, Clarke G. More than just a number: the gut microbiota and brain function across the extremes of life. Gut Microbes. 2024;16(1):2418988.
41. Kimmel MC, Verosky B, Chen HJ, Davis O, Gur TL. The maternal microbiome as a map to understanding the impact of prenatal stress on offspring psychiatric health. Biol Psychiatry. 2024;95(4):300–9.
42. Sun Z, Lee-Sarwar K, Kelly RS, Lasky-Su JA, Litonjua AA, Weiss ST, et al. Revealing the importance of prenatal gut microbiome in offspring neurodevelopment in humans. eBioMedicine [Internet]. 2023;90. Available at: https://www.thelancet.com/journals/ebiom/article/PIIS2352-3964(23)00056-7/fulltext.
43. Yeramilli V, Cheddadi R, Shah J, Brawner K, Martin C. A review of the impact of maternal prenatal stress on offspring microbiota and metabolites. Meta. 2023;13(4):535.
44. Zhang X, Li Y, Pei Y, Yu C, Zhang X, Cao F. Association between maternal stress patterns and neonatal meconium microbiota: a prospective cohort study. J Affect Disord. 2025;383:59–68.
45. Osadchiy V, Martin CR, Mayer EA. The gut–brain axis and the microbiome: mechanisms and clinical implications. Clin Gastroenterol Hepatol. 2019;17(2):322–32.
46. Cerdó T, Nieto-Ruíz A, García-Santos JA, Rodríguez-Pöhnlein A, García-Ricobaraza M, Suárez A, et al. Current knowledge about the impact of maternal and infant nutrition on the development of the microbiota–gut–brain axis. Annu Rev Nutr. 2023;43:251–78.
47. Sherman MP, Zaghouani H, Niklas V. Gut microbiota, the immune system, and diet influence the neonatal gut–brain axis. Pediatr Res. 2015;77(1):127–35.
48. Mady EA, Doghish AS, El-Dakroury WA, Elkhawaga SY, Ismail A, El-Mahdy HA, et al. Impact of the mother's gut microbiota on infant microbiome and brain development. Neurosci Biobehav Rev. 2023;150:105195.

Oxytocin: The Protective Factor Against High Levels of Maternal Stress and Its Adverse Consequences

11

Kerstin Uvnäs Moberg, Magdalena Bolling, and Maria Petersson

Abstract

Oxytocin, an ancient substance from an evolutionary perspective, is produced in many locations and exerts a multitude of peripheral and central effects. It is produced in neurons of the supraoptic nucleus (SON) and paraventricular nucleus (PVN) within the hypothalamus. Oxytocin from magnocellular neurons of these nuclei is transported to the posterior pituitary and released into the circulation to exert hormonal effects. Oxytocin from the parvocellular neurons of the PVN release oxytocin within the brain to act as a neurotransmitter. Oxytocin is also produced in various peripheral organs, where it exerts local paracrine effects.

Female reproduction includes oocyte maturation, ovulation, fertilization, labor, birth, and breastfeeding. These diverse physiological processes are all facilitated by oxytocin. Oxytocin released into the circulation from the SON and PVN induces contractions of the uterine myometrium during labor and contractions of the myoepithelial cells in the mammary glands to induce milk ejection during breastfeeding. Oxytocin released from the parvocellular neurons within the brain increases the propensity for social interaction; decreases fear, pain, stress, and inflammation; and enhances calm and well-being as well as processes related to growth and restoration (the calm and connection response). This pattern of oxytocin effects, with some modifications, is induced

K. Uvnäs Moberg (✉)
Department of Animal Environment and Health, Section of Anthrozoology and Applied Ethology, Swedish University of Agricultural Sciences, Skara, Sweden

M. Bolling
Degree Programme in Nursing, Sophiahemmet University, Stockholm, Sweden

M. Petersson
Department of Endocrinology, Karolinska University Hospital and Department of Molecular Medicine and Surgery, Karolinska Institutet, Stockholm, Sweden

R. A. Caparros-Gonzalez (ed.), *Maternal Stress during Pregnancy and Postpartum*, https://doi.org/10.1007/978-3-032-09245-8_11

during all the different phases of female reproduction, i.e., pregnancy, labor, and breastfeeding. Skin-to-skin treatment between mother and newborn immediately after birth could be regarded as part of labor and is associated with a strong activation of oxytocin release in both mother and newborn, in particular of the parvocellular neurons that mediate the calm and connection response. The skin-to-skin contact relieves the stress of giving birth and of being born in mothers and newborns, respectively. The oxytocin release induced during skin-to-skin treatment is induced by activation of sensory cutaneous nerves originating in the chest region.

The central oxytocinergic effect pattern can be promoted/induced in situations perceived by the mother as supportive and safe, such as being in the presence of a trusted individual in a familiar environment. Conversely, oxytocin release is not stimulated in situations, which the mother perceives as unsupportive and unsafe. The oxytocin release induced by labor, breastfeeding, and skin-to-skin contact may even be inhibited under these circumstances.

Different types of stress can hinder reproduction, causing infertility and somatic as well as psychological complications during pregnancy and birth. High stress levels during pregnancy and labor may give rise to maternal mental health issues including maternal depression, anxiety, and posttraumatic stress disorder (PTSD). Additionally, stress can negatively impact fetal growth and development.

Specific clinical practices have been linked to better outcomes for mothers and babies in both the short and long-term perspective, including a reduced incidence of maternal mental issues. These practices include continuity of care which allows the mother to meet the same midwife during pregnancy, giving birth in a familiar environment, and having a supportive individual present during labor. Postpartum skin-to-skin contact, as well as other forms of extra touch and massage, may further contribute to positive outcomes. Additionally, well-functioning social relationships and social networks have been shown to be beneficial. All these practices are associated with an enhanced release/function of oxytocin.

In order to decrease the risk of stress reactions and of stress-related short - and long-term negative consequences for mother and baby, it is of importance to optimize oxytocin release during pregnancy, labor/birth, skin-to-skin contact, and breastfeeding. The use of the clinical practices that enhance oxytocin function which have been associated with a positive outcome and experience of labor and birth and which decrease the risk of maternal depression, anxiety, and PTSD should be recommended. Administration of synthetic oxytocin might be used in the future to prevent or treat short- and long-term negative consequences of stress during pregnancy and birth, but further studies are needed to prove this.

Keywords

Oxytocin · Antistress effects · Growth promotion · Reproduction · Pregnancy · Birth · Breastfeeding · Skin-to-skin · Sensory stimulation · Stress · Depression · PTSD · SGA

11.1 Introduction: Oxytocin and Female Reproduction

Oxytocin is a reproductive substance in a very broad sense and is involved in many aspects of female reproduction. It promotes fertility in several ways, and it facilitates oocyte maturation, ovulation, tubal transport of the eggs and implantation of the fertilized egg/embryo as well as growth of the fetus [1–6]. Oxytocin helps to adapt maternal physiology and behavior to the needs of pregnancy. During birth, oxytocin facilitates expulsion of the fetus by stimulating contractions of the uterine muscles. These effects are reinforced by pain, fear, and stress relieving effects exerted by oxytocin released in the brain [7]. Skin-to-skin contact between parent and child after birth is linked to a substantial release of oxytocin and an intense reduction of pain, fear, and stress levels and as well as to an increase of well-being, which facilitates bonding to the newborn [8]. Additionally, physiological functions related to promotion of growth are activated [9]. During breastfeeding circulating oxytocin is responsible for milk ejection. In addition, oxytocin reduces stress levels and adapts metabolic functions through peripheral and central actions [10, 11].

It follows from what is stated above that the release of oxytocin and oxytocin-mediated effects are of prime importance for an optimal function of female reproduction. Pregnancy, vaginal birth, skin-to-skin contact postpartum, and breastfeeding are all associated with a substantial release of oxytocin [7, 8, 10].

Fear, pain, and stress counteracts oxytocin release and may therefore hamper the function of the different phases of reproduction [12]. Severe stress may also increase the risk of maternal mental problems during pregnancy and postpartum, such as depression and PTSD [13]. As oxytocin reduces stress levels, stress can to a certain extent be reversed by enhancing the release of endogenous oxytocin [12]. Thereby the normal physiological functioning may be restored and the risk of long-term postpartum mental issues decreased.

The oxytocinergic effects may be reinforced by extra activation of cutaneous afferent nerves that trigger oxytocin release and its effects [14, 15]. In addition, familiar individuals and environments facilitate oxytocin release during the different phases of female reproduction. By contrast the presence of unfamiliar individuals and environments may unconsciously be interpreted as unsafe and is associated with a blockade of oxytocin release and effects [16, 17].

In this chapter, we will describe the basic function of the oxytocin system with a particular focus on the effects exerted during female reproduction. We will also describe how fear, stress, pain, and an unsafe environment may inhibit oxytocinergic activity and how oxytocin can counteract stress induced inhibition of oxytocin levels and effects. Finally, we will describe some of the clinical interventions that have been scientifically proven to facilitate different aspects of female reproduction and link them to an enhanced activity in the oxytocin system.

11.2 The Oxytocin System

11.2.1 Oxytocin

Oxytocin was originally (around 1900) discovered as the hormone responsible for stimulation of myometrial contractions during birth and of contractions of the mammary myoepithelial cells in connection with breastfeeding [18–20]. It has since then been discovered that oxytocin is not only a circulating hormone but also a neurotransmitter in the brain and a paracrine substance in peripheral organs [21]. The effect spectrum of oxytocin has been broadened, and in addition to the classical endocrine effects, we nowadays know that oxytocin has important central physiological and behavioral effects [16, 21, 22].

11.2.1.1 Chemistry of Oxytocin

Oxytocin is a peptide composed of nine amino acids, closely related in structure to antidiuretic hormone (ADH) also known as vasopressin [23, 24]. From an evolutionary standpoint, both substances are ancient, with variants present in primitive organisms. Similarly, the oxytocin receptor, a G-protein-coupled receptor, bearing resemblances to the vasopressin receptors, is archaic and has been well conserved throughout evolution [16, 21, 22].

11.2.1.2 The Oxytocinergic System

The majority of oxytocin is produced in neurons in the supraoptic (SON) and the paraventricular (PVN) nuclei of the hypothalamus. The hypothalamic oxytocin system comprises two parts: the magnocellular neurons of the SON and PVN which project to the posterior pituitary, wherefrom oxytocin passes into the circulation, and the parvocellular neurons in the PVN wherefrom oxytocinergic nerves project to several important regulatory areas within the brain and the brainstem. In addition, these regulatory areas receive innervation from axon-collaterals emanating from the magnocellular oxytocin neurons projecting to the posterior pituitary [21, 25–29].

The release of oxytocin into the circulation and from the oxytocinergic pathways in the brain may be activated together, or separately. In this way, oxytocin may coordinate different oxytocinergic effect patterns. Together the peripheral and central effects of oxytocin may be referred to as the oxytocinergic system [9].

11.2.2 Effects of Oxytocin

11.2.2.1 Effects of Circulating Oxytocin

Oxytocin is released into the bloodstream to stimulate contractions of the uterine myometrium and the myoepithelial cells in the mammary glands, thereby stimulating labor and milk ejection. These effects will be examined in greater detail in Sect. 11.3.

11.2.2.2 Effects of Oxytocin Through Neuronal Networks in the Brain

11.2.2.2.1 Oxytocin and Social Interaction and Well-Being

Social interaction can be divided into two distinct phases: the approach phase and the calming/relaxing phase, which both involve oxytocin from the PVN and SON. The structure of the social approach system, which involves gentle touch, activation of tachykinin neurons as well as a release of oxytocin and dopamine, has been extensively detailed [30, 31]. The calming/relaxing/antistress effects in response to touch and physical closeness during social interactions are induced by activation of cutaneous sensory nerves that activate a different subset of oxytocinergic nerves [12, 14, 15, 32]. These effects will be discussed in more depth below.

11.2.2.2.2 Oxytocin and Reduction of Fear, Pain, Stress, and Inflammation

The amygdala is activated in response to stressful stimuli. Corticotrophin-releasing factor (CRF) containing neurons originating in the amygdala projects to the locus coeruleus (LC), where CRF activates noradrenergic fibers. Then noradrenergic fibers, which project to the PVN, activate the CRF neurons which control the activity in the hypothalamo-pituitary-adrenal (HPA) axis and which participate in the regulation of the sympathetic nervous system [12].

Oxytocin inhibits the activity of the stress system by several mechanisms. Oxytocin reduces fear, by an effect in the amygdala. The central nucleus of the amygdala receives oxytocinergic fibers from the SON and PVN which decrease the alerting function of the amygdala by activating GABA-receptors. In addition, oxytocin from the SON and PVN inhibits the CRF-mediated activation of noradrenergic fibers in the LC and the noradrenergic activation of CRF neurons in the PVN thereby decreasing the activity in the stress system [12].

Furthermore, the activity of the HPA axis is modulated by oxytocinergic mechanisms at multiple levels. Oxytocin inhibits the secretion of CRF via a GABA receptor-mediated inhibition of the neurons that produce CRF in the PVN. Additionally, oxytocinergic fibers project to the median eminence, as well as to the anterior pituitary where they inhibit CRF-induced secretion of adrenocorticotrophic hormone (ACTH). Consequently, the release of cortisol from the adrenal gland is diminished [12].

Oxytocinergic fibers to the locus coeruleus (LC), preganglionic sympathetic ganglia, and the rostral ventrolateral medulla (RVLM) contribute to the inhibition of sympathetic nerve activity [12].

The pain-relieving effects of oxytocin are mainly mediated by oxytocinergic neurons that project to the amygdala, the periaqueductal grey (PAG), and the dorsal horns of the spinal cord. These effects are primarily mediated through the activation of opioidergic mu receptors and serotonin receptors. However, GABA-receptors may be involved as well [33, 34].

Oxytocin also exerts potent anti-inflammatory effects, where, for example, the levels of several cytokines are decreased. The anti-inflammatory effects of oxytocin are exerted within the PAG and the amygdala and also within the periphery where oxytocin in addition modulates immune responses, for example, through stimulating T cell-mediated immunity [34, 35].

11.2.2.2.3 Oxytocin and Stimulation of Growth and Activation of the Endocrine System of the Gastrointestinal Tract

Oxytocinergic fibers project to the nucleus tractus solitarius (NTS) and the dorsal vagal motor nucleus (DMX) in the brainstem [25–27]. This connection is significant because it allows the oxytocin system to activate vagal/parasympathetic pathways, which influence the activity of the endocrine system of the gastrointestinal tract, thereby stimulating digestive processes, anabolic metabolism, and growth. The impact of the endocrine system of the gastrointestinal tract on anabolic functions and growth is particularly crucial during early development. A key mechanism by which oxytocin influences the endocrine system of the gastrointestinal tract is through a vagally mediated inhibition of the extensive somatostatin system in the gastrointestinal tract, which suppresses digestive and metabolic/anabolic functions [9]. Consequently, oxytocin enhances the function of the endocrine system of the gastrointestinal tract by reducing the inhibitory somatostatinergic tone. This connection between oxytocin and the vagal system is fundamentally important during reproductive processes and in early life as it facilitates growth and restorative functions [9]. Additionally, there are oxytocin receptors in several of the hypothalamic brain areas that are involved in feeding and satiety. For example, oxytocin receptors are present in both the ventromedial hypothalamic nucleus and the arcuate nucleus [36].

11.2.2.2.4 The CRF System and the Oxytocin System Oppose Each Other

The oxytocinergic system and the CRF system originating from the PVN form a Yin Yang system, as they exert opposing effects. When the CRF system is activated, stress levels rise through the HPA axis and the sympathetic nervous system, while vagal nerve activity is reduced, inducing a mini variant of the "fight or flight response." Conversely, activation of the oxytocinergic fibers inhibits both the HPA axis and the sympathetic nervous system thereby decreasing stress levels. In addition, it enhances the activity of the vagal fibers which are connected to the endocrine system of the gastrointestinal tract, thereby promoting growth and restoration. This effect pattern will be referred to as the "calm and connection response." As the CRF and oxytocin fibers, exerting opposite effects, run in parallel to the regulatory areas mentioned above, the system receiving the strongest stimulation will dominate, and in addition it will diminish the effect of the other system [9, 12, 14].

11.2.3 Activation of Oxytocin Release

11.2.3.1 Oxytocin Release by Hormones

Oxytocin is released by other hormones and by sensory stimulation. Estrogen is the most important endocrine stimulator of oxytocin synthesis and release and also of the synthesis/function of oxytocin receptors. The role of estrogen will be discussed in more detail in Sect. 11.3 of this chapter.

11.2.3.2 Oxytocin Release in Response to Sensory Stimulation

11.2.3.2.1 Activation of Oxytocin Release in Response to the Ferguson and Suckling Reflex

The Ferguson reflex and the suckling reflex are activated in connection with labor/birth and lactation, respectively. Both these types of sensory stimulation give rise to a pulsatile release of oxytocin, which is associated with coordinated electrical activity in the magnocellular neurons of the SON and PVN. The Ferguson reflex is mediated by somatic sensory afferents and parasympathetic afferents from the uterus and the suckling reflex by a special type of sensory, cutaneous nerves from the nipples [7, 10, 21]. Oxytocin may also be released in response to the activation of sensory nerves from the skin, in particular in response to stroking, light pressure, and warmth. This oxytocin release is, however, never pulsatile and may particularly involve the parvocellular neurons in the PVN [9, 14, 15, 32].

11.2.3.2.2 Food Intake Releases Oxytocin via Activation of Vagal Nerve Afferents

The release of oxytocin is also promoted by food intake. The gastrointestinal hormone cholecystokinin is released from the mucosa in the duodenum in particular in response to proteins and fat. Cholecystokinin activates afferent vagal nerve activity which in turn stimulates the release of oxytocin [9].

Vagally mediated information about food intake is mandatory for oxytocin release. This was demonstrated in experiments in which the abdominal vagal nerve was cut in lactating animals. Within a few days, oxytocin levels did not rise in response to suckling, the levels of prolactin which stimulates milk production decreased, and milk production eventually disappeared. In this situation the lack of the calorie-dependent vagal input to the brain was interpreted as starvation (in spite of the fact that the dams continued to eat). As a life-saving measure, oxytocin levels and milk production were inhibited [36, 37].

Interestingly, oxytocin levels in human mothers are positively related to the weight of the newborn and inversely correlated with maternal somatostatin levels, the gastrointestinal hormone that blocks the activity of the endocrine system of the gastrointestinal tract, which is of such prime importance for processes related to reproduction and growth (see above). This effect is achieved by oxytocinergic mechanisms in the brain. One important mechanism by which oxytocin increases the function of the endocrine system of the gastrointestinal tract is by decreasing the activity of the somatostatin brake via effects of oxytocin released within the DMX and NTS. In this way, the ratio between oxytocin and somatostatin levels becomes an important measure of anabolic activity [9, 37, 38].

Warm pleasant temperature, e.g., mediated by skin contact, stimulates oxytocin release, and its effects. Interestingly, the skin overlying the chest is innervated by a particular type of afferent sensory fibers which join the afferent vagal nerves and stimulate the release of oxytocin [8, 39, 40]. Perhaps both mother and newborn experience and interpret warm chest skin temperature of "the other" as a sign of vitality and thereby safety. Cold skin temperature may on the other hand be interpreted as a sign of "lack of energy" and may in analogy to lack of food via a decreased activity in vagal afferents inhibit oxytocin release. Without information about available resources (lack of food or lack of warmth) the production and release of oxytocin is blocked [8, 9].

11.2.3.2.3 Activation of the Oxytocin and the CRF System by Stimulation of Cutaneous Sensory Nerves

Stimulation of sensory nerves from the skin affects the CRF and the oxytocin systems in the PVN. Painful (noxious) stimulation gives rise to activation of the CRF neurons via axon collaterals, which project to the PVN within the hypothalamus, from pain-mediating fibers, before these nerves reach the thalamus and the sensory cortex, where the sense of pain is recognized. In addition, the oxytocin or "the calm and connection system" can be activated by sensory fibers responding to light pressure, stroking, and warm, pleasant temperature (non-noxious stimulation). In analogy with the pain mediating fibers, the fibers inducing "the calm and connection response" stimulate the release of oxytocin by axon reflexes from sensory nerves, before they reach their terminal areas. Note that these basic, almost archaic reaction patterns, triggered by activation of cutaneous sensory nerves, are induced at a very basal level in the brain, i.e., before the conscious experience of fear, stress or pain, or calm/relaxation. CRF and oxytocin release induced by cutaneous sensory stimulation and their respective effect patterns can, however, be reinforced at a later stage in response to the emotional experience of either type of stimulation [9, 12, 14].

11.2.3.2.4 Activation via the Amygdala Hippocampal Pathway

The CRF and parvocellular oxytocin neurons in the PVN also receive innervation from the hippocampus/amygdala/bed nucleus of the stria terminalis (BNST), which can result in "the fight-flight" or "the calm and connection responses." Stimuli reflecting danger, unsafety, and distrust will trigger CRF secretion and mental stimuli reflecting safety, trust, and support, but also resources and warmth will trigger oxytocin secretion [12, 16, 17].

The signaling in the hippocampal/amygdala/BNST pathway also serves as a gating mechanism for other types of oxytocin release by sensory stimulation. If the central oxytocinergic pathway is activated, the oxytocin-mediated effects induced by stimulation of sensory nerves will be reinforced. By contrast, if the surrounding is interpreted as unsafe, even by minor stressors such as unfamiliarity, the oxytocin release induced by sensory stimulation from peripheral sensory nerves, e.g., the suckling and Ferguson reflexes, will be reduced [41–44]. In situations of danger, the oxytocin effect profile may be completely turned around and oxytocin may induce defense and stress effects [45, 46].

11.3 Oxytocin and Its Effects During Pregnancy, Parturition, and Postpartum

11.3.1 Pregnancy

11.3.1.1 Role of Estrogen

During pregnancy, plasma oxytocin levels increase three- to fourfold, primarily due to elevated estrogen levels. Estrogen significantly increases the number of oxytocin receptors in the uterine mucosa, reaching a peak at term where the receptor count can rise by 100 to 1000 times compared to pre-pregnancy levels. In addition, central oxytocin receptors are upregulated by estrogen thereby facilitating oxytocin-mediated maternal adaptive behaviors [47–50].

Estrogen increases the activity of certain oxytocinergic nerve bundles originating from the PVN which influence some aspects of vagal (parasympathetic) and of sympathetic nervous activity. The oxytocin-mediated activation of vagal nerve activity enhances the function of the endocrine system of the gastrointestinal tract which enables the efficient utilization of ingested calories for metabolic and anabolic functions, thereby potentially supporting early maternal weight gain. Generally, a mother's weight increases by 3–4 kg during the first trimester of pregnancy without a notable increase in fetal weight. The decreased activity in the sympathetic nervous system may be associated with the pronounced reduction in maternal blood pressure that takes place in early pregnancy [38] (perhaps involving an oxytocin-induced increase in nitric oxide (NO) [51]. Later during pregnancy, the mother develops further physiological adaptations that facilitate the transfer of nutrients to the fetus.

11.3.2 Labor and Birth

Oxytocin induces numerous effects that facilitate labor and birth, operating through its circulating impact on the myometrium as well as via various neural mechanisms in the brain.

11.3.2.1 Release of Oxytocin into the Circulation

During pregnancy, the occurrence of oxytocin pulses is inhibited by an opioidergic mechanism. This inhibition is lifted with the onset of labor due to decreasing levels of the neurosteroid pregnanolone, a metabolite of progesterone [21]. The reduction of this opioidergic inhibition allows oxytocin levels to pulse, which subsequently initiates myometrial contractions via activation of oxytocin receptors on the uterine muscles. The frequency and magnitude of oxytocin pulses gradually increase, reaching 3 pulses per 10 min just before birth [52, 53].

Additionally, oxytocin is released from a subset of oxytocin producing cells in the decidua and membranes. This locally produced oxytocin activates a subset of oxytocin receptors that stimulate the production and release of prostaglandins and other inflammatory substances from special cells in the decidua and membranes. These substances promote labor by reinforcing contractions and facilitating cervical dilation through tissue breakdown [54].

11.3.2.1.1 The Ferguson Reflex

The release of oxytocin during labor is reinforced by the Ferguson reflex, which is triggered by the pressure exerted by the fetus on the cervix, thereby activating most importantly parasympathetic sensory nerves. Consequently, a positive feed-forward reflex is initiated; as oxytocin release increases, contractions become stronger, further enhancing the release of oxytocin [21].

11.3.2.2 Release of Oxytocin in the Brain

11.3.2.2.1 Parasympathetic Nervous Activity Induces Uterine Contractions

The autonomic nervous system plays an important role in the process of labor. A subset of parvocellular oxytocinergic fibers from the PVN innervates parasympathetic/cholinergic ganglia in the lumbosacral region. Stimulation of parasympathetic nerves results in myometrial contractions and an increase in local blood flow. The release of oxytocin into the circulation and the activation of oxytocinergic nerves to the lumbosacral region are coordinated and thereby their effect on myometrial contractions. Activation of the sympathetic nervous system induces a distinct type of contraction that is more prolonged and presumably more painful and associated with reduced uterine blood flow [55].

The fact that the autonomic nervous system may induce uterine contractions by itself could explain why some animal studies suggest oxytocin is not necessary for labor. In such cases, the autonomic nervous system might be responsible for the stimulation of myometrial contractions [56].

Experimental studies have shown that uterine contractions can be induced either by oxytocin infusions or autonomic nerve stimulation alone in a dose-dependent manner. Researchers identified a dose of oxytocin and a type of nerve stimulation that did not induce contractions on their own. However, when these two inactive treatments were combined, uterine contractions resumed. These findings imply that parasympathetic, cholinergic nerve activity additionally influences oxytocin receptors in the myometrium, making them more sensitive to oxytocin [54, 57, 58].

The possibility of enhancing the effect of circulating oxytocin on uterine contractions via an increased function of oxytocin receptors has notable clinical implications, as mental support and physical touch and closeness in connection with birth increase parasympathetic nervous activity via oxytocinergic fibers from the PVN. This may explain why social support during birth promotes labor and even shortens the duration of labor [59]. This phenomenon will be further discussed in Sect. 11.5.

11.3.2.2.2 Maternal Behavior and Bonding

Oxytocin released within the brain during labor plays a crucial role in facilitating the development of maternal behavior. Experimental studies in sheep have demonstrated that mothers administered oxytocin antagonists or epidural anesthesia, which block or counteract the Ferguson reflex, did not develop maternal behavior and bonding with their offspring unless additional oxytocin was administered, or additional oxytocin release was triggered [46, 60].

11.3.2.2.3 Decreased Fear, Pain, and Stress and Increased Well-Being and Bonding

During labor, oxytocinergic fibers that decrease levels of fear, stress, and pain are activated in response to the Ferguson reflex. Additionally, the reward center and the release of dopamine are activated, particularly toward the end of labor. Dopamine is released to promote the mother's well-being and facilitates bonding between the mother and her newborn [7, 54].

Women do not express a preprogrammed maternal behavior, like other mammals do. However, studies in women demonstrate that vaginal birth promotes the interest in social interaction and closeness and decreases the levels of anxiety, as expressed in personality inventories. These effects are not observed in mothers who had an acute Cesarean section, which does not involve oxytocin release. Epidural analgesia, which partially blocks the Ferguson reflex, is also associated with a reduced development of these maternal mental adaptations [7, 54, 61–63].

11.3.2.2.4 Afferent Stimulation of Sympathetic Nerves Causes Stress, Fear, and Pain

Afferent sympathetic nerves are activated during labor and birth. These nerves undergo intense stimulation, particularly in response to prolonged and frequent contractions of the myometrium. Such contractions give rise to reduced levels of oxygen, nutrients, and a lowered pH in the myometrial tissue and are associated with activation of CRF release in the PVN with enhanced sympathetic nerve activity and reduced levels of oxytocin. This can result in increased perception of pain and in elevated levels of fear and stress, which may in turn negatively impact the oxytocin release and the progress of labor [7, 21, 54].

11.3.2.2.5 The Afferent Parasympathetic (Ferguson) and Sympathetic Nerve Activity Counteract and Inhibit Each Other's Activity

As discussed in the previous section, the balance between the activity of CRF neurons and oxytocin neurons from the PVN is crucial for regulating levels of fear, pain, and stress. When Ferguson afference is stronger compared to sympathetic afference input, oxytocinergic activity is enhanced, which positively impacts the progress of labor and reduces the experience of fear, stress, and pain [7, 12, 21, 54].

The balance between the activity in the CRF, the sympathetic nervous system, and the oxytocinergic system not only influences the progress of labor but also affects the overall experience of birth. When oxytocinergic activity is high, the birth experience tends to be more positive. This may be attributed to a decreased activity in systems associated with fear, pain, and stress, as well as to an activation of dopaminergic mechanisms and the reward system. It is also known that oxytocin influences the experience of birth in the long term, as it causes an amnesic effect or a diminishment of the memory of birth pain [7, 12, 21, 54, 64]. Supportive evidence comes from studies indicating that mothers who have received analgesia during childbirth—linked to a reduced activation of central oxytocinergic mechanisms—do not experience this reduction in pain perception after birth to the same extent as mothers who have given birth without such interventions [65].

A subpopulation of oxytocinergic fibers projecting from the PVN to the amygdala has been shown to block mechanisms by which the experience of labor pain is transferred into memories via hippocampal mechanisms [66, 67]. In this way, the release of oxytocin during labor may actively counteract the formation of negative memories of childbirth that might otherwise occur. These data suggest that normal physiological birth involves oxytocinergic mechanisms, which reduce the likelihood of negative experiences during birth and of negative memories of childbirth. The activation of such oxytocin-dependent protective mechanisms may lower the risk of postpartum maternal mental health issues such as postpartum depression and PTSD.

11.3.2.2.6 The Fetus

The frequency and strength of contractions during labor are also significant from the perspective of the fetus. Increased frequency and longer duration of contractions can reduce blood flow to the fetus, which might negatively impact its behavior and physiology.

The fetus has its own oxytocin system which is activated during birth. Babies born by vaginal delivery have higher levels of oxytocin in the umbilical cord than those born by planned Cesarean section, demonstrating that fetal oxytocin is released during labor. Research indicates that the fetus benefits from oxytocin-mediated pain relief and anti-inflammatory effects during labor. In fact, the higher the newborn's stress levels are, the higher its oxytocin levels, indicating that oxytocin levels adapt to stress levels [7, 53, 68, 69].

11.3.3 Skin-to-Skin Contact After Birth

Skin-to-skin contact between mothers and newborns is part of the normal physiological process of birth, and it is associated with stimulation of oxytocin release in both. When placed on the mother's chest, the newborn exhibits an innate crawling behavior and begins suckling within 90 min after birth [70]. Both the newborn's tactile interaction with the mother and the suckling stimulate maternal oxytocin release, which in turn enhance maternal interaction and caregiving behaviors toward the newborn [8, 10, 71–73]. Essentially, the newborn seeks both nourishment and care through this instinctive approach.

Maternal chest skin temperature begins to fluctuate during skin-to-skin contact, due to oxytocin-induced dilation of the cutaneous blood vessels. This, together with an increase in skin temperature, activates the newborn's oxytocin system in a temperature-dependent manner. The more the mother's temperature fluctuates and rises, the greater the newborn's rise in skin temperature and reduction in stress levels [74].

Skin-to-skin contact is linked to a reduction in fear, pain, stress, and inflammation in both parents and newborns. Furthermore, the reward center with dopamine release promotes bonding between mother and newborn. Activation of vagal/parasympathetic mechanisms enhances maternal milk production and supports infant growth, as discussed in detail in the preceding section. All these effects are mediated by oxytocin released from parvocellular neurons in the PVN in response to the activation of cutaneous sensory nerves in response to physical closeness between the parent and newborn [8, 71–75].

The significant release of oxytocin during postpartum skin-to-skin contact alleviates the stress associated with childbirth for both mother and child [71–75]. This practice is also vital for long-term development in both mother and newborn by enhancing social interaction skills and the ability to manage stress over time [76]. Additionally, postpartum skin-to-skin contact mediates protection against future negative maternal mental health conditions, such as maternal depression [76–79].

11.3.4 Breastfeeding

Although breastfeeding is not the central topic of this article, it is important to note that breastfeeding not only stimulates milk ejection and production but is also linked to significant antistress effects, and it promotes growth and well-being for both mother and newborn [10, 11]. The substantial and repeated release of oxytocin within the brain during breastfeeding has long-term antistress benefits for the mother and reduces the risk of postpartum maternal mental health issues. In addition, breastfeeding decreases the mother's future risk of developing cardiovascular disease such as type 2 diabetes, stroke, heart infarction, and hypertension [10, 11, 80].

11.4 Stress and Female Reproduction

11.4.1 Pregnancy

Fertilization does not occur in case the maternal fat depots are too small, and pregnancy is a demanding process from a nutritional perspective. Around 100,000 extra calories are needed during pregnancy. A number of maternal physiological and metabolic "saving" mechanisms are activated during pregnancy to optimize digestion and storing of ingested nutrients. In case the pregnant mother receives too little energy, the CCK-mediated facilitation of oxytocin release is withdrawn. The mother may reduce her own energy expenditure in order to provide the fetus with nutrition. If this "strategy"is not sufficient, she may reduce the transfer of nutrients to the fetus with negative consequences for fetal growth and development [9, 12, 38]. As a worst-case scenario, premature labor might be induced.

It is not uncommon for mothers to experience stress during pregnancy. Some reasons for maternal stress during pregnancy are described in other chapters of this book. Irrespective of the type of stressor the "same" maternal stress system is activated. This may include activation of the CRF neurons in the amygdala, which then enhances noradrenergic activity in the locus coeruleus (LC) including activation of the parvocellular CRF neurons in the PVN and consequent activation of the HPA axis and the sympathetic nervous system. Such activation of the stress system will give rise to a decreased function of the central oxytocinergic neurons and a decrease in the endocrine system of the gastrointestinal tract and anabolic metabolism and growth in a broad sense [9, 11, 12, 38]. At the same time, it may increase sympathetic nervous tone which may induce a decrease in blood flow to the placenta and the fetus. In this way retardation of fetal growth may occur, and in addition the fetal cortisol levels may rise [81]. Fetal stress will be discussed in another chapter of this book.

11.4.1.1 Premature Birth as a Consequence of Stress During Pregnancy

Many animal species end their pregnancies in response to extreme stress. The stressors may involve dangers in the environment, lack of food, or even abandonment. In some species, the mothers may abort or even absorb their fetuses in order to save themselves. It is possible that also human mothers may give birth prematurely as a response to overwhelming environmental or severe nutritional stress.

The mechanism behind premature labor is not fully known, but it has been suggested that the stress-related release of cortisol together with an increase in cytokines may induce a change in the estradiol/progesterone ratio and a premature disruption of the opioidergic inhibition of the pulsatile oxytocin release, a prerequisite for initiation of birth [21, 81].

11.4.1.2 Familiarity and Safety Versus Unfamiliarity and Unsafety

Continuous interaction with familiar and trusted individuals within and outside the family is associated with repeated activation of the oxytocinergic system. Such interaction may involve physical touch as well as a direct effect on oxytocin release by the presence of familiar individuals and surroundings [9, 17]. Specific nerve fibers have been identified in the frontal cortex, which respond to such stimuli [16]. In contrast, unfamiliar individuals and environments induce stress and may even cause an inhibition of the release of oxytocin induced by sensory stimulation, during labor, birth, suckling, and skin-to-skin contact [41–45].

11.4.2 Labor-Birth

Complicated, long-lasting labor, often associated with frequent and intense myometrial contractions, may be associated with myometrial hypoxia. As a consequence, afferent sympathetic nervous fibers will be activated, and the mother may experience severe pain, fear, and stress, and she may become exhausted. In addition, the activity in the oxytocinergic system with its fear, pain, and stress-reducing capacity will be counteracted, which will contribute to the mother's negative experiences of birth and potentially negatively impact the process of birth. Memories of the experience of pain, fear, and stress may in some cases be translated into mental depression or anxiety disorders postpartum [7, 12, 13, 54].

A difficult labor/birth may be associated with damage to the fetus, e.g., due to hypoxia caused by reduced placental circulation.

11.4.3 Absence of Skin-to-Skin Contact and Social Interaction Postpartum

Separation between mother and newborn causes distress in the newborn. For example, a newborn baby that is put in skin-to-skin after birth doesn't cry, whereas separated babies do until they are placed in skin-to-skin contact [82]. Obviously, the need for closeness is strong in newborns after birth. Without the skin-to-skin contact after birth, much less oxytocin will be released with a consequent reduction of oxytocin-induced effects in both parents and newborns in the postpartum period. The psychophysiological "deficiency state" induced in newborns who are not allowed skin-to-skin contact immediately after birth with possible negative long-term effects has been labeled toxic stress [83, 84].

11.4.3.1 Lack of Physical Contact in Infancy

A similar long-term deficiency state may be induced in infants who are deprived of physical and social contact during infancy. Such deprivation may significantly impact the development of social functioning and the ability to handle stress in the child. Additionally, growth and development may be delayed, and the risk for serious infections may increase [84, 85].

Consequences of oxytocin deficiencies are shown in the table below (Table 11.1).

Table 11.1 Consequences of oxytocin deficiency

Absence of skin-to-skin contact between mother and newborn postpartum
No skin-to-skin induced release of oxytocin
Reduced oxytocin-induced stimulation of social interaction between mother and infant
Delayed bonding between mother and infant
Reduced oxytocin-induced reduction of levels of pain, fear, stress, and inflammation
Reduced oxytocin-induced increase of well-being
Delayed weight gain and growth
Delayed onset of suckling, reduced milk production, and shorter duration of breastfeeding
Sleep problems
Reduced long-term stimulation of social interactive skills in mother and newborn and of reduction of stress levels in the newborn
Absence of breastfeeding
Reduced stimulation of the oxytocin system and of consequent oxytocin-mediated effects, e.g., protection against maternal postpartum depression and anxiety disorders
Absence of physical interaction during the first years of life
Failure to thrive
Reduced weight gain
Hampered development of social skills
Enhanced stress levels
High mortality due to infections

11.5 Maternal Depression, Anxiety, and PTSD

11.5.1 General Aspects of Depression and Anxiety-Related Disorders Including Posttraumatic Stress Disorder (PTSD)

11.5.1.1 Depression

Depression is more common in women than in men. Studies have shown that around 15–20% of all women will have a depression at some point during their lifetime. The pathophysiology of depression has been debated and is likely multifactorial. Factors such as heredity, previous life events, stress, diseases, endocrine disorders, and previous experience of trauma might all be involved. Many neurotransmitter systems in the brain have been connected to depression, serotonin, noradrenaline, and dopamine being the three most well-known and most medical treatments for depression are designed to modify the function of these systems. Other neurotransmitters, such as glutamate, GABA, and oxytocin have also been suggested to play a role in the expression of depression. In addition, the female sex steroids are associated with depression and mood changes. For example, progesterone has been associated with premenstrual syndrome, whereas its precursor, pregnanolone, and its metabolite, allopregnanolone, both seem to give rise to antidepressant effects [86].

Bipolar disorder is characterized by changes in mood from deep depression to mania and experiences of tirelessness. Unbalances of the same neurotransmitters as discussed in relation to depression seem to be involved in bipolar disorder. Bipolar disorder might deteriorate during pregnancy [86].

11.5.1.2 Anxiety-Related Symptoms and Disorders

Anxiety-related disorders are characterized by avoidance, fear, physical symptoms such as heart palpitations and sweating, and sometimes also panic attacks. There is a close relation to different degrees of obsessions and even obsessive-compulsive disorders (OCD). Disturbances in the function of serotonin and dopamine are involved in these disorders too, but especially an imbalance between glutamate and GABA seems to be important here. Pharmacological treatment is similar to that used in depression but also involves benzodiazepines, which affect GABA receptors.

11.5.1.3 PTSD

Posttraumatic stress disorder may ensue following experience of particularly traumatic situations. Typical physiological symptoms include difficulties to sleep, high blood pressure, tachycardia, mood changes, irritability, and memory impairment, as well as the characteristic flashbacks of memories and avoidance of things and situations which could be related to the earlier trauma. Aberrations in the function of several neurotransmitter systems such as noradrenaline and serotonin have been implicated, along with a changed reactivity of the HPA axis.

Some studies indicate that women with PTSD and other general anxiety disorders may improve during pregnancy. However, they have an increased risk of developing gestational diabetes and preeclampsia. They also have an increased risk of giving birth to babies that are small for gestational age (SGA) [87].

11.5.1.4 Role of Oxytocin

Plasma levels of oxytocin are lower in women with anxiety-like disorders including PTSD and sometimes in women with depression than in healthy controls [88]. These data suggest that the function of the oxytocin system is deficient in these mental diseases.

In animal studies, oxytocin administration has been found to have anti-depressant, anxiolytic, and stress-reducing effects. Oxytocin induces effects comparable to those produced by the administration of serotonin reuptake inhibitors (SSRIs). These effects of oxytocin may be mediated by an increase in serotonin and dopamine levels. Conversely, the administration of selective serotonin reuptake inhibitors (SSRIs) may lead to an increase in oxytocin levels through the activation of 5-HT1 receptors. The symptom relief observed in patients with obsessive-compulsive disorder (OCD) treated with SSRIs can in part be attributed to the increased secretion of oxytocin resulting from elevated serotonin levels [89].

Intranasal administration of oxytocin has in some studies been reported to improve the symptoms of depression [90].

11.5.2 Maternal Blues, Depression, and PTSD in the Postpartum Period

The postpartum period is associated with an increased risk of development of certain maternal mental disorders such as maternal blues and maternal depression as well as anxiety disorders and PTSD.

11.5.2.1 Maternal Blues

Maternal blues, also called postpartum blues, is common and occurs in up to 85% of all women postpartum. The symptoms are mild and characterized by sadness and they decline within 2 weeks. Postpartum blues is associated with the sudden drop in the levels of sex steroid hormones which are substantially increased during pregnancy. In addition, oxytocin levels, which are increased in response to the high estrogen levels during pregnancy and peak during parturition, may decline postpartum. The fatigue associated with delivery in the early postpartum period also contributes to the development of postpartum blues.

11.5.2.1.1 Effects of Oxytocin

Skin-to-skin contact between the mother and the newborn immediately after birth, as well as frequent breastfeeding, situations which are linked to oxytocin release in the mother, has been shown to decrease the risk of postpartum blues [77, 79, 80]. In addition, intranasal administration of oxytocin has been shown to relieve the symptoms of maternal blues [91]. The fact that both skin-to-skin contact between mother and newborn and breastfeeding, which are associated with elevated oxytocin levels, and intranasal administration of exogenous oxytocin relieves the symptoms of maternal blues underscores the important role of oxytocin as a treatment for maternal blues.

11.5.2.2 Postpartum Depression

The incidence of postpartum depression is about 10–15% of all women giving birth [92]. This type of depression usually begins within 2–3 months postpartum and is characterized by more severe symptoms compared to maternal blues. The symptoms are the same as in general depression, together with anxiety and worries about the child and/or about harming the child. The symptoms can persist for months and even years if not treated [93]. It is important to treat maternal depression, as it has been shown to negatively impact the mother's interaction and bonding with her child and the psychological development of the child. First-line treatment options are counseling and psychotherapy. Second-line treatment is the same as for general depression but clinical studies with allopregnanolone treatment are ongoing [93, 94].

11.5.2.2.1 Role and Effects of Oxytocin

An important role of oxytocin in postpartum depression has been demonstrated in animal experiments. In a model of postpartum depression, a reduction of both oxytocin immunoreactivity and oxytocin receptors was demonstrated within the ventrotegmental area. High maternal oxytocin levels indicating a high production of oxytocin seem to protect against maternal blues and postpartum depression. For example, low plasma levels of oxytocin in the last trimester of pregnancy were found to be associated with an increased risk of developing postpartum depression. In addition, in postpartum mothers, oxytocin levels correlated negatively with both anxiety as well as depression scores [94–97].

Stimulation of endogenous oxytocin release by physical contact and support during pregnancy and labor and by skin-to-skin contact after birth as well as breastfeeding has been shown to reduce the occurrence of maternal depression [77–80, 96]. However, administration of intranasal oxytocin spray has not shown convincing effects in the treatment of postpartum depression [90, 97].

11.5.2.3 Postpartum PTSD

A specific type of postpartum traumatic stress disorder may follow a traumatic childbirth, when the mothers have experienced birth as linked to strong experiences of fear, pain, and stress. As intense stress may inhibit oxytocin release and production [12], it is easy to assume that the release of endogenous oxytocin might have been disrupted during a traumatic childbirth. Factors that have been shown to protect against maternal postpartum PTSD include the mother's self-determination, administration of pain relief, as well as support by a doula [98].

Previous experiences of stress, in particular during pregnancy, predispose for PTSD postpartum. Animals that had been exposed to stress during pregnancy had higher corticosterone levels during lactation. The animals were primed for a defensive reaction which impacted lactation and nurturing of the offspring [99].

11.5.2.4 Treatment of Postpartum Depression and PTSD with Oxytocin

As already discussed, women with general PTSD may improve during pregnancy and breastfeeding, suggesting that the rise of oxytocin during these phases of reproduction exerts positive effects on the symptoms of PTSD.

In addition, mothers with low oxytocin levels and high levels of methylation of the oxytocin receptors (indicating low oxytocin receptor function) had increased incidence of postnatal depression as well as symptoms of anxiety [100].

Given the fact that a stressful event often precedes the development of both maternal depression and PTSD and that stress inhibits oxytocin production and release, it is reasonable to assume that the activity of the oxytocin system is hampered in these conditions [12]. Indeed, oxytocin levels have been shown to be reduced in PTSD and sometimes in maternal depression, as evidenced by several studies [88]. A low function in the oxytocin system would inevitably be linked to reduced levels of social interaction, well-being and mood, increased levels of fear, pain, stress, and inflammation, which are all part of the oxytocin effect spectrum.

Therefore, it might be assumed that administration of exogenous oxytocin could alleviate the symptoms of depression and anxiety, including PTSD. Some studies, but definitely not all, show that administration of oxytocin as a nasal spray decreases stress levels and symptoms of depression [90]. Given the questionable penetration of oxytocin over the blood-brain barrier into the brain after intranasal administration and the ability of oxytocin, probably via different receptor populations, to exert opposing effects on some stress-related variables, these contrasting findings are not surprising [54]. In some individuals, oxytocin spray may give rise to functional oxytocin levels in the brain and thereby therapeutic effects and in some not.

In conclusion, several of the effects of oxytocin may contribute to the positive effects on maternal postpartum mental disorders, not only the antistress effects but also the anti-inflammatory effects and in addition the stimulation of the reward center and dopamine release [12, 16, 21]. Some antidepressive agents including serotonin uptake inhibitors exert part of their effect by oxytocin release, as there is a close relationship between oxytocin and serotonin function [89].

An alternative way to obtain the protective/healing oxytocin effects is to allow and promote maximal amount of physical contact and social support during all the phases of female reproduction, i.e., during pregnancy, birth, skin-to-skin contact after birth, and breastfeeding. It is also important to optimize the release and function of the oxytocin system during these different phases by providing an environment that is perceived as familiar and safe. By keeping these interventions in mind, we may be able to prevent stress during pregnancy and birth and thereby minimize the development of postpartum depression and anxiety disorders.

11.6 Clinical Practices That Support Female Reproduction and Prevent Negative Long-Term Consequences in Mothers and Newborns by Enhancing Oxytocin Release and Effects

It can be anticipated from the previous paragraphs that the effects of several of the stressors that negatively impact the different phases of female reproduction can be diminished or counteracted by oxytocin. Spontaneous release of endogenous oxytocin during the different phases of female reproduction, pregnancy, vaginal birth, skin-to-skin contact postpartum, and breastfeeding plays an important role. In addition, the physiological release of maternal oxytocin can be reinforced. This can, e.g., be achieved by some clinical practices, such as attendance of the mother by the same midwife during pregnancy and the presence of a supportive and trusted person during birth, and by providing extra massage to the mother during pregnancy or by baby massage postpartum. Oxytocin release and effects can also be promoted by minimizing the exposure to stress, which inhibits oxytocin release. Even slight stressors, such as unfamiliar places and individuals, which may be experienced as unsafe by the mother, should be avoided as they are associated with inhibition of oxytocin release.

11.6.1 Optimizing Physiological Release of Oxytocin to Facilitate Pregnancy and Labor and to Prevent Long-Term Negative Consequences in Mother and Infant Postpartum

11.6.1.1 Vaginal Birth

The release of oxytocin into the circulation with effects on uterine contractions and the release of oxytocin into the brain with behavioral and physiological effects were described in detail in Sect. 11.3. Women who have had a vaginal birth describe themselves as more socially interactive and less anxious after birth as observed by personality inventories, and these effects correlate with maternal oxytocin release in response to breastfeeding 2 days after birth [7, 61–63].

11.6.1.1.1 Medical Interventions During Birth

The use of medical interventions such as planned Cesarean section, epidural analgesia, and oxytocin infusions to initiate or augment labor is becoming more common. These interventions are aimed at increasing the survival of mother and fetus and at reducing pain during labor. However, such interventions may also influence the function of the endogenous oxytocin system with some negative behavioral and physiological consequences.

11.6.1.1.2 Cesarean Section

Cesarean section may be life-saving for mother and baby. A planned Cesarean section is, however, not associated with a physiological birth process and therefore not with the normal release of oxytocin either into the circulation or into the brain. Oxytocin levels are lower following Cesarean section in both mothers and babies than after vaginal delivery [101]. As mentioned above some physiological and psychological adaptations have been observed in women who have given birth vaginally. These adaptations are not observed in mothers, who had a planned Cesarean section. The Cesarean section mothers, e.g., describe themselves as less calm and interested in social interaction and more detached in comparison to mothers who had a vaginal delivery [63].

In addition, mothers who have given birth by a planned Cesarean section release less oxytocin in response to skin-to-skin contact with their babies after birth [102], release less oxytocin and prolactin in response to breastfeeding, breastfeed less often, and feel less healthy postpartum compared to women who have had a vaginal delivery suggesting a reduced function of the oxytocinergic system [62, 103].

11.6.1.1.3 Epidural Analgesia

Epidural analgesia can potentially stimulate the progress of labor by reducing maternal fear, pain, and stress levels. However, neuraxial analgesia not only blocks the sensation of pain but also partially inhibits the Ferguson reflex, which is associated with oxytocin release into the circulatory system and the brain. Mothers who receive epidural analgesia tend to exhibit fewer personality changes toward calmness and social interaction and experience reduced prolactin release during suckling, compared to mothers who undergo vaginal birth [7, 54, 61]. Due to potential delays in labor progress caused by epidural analgesia, synthetic oxytocin infusions are often administered.

11.6.1.1.4 Infusion of Synthetic Oxytocin

Infusions of exogenous oxytocin are often given to initiate and/or to augment labor, and it may under some conditions shorten the duration of labor by 2 h. In contrast to oxytocin levels in connection with physiological birth, oxytocin levels in response to infusions of synthetic oxytocin are not pulsatile but sustained. Oxytocin infusions maximally increase plasma levels of oxytocin two- to threefold. Since oxytocin penetrates the blood-brain barrier in negligible amounts, the central effects of oxytocin are not induced to the same degree as during vaginal birth [7, 54, 68].

Oxytocin infusions often result in more intense and prolonged myometrial contractions. The perception of birth can be less positive when oxytocin infusions are administered, potentially due to the increased pain from contractions. As a result, epidural analgesia is frequently provided alongside synthetic oxytocin to manage pain. Rather unexpectedly, infusions of synthetic oxytocin during labor have been shown to promote the expression of psychological adaptations toward more social interactive behavior and reduced anxiety after birth [7, 54, 61, 104]. When administered in connection with an epidural analgesia, these infusions reintroduce some of the maternal mental adaptations that are typically lacking in such conditions [61]. Additionally, the release of oxytocin in response to skin-to-skin contact, which is usually reduced in mothers who undergo a planned Cesarean section, is reinstated [102]. The administration of oxytocin infusions can be viewed as a pharmacological replacement for the insufficient endogenous release of oxytocin in mothers who have undergone planned Cesarean sections or received epidural analgesia during childbirth.

11.6.1.2 Skin-to-Skin Contact Between Parents and Newborn Postpartum

This practice involves the release of oxytocin through the activation of cutaneous sensory nerves, which triggers a significant release of oxytocin into both the circulation and the brain from parvocellular neurons in the PVN. As noted in Sect. 11.3, skin-to-skin contact between parents and their newborns is linked to several adaptive psychophysiological behaviors. Such contact enhances social interaction, alleviates pain, and induces substantial antistress effects for both the mother and the newborn [8, 39, 71–76, 103]. By decreasing activity in the HPA axis and certain aspects of the sympathetic nervous system, skin-to-skin contact mitigates the stress associated with childbirth [39]. Concurrently, such contact promotes growth through vagal/parasympathetic pathways mediated by the endocrine system of the gastrointestinal tract [8, 9]. Furthermore, the weight loss seen after birth is more quickly reversed into weight gain after skin-to-skin contact, and the newborns increase more in weight per ingested calorie [75]. In addition, early or immediate skin-to-skin contact after Cesarean section improves breastfeeding rates as well as exclusive breastfeeding rates [105].

11.6.1.2.1 Bonding and Maternal Protection

Marshall Klaus noted in his pioneering studies that mothers who had been separated from their infants after birth were less watchful during examination than mothers who had been close to their infants. He pointed out that early contact between mothers and babies promoted the interaction between them, and he introduced practices with skin-to-skin contact and closeness between mother and newborns after birth [106].

It is of importance to understand that the effect of bonding has two opposing but complementary sides. During interaction with the newborns, the mothers who have had early skin-to-skin contact with their newborns feel happier and interact more with their newborns compared to mothers who have been separated from their babies. On the other hand, these mothers experience more anxiety when separated from their newborns, an expression of the protective aspect of maternal behavior or bonding to the infant [76].

11.6.1.2.2 Long-Term Positive Effects

The period immediately after birth, the "early sensitive period" as coined by Marshall Klaus and John Kennell, is also important in the sense that the effects induced by skin-to-skin become long-lasting [106]. Positive effects on social interaction and reduced stress levels can be observed for 1 year after the treatment [76]. If skin-to-skin contact is performed repeatedly with full-term infants, positive effects regarding interaction between mother and infant and also stress reduction have been observed several years later [78]. The reduction of stress levels caused by skin-to-skin practices has been linked to decreased risk for development of maternal depression and anxiety disorders later on in the postpartum period [77–79].

11.6.1.2.3 Kangaroo Care

If the newborns are premature and treated with Kangaroo care, the positive growth promoting effects of skin-to-skin treatment become particularly prominent. Kangaroo care has been associated with more rapid weight gain growth and development of the infants [8, 9, 72, 75, 83, 84, 107]. All these effects can be attributed to activation of the oxytocin-mediated calm and connection system in response to repeated activation of the cutaneous nerves, in the chest region in particular, that trigger oxytocin release [40].

11.6.1.2.4 Oxytocin Induces Long-Term Effects

One aspect of the oxytocin effect spectrum that warrants further discussion is its capacity to induce long-term outcomes. In animal studies, oxytocin has been demonstrated to decrease the activity within the HPA axis and the sympathetic nervous system and to stimulate the activity in the endocrine system of the gastrointestinal tract via an increased responsiveness in alpha 2-adrenoreceptors and to decrease pain threshold via activation of opioidergic mu receptors. These effects can be turned into long lasting effects if the oxytocin treatment is repeated [108]. If newborn pups are administered oxytocin injections or exposed to extra sensory stimulation repeatedly after birth, they become less sensitive to pain, and their stress levels are lower as expressed by lower cortisol levels and lower blood pressure for life. Even elevated cortisol levels caused by nutritional stress, i.e., restricted food intake during pregnancy, are normalized by oxytocin. Also, the function of alpha 2-adrenoceptors is increased [5, 6, 12, 108].

As described in this article, a similar effect pattern consisting of antistress effects and promotion of social interaction and growth is induced in response to skin-to-skin contact after birth. In addition, these effects become long-lasting [8, 9, 15, 16, 32, 76, 78, 106]. Together these data suggest a biological window after birth during which basic psychophysiological functions can be influenced in the long-term. Further, the data suggest that oxytocin may play an important role in these adaptations. It is not known by which mechanisms these effects are obtained. A possible explanation would be a decrease in the level of methylation of the oxytocin or oxytocin receptor gene, thereby enhancing oxytocin production and oxytocin receptor sensitivity. Indeed, a decreased methylation of the oxytocin/oxytocin receptor gene has been demonstrated in clinical studies following skin-to-skin contact [109–111].

11.6.1.2.5 Continued Physical Contact Between Mother/Father (or Other Caregivers) and Infants

Physical contact remains crucial during infancy. The mechanisms activated through skin-to-skin contact post-birth are similarly triggered by various forms of touch and close physical interaction in infants [38, 85]. Such contact stimulates the oxytocin-linked, vagally mediated activation of the endocrine system within the gut (8,9). As previously discussed, the lack of touch and physical contact can cause growth retardation in infants and children, as well as hinder the development of social competence, leading to failure to thrive syndrome [8, 9, 38, 85].

11.6.1.3 Breastfeeding

During breastfeeding oxytocin is released in a pulsatile way in high amounts into the circulation but also into the brain. Prolactin release and the activity in the calm and connection system are reinforced, whereas the activity in the fight and flight system is decreased. Breastfeeding is therefore linked to powerful antistress effects at the same time as the vagally innervated endocrine system of the gastrointestinal tract is induced. This adaptation helps the mother optimally handle her energy balance to allow milk production in the long term [8–11, 38, 85].

Women who breastfeed exclusively for a long time are exposed to extremely large amounts of oxytocin, which is reflected in long-term antistress effects in the mother with a decreased risk of developing type 2 diabetes, hypertension, heart infarction, and stroke [11, 80, 112, 113]. The risk of developing postpartum blues, postpartum depression, and anxiety is decreased by breastfeeding, unless the mother finds breastfeeding problematic. All of the postpartum maternal mental issues are more frequent if the mother is not exclusively breastfeeding or stops breastfeeding before 2 months postpartum [10, 11, 80, 113, 114].

Suckling also releases oxytocin in the newborn. Touching of the oral mucosa activates sensory nerves, which induce oxytocin release from the parvocellular neurons in the PVN. This mechanism is linked to reduced stress levels and to stimulation of growth (the calm and connection system) [8–10, 12, 14, 15, 32, 85]. The latter effects probably involve a release of growth factors as well as an inhibition of the somatostatinergic system that blocks the activity of the endocrine system of the gastrointestinal tract [9, 38, 85]. In this way both suckling and touching of the skin promote the rate of growth in infants [38, 85].

11.6.2 Clinical Practices That Reinforce Physiological Release of Oxytocin

11.6.2.1 Touch or Extra Cutaneous Sensory Stimulation Such as Massage

Touch stimulates oxytocin release from the SON and PVN, e.g., via activation of axon collaterals from cutaneous sensory nerves. A pronounced release of oxytocin is induced from parvocellular neurons from the PVN, which will lead to an enhanced expression of the calm and connection reaction with decreased stress levels [8, 32, 38, 71–75, 108]. One way to enhance the stimulation of the cutaneous sensory nerves linked to oxytocin release is to apply light massage or tactile stimulation on the skin. Massage given to stressed pregnant women has been shown to reduce stress levels in mother and fetus and also to increase the weight of the newborn and to prolong pregnancy. Baby massage, i.e., massage of the newborn performed by the mother after birth gives rise to improved growth of the newborns and better interaction and bonding between mother and newborn. In addition, maternal depressed mood postpartum is antagonized [115–121].

11.6.2.2 Presence of a Supportive Person or Doula During Labor

The presence of a supportive person, a midwife or a doula, during birth has many positive effects. It may shorten the duration of labor by approximately 2 h, it, e.g., decreases the use of medical interventions and makes the mother's experience of birth more positive.

Mothers who had continuous support during birth also breastfeed more often [122–126].

The concept of support during birth is related to the much broader psychological concept of social support which has been shown to be linked to stress buffering effects and oxytocin release in humans [127].

The doula interacts with the birthing mothers in several ways, e.g., by touch and massage, which activate sensory nerves in the skin, which are associated with oxytocin release. In addition, the presence of the doula is linked to activation of the parvocellular oxytocinergic system via projections from the frontal cortex, amygdala, and BNST [8, 9, 12, 14, 16, 17]. When these pathways are activated, there will an enhanced expression of the calm and connection reaction with a strong reduction in fear, pain, and stress together with activation of facilitative processes linked to restoration and growth [8, 9, 12, 14, 16, 17].

The positive effect on the progress of labor caused by the presence of a supportive person during birth or a doula might be expected to be caused by an increased release of oxytocin into the circulation with consequent activation of uterine contractility. However, touch does not give rise to a pulsatile release of oxytocin levels, and the presence of a supportive person during birth has not been shown to be associated with oxytocin pulses in the circulation [128]. It may be suggested that doula-induced facilitation of labor is instead mediated by activation parvocellular oxytocinergic nerves, which project to the parasympathetic plexus in the lumbosacral region. Activation of parasympathetic, cholinergic neurons may enhance the function of oxytocin receptors in the uterine myometrium, as described in Sect. 11.3. In this way, a doula could potentially increase the contractile effect of oxytocin without elevating circulating oxytocin levels [54–58].

11.6.2.3 Social Contacts Are Linked to Maternal Safety and Trust

Continuous interaction with trusted individuals within and outside the family is associated with repeated activation of the oxytocinergic system. Such interaction may involve physical touch or just "anticipation of touch" in a familiar environment and among familiar individuals. Studies have also demonstrated that the incidence of postpartum depression is lower in women who have relationships with trusted individuals [80].

The positive or oxytocin enhancing effect of repeated interaction with familiar and trusted individuals may explain why pregnant women who were allowed to see the same midwife during pregnancy were found to have better outcomes. They gave birth prematurely less often than those mothers without continuity care. Birth was less problematic, e.g., shown by less need for medical interventions in connection with birth [129].

11.6.2.4 Avoidance of Unfamiliar Individuals and Environment

Exposure to unfamiliar individuals and environments may cause stress and an inhibition of the release of oxytocin, e.g., in response to sensory stimulation during labor, birth, suckling, and skin-to-skin contact.

Some reports indicate that the risk of premature birth was reduced during the societal lockdown associated with the COVID-19 pandemic in some Scandinavian countries [130]. This protective effect may possibly be interpreted as a consequence of a changed proportion between exposure to familiar and unfamiliar environments/people. Going to work is inevitably linked to exposure to unfamiliar people and environments. As the mothers stayed at home and didn't go to work, the time during which they were exposed to familiar people in a safe environment increased. In other words, by staying at home, the pregnant women were exposed to fewer stressors and to less time in unfamiliar environments together with unfamiliar people. As mentioned above, unfamiliarity may unconsciously and at a very primitive physiological regulatory level be interpreted as unsafety, which is known to be linked to inhibition of certain types of oxytocin release.

Other studies, however, have shown the opposite that premature birth rates increased during the COVID-19 pandemic. It is reasonable to think that the pandemic affected women differently depending on social and environmental circumstances, which may even vary between countries. Some women became stressed because of the isolation during the pandemic, the fear of getting infected during pregnancy, and the fear of not getting proper care, when giving birth. The incidence of postpartum depression during the pandemic increased in the whole population, suggesting a negative effect caused by isolation [131, 132].

11.6.2.5 Appropriate Food Intake

As described in the previous section, there is a tight link between female reproduction, energy intake, and energy stores. Food intake and satiety increase oxytocin levels and activity within the parasympathetic nervous system. In addition, food deprivation disturbs the function of the gonadotrophin-axis and thereby reduces fertility. During pregnancy the risk of premature birth and giving birth to a child with SGA increases, and food deprivation postpartum may lead to difficulties with breastfeeding.

11.7 Summary/Conclusion

This article summarizes the stress-reducing, healing, and protective effects of the oxytocin system during female reproduction. The role of touch, physical closeness, and social interaction for an optimal stimulation of oxytocin release has been highlighted (Table 11.2).

Pregnancy, labor/birth, skin-to-skin contact, and breastfeeding are associated with oxytocin release/function that activates and facilitates behavioral and physiological functions needed during these different phases of female reproduction. Some clinical practices known to ameliorate the outcome of pregnancy and birth actually act by reinforcing the function of endogenous oxytocin.

Table 11.2 Practices or interventions that stimulate/protect oxytocin release and effects

Extra massage to pregnant mothers
Care by the same midwife during pregnancy
Presence of supportive persons during birth
Warm bath and/or water birth
Skin-to-skin contact after birth
Extra massage between mothers and their newborns (baby massage)
Breastfeeding
Frequent physical contact
Social interaction
Avoidance of stress
Avoidance of unfamiliar environments, people, and situations that may be experienced as dangerous and unsafe

We have focused on the positive effects of oxytocin in this article. Oxytocin is, however, not a solo player. The oxytocin system interacts with both serotoninergic, dopaminergic, and noradrenergic pathways and in addition with opioid-, GABA-, and alpha 2-adrenoreceptors. Oxytocin may influence the activity of these other signaling systems, or they may influence oxytocin release/function, or alternatively they may constitute parallel systems. Still data from animal experiments and also from clinical studies demonstrate that activation of endogenous and sometimes administration of exogenous oxytocin do give rise to the entire effect pattern of oxytocin. We hypothesize that this is because the oxytocin system is located deep down in the brain and is in close contact with the surrounding via sensory nerves. It responds to relatively mild stimuli, e.g., touch, light pressure, and warmth of the skin/mucosal linings or analogous stimuli via the CNS. In this way the parvocellular oxytocin nerves from the PVN activates the integrated "calm and connection response," which will facilitate many aspects of behaviors or physiological functions, which are of importance for all phases of female reproduction. Administration of exogenous oxytocin via nasal spray may exert some positive effects but has functional limitations due to restricted penetration into the brain and in addition to possible simultaneous activation of oxytocin receptors with opposite functions.

References

1. Mitchell MD, Haynes PJ, Anderson AB, Turnbull AC. Oxytocin in human ovulation. Lancet. 1980;316:704.
2. Gelety TJ, Chaudhuri G. Prostaglandins in the ovary and fallopian tube. Baillieres Clin Obstet Gynaecol. 1992;6:707–29.
3. Beretsos P, Loutradis D, Koussoulakos S, Margaritis LH, Kiapekou E, Mastorakos G, Papaspirou I, Makris N, Makrigiannakis A, Antsaklis A. Oxytocin receptor is differentially expressed in mouse endometrium and embryo during blastocyst implantation. Ann N Y Acad Sci. 2006;1092:466–79.
4. Furuya K, Mizumoto Y, Makimura N, Mitsui C, Murakami M, Tokuoka S, Ishikawa N, Nagata I, Kimura T, Ivell R. A novel biological aspect of ovarian oxytocin: gene expression of oxytocin and oxytocin receptor in cumulus/luteal cells and the effect of oxytocin on embryogenesis in fertilized oocytes. Adv Exp Med Biol. 1995;395:523–8.
5. Sohlström A, Olausson H, Brismar K, Uvnäs Moberg K. Oxytocin treatment during early life influences reproductive performance in ad libitum fed and food-restricted female rats. Biol Neonate. 2002;81:132–8.
6. Sohlström A, Carlsson-Skwirut C, Bang P, Brismar K, Uvnäs Moberg K. Effects of oxytocin treatment early in pregnancy on fetal growth in ad libitum-fed and food-restricted rats. Pediatr Res. 1999;46:339–44.
7. Uvnäs Moberg K, Ekström-Bergström A, Berg M, Buckley S, Pajalic Z, Hadjigeorgiou E, Kotłowska A, Lengler L, Kielbratowska B, Leon-Larios F, Magistretti CM, Downe S, Lindström B, Dencker A. Maternal plasma levels of oxytocin during physiological childbirth—a systematic review with implications for uterine contractions and central actions of oxytocin. BMC Pregnancy Childbirth. 2019;19:285.
8. Uvnäs Moberg K, Handlin L, Petersson M. Neuroendocrine mechanisms involved in the physiological effects caused by skin-to-skin contact—with a particular focus on the oxytocinergic system. Infant Behav Dev. 2020;61:101482.

9. Uvnäs Moberg K. Oxytocin in growth, reproduction, restoration and health. Comprehens Psychoneuroendocrinol. 2024;20:100268.
10. Uvnäs Moberg K, Ekström-Bergström A, Buckley S, Massarotti C, Pajalic Z, Luegmair K, Kotlowska A, Lengler L, Olza I, Grylka-Baeschlin S, Leahy-Warren P, Hadjigeorgiu E, Villarmea S, Dencker A. Maternal plasma levels of oxytocin during breastfeeding—a systematic review. PLoS One. 2020;15:e0235806.
11. Uvnäs Moberg K. Oxytocin: the biological guide to motherhood. Amarillo: Praeclarus Press; 2014.
12. Uvnäs Moberg K, Gross MM, Calleja-Agius J, Turner JD. The Yin and Yang of the oxytocin and stress systems: opposites, yet interdependent and intertwined determinants of lifelong health trajectories. Front Endocrinol. 2024;15:1272270.
13. Suarez A, Yakupova V. Effects of postpartum PTSD on maternal mental health and child socioemotional development—a two-year follow-up study. BMC Pediatr. 2024;24:789.
14. Uvnäs Moberg K, Petersson M. Physiological effects induced by stimulation of cutaneous sensory nerves, with a focus on oxytocin. Curr Opin Behav Sci. 2022;43:159–66.
15. Stock S, Uvnäs Moberg K. Increased plasma levels of oxytocin in response to afferent electrical stimulation of the sciatic and vagal nerves and in response to touch and pinch in anaesthetized rats. Acta Physiol Scand. 1988;132:29–34.
16. Jurek B, Neumann ID. The oxytocin receptor: from intracellular signaling to behavior. Physiol Rev. 2018;98:1805–908.
17. Uvnäs Moberg K, Arn I, Magnusson D. The psychobiology of emotion: the role of the oxytocinergic system. Int J Behav Med. 2005;12:59–65.
18. Dale HH. On some physiological actions of ergot. J Physiol. 1906;34:163–206.
19. Ott I, Scott JC. The action of infundibulin upon the mammary secretion. Proc Soc Exp Biol Med. 1910;8:48–9.
20. Schafer EA, Mackenzie K. The action of animal extracts on milk secretion. Proc R Soc London Ser B, Containing Papers of a Biological Character. 1911;84:16–22.
21. Burbach JPH, Young LJ, Russell JA. Oxytocin: synthesis, secretion, and reproductive functions. In: Neill JD, editor. Knobil and Neill's physiology of reproduction. 3rd ed. Amsterdam: Elsevier; 2006. p. 3055–128.
22. Gimpl G, Fahrenholz F. The oxytocin receptor system: structure, function, and regulation. Physiol Rev. 2001;81:629–83.
23. Du Vigneaud V, Ressler C, Roberts CW, Katsoyannis PG, Gordon S. The synthesis of an octapeptide amide with the hormonal activity of oxytocin. J Am Chem Soc. 1953;75:4879–80.
24. Du Vigneaud V, Ressler C, Trippett S. The sequence of amino acids in oxytocin, with a proposal for the structure of oxytocin. J Biol Chem. 1953;205:949–57.
25. Buijs RM. Vasopressin and oxytocin—their role in neurotransmission. Pharmacol Ther. 1983;22:127–41.
26. Sawchenko PE, Swanson LW. Relationship of oxytocin pathways to the control of neuroendocrine and autonomic function. In: Amico J, Robinson AG, editors. Oxytocin: clinical and laboratory studies: proceedings of the second international conference on oxytocin. Excerpta Medica; 1985.
27. Sofroniew MV. Morphology of vasopressin and oxytocin neurones and their central and vascular projections. Prog Brain Res. 1983;60:101–14.
28. Knobloch HS, Charlet A, Hoffmann LC, Eliava M, Khrulev S, Cetin AH, Osten P, Schwarz MK, Seeburg PH, Stoop R, Grinevich V. Evoked axonal oxytocin release in the central amygdala attenuates fear response. Neuron. 2012;73:553–66.
29. Stoop R, Hegoburu C, Van Den Burg E. New opportunities in vasopressin and oxytocin research: a perspective from the amygdala. Annu Rev Neurosci. 2015;38:369–88.
30. Petersson M, Uvnäs Moberg K. Interactions of oxytocin and dopamine-effects on behavior in health and disease. Biomedicine. 2024;12:2440.
31. Yu H, Miao W, Ji E, Huang S, Jin S, Zhu X, Liu MZ, Sun YG, Xu F, Yu X. Social touch-like tactile stimulation activates a tachykinin 1-oxytocin pathway to promote social interactions. Neuron. 2022;110:1051–1067.e7.

32. Takahashi T. Sensory stimulation of oxytocin release is associated with stress management and maternal care. Front Psychol. 2021;11:588068.
33. Boll S, Almeida de Minas AC, Raftogianni A, Herpertz SC, Grinevich V. Oxytocin and pain perception: from animal models to human research. Neuroscience. 2018;387:149–61.
34. Nishimura H, Yoshimura M, Shimizu M, Sanada K, Sonoda S, Nishimura K, Baba K, Ikeda N, Motojima Y, Maruyama T, Nonaka Y, Baba R, Onaka T, Horishita T, Morimoto H, Yoshida Y, Kawasaki M, Sakai A, Muratani M, Conway-Campbell B, Lightman S, Ueta Y. Endogenous oxytocin exerts anti-nociceptive and anti-inflammatory effects in rats. Commun Biol. 2022;5:907.
35. Buemann B, Uvnäs Moberg K. Oxytocin may have a therapeutical potential against cardiovascular disease. Possible pharmaceutical and behavioral approaches. Med Hypotheses. 2020;138:109597.
36. Iovino M, Messana T, Marucci S, Triggiani D, Giagulli VA, Guastamacchia E, Piazzolla G, De Pergola G, Lisco G, Triggiani V. The neurohypophyseal hormone oxytocin and eating behaviors: a narrative review. Hormones. 2024;23:15–23.
37. Lindén A, Eriksson M, Hansen S, Uvnäs Moberg K. Suckling-induced release of cholecystokinin into plasma in the lactating rat: effects of abdominal vagotomy and lesions of central pathways concerned with milk ejection. J Endocrinol. 1990;127:257–63.
38. Uvnäs Moberg K. The gastrointestinal tract in growth and reproduction. Sci Am. 1989;261:78–83.
39. Bystrova K, Widström AM, Matthiesen AS, Ransjö-Arvidson AB, Welles-Nyström B, Wassberg C, Vorontsov I, Uvnäs Moberg K. Skin-to-skin contact may reduce negative consequences of "the stress of being born": a study on temperature in newborn infants, subjected to different ward routines in St. Petersburg. Acta Paediatr. 2003;92:320–6.
40. Eriksson M, Lindh B, Uvnäs Moberg K, Hökfelt T. Distribution and origin of peptide-containing nerve fibres in the rat and human mammary gland. Neuroscience. 1996;70:227–45.
41. Ueda T, Yokoyama Y, Irahara M, Aono T. Influence of psychological stress on suckling-induced pulsatile oxytocin release. Obstet Gynecol. 1994;84:259–62.
42. Bruckmaier RM, Wellnitz O, Blum JW. Inhibition of milk ejection in cows by oxytocin receptor blockade, alpha-adrenergic receptor stimulation and in unfamiliar surroundings. J Dairy Res. 1997;64:315–25.
43. Dejneka J, Samborski Z, Raułuszkiewicz S, Marcinkowski K. Wpływ stresu na motoryke macicy u krów [Effect of stress on uterine contraction in cows]. Pol Arch Weter. 1981;23:71–8.
44. Newton N. The relation of the milk-ejection reflex to the ability to breast feed. Ann N Y Acad Sci. 1992;652:484–6.
45. Mezzacappa ES, Kelsey RM, Myers MM, Katkin ES. Breast-feeding and maternal cardiovascular function. Psychophysiology. 2001;38:988–97.
46. Neumann ID, Landgraf R. Balance of brain oxytocin and vasopressin: implications for anxiety, depression, and social behaviors. Trends Neurosci. 2012;35:649–59.
47. Fuchs AR, Fuchs F, Husslein P, Soloff MS, Fernström MJ. Oxytocin receptors and human parturition: a dual role for oxytocin in the initiation of labor. Science. 1982;215:1396–8.
48. Fuchs AR, Fuchs F, Husslein P, Soloff MS. Oxytocin receptors in the human uterus during pregnancy and parturition. Am J Obstet Gynecol. 1984;150:734–41.
49. Fuchs AR, Periyasamy S, Alexandrova M, Soloff MS. Correlation between oxytocin receptor concentration and responsiveness to oxytocin in pregnant rat myometrium: effects of ovarian steroids. Endocrinology. 1983;113:742–9.
50. Bale TL, Pedersen CA, Dorsa DM. CNS oxytocin receptor mRNA expression and regulation by gonadal steroids. Adv Exp Med Biol. 1995;395:269–80.
51. Petersson M. Cardiovascular effects of oxytocin. Prog Brain Res. 2002;139:281–8.
52. Fuchs AR, Romero R, Keefe D, Parra M, Oyarzun E, Behnke E. Oxytocin secretion and human parturition: pulse frequency and duration increase during spontaneous labor in women. Am J Obstet Gynecol. 1991;165:1515–23.
53. Fuchs AR, Fuchs F. Endocrinology of human parturition: a review. Br J Obstet Gynaecol. 1984;91:948–67.

54. Uvnäs Moberg K. The physiology and pharmacology of oxytocin in labor and in the peripartum period. Am J Obstet Gynecol. 2024;230:S740–58.
55. Sato Y, Hotta H, Nakayama H, Suzuki H. Sympathetic and parasympathetic regulation of the uterine blood flow and contraction in the rat. J Auton Nerv Syst. 1996;59:151–8.
56. Nishimori K, Young LJ, Guo Q, Wang Z, Insel TR, Matzuk MM. Oxytocin is required for nursing but is not essential for parturition or reproductive behavior. Proc Natl Acad Sci USA. 1996;93:11699–704.
57. Theobald GW, Lundborg RA. Changes in myometrial sensitivity to oxytocin provoked in different ways. J Obstet Gynaecol Br Commonw. 1962;69:417–27.
58. Theobald GW. Nervous control of uterine activity. Clin Obstet Gynecol. 1968;11:15–33.
59. Kennell JH, Klaus MH. Continuous nursing support during labor. JAMA. 2003;289:175–6.
60. Kendrick KM, Keverne EB, Hinton MR, Goode JA. Cerebrospinal fluid and plasma concentrations of oxytocin and vasopressin during parturition and vaginocervical stimulation in the sheep. Brain Res Bull. 1991;26:803–7.
61. Jonas W, Nissen E, Ransjö-Arvidson AB, Matthiesen AS, Uvnäs Moberg K. Influence of oxytocin or epidural analgesia on personality profile in breastfeeding women: a comparative study. Arch Womens Ment Health. 2008;11:335–45.
62. Nissen E, Uvnäs Moberg K, Svensson K, Stock S, Widström AM, Winberg J. Different patterns of oxytocin, prolactin but not cortisol release during breastfeeding in women delivered by caesarean section or by the vaginal route. Early Hum Dev. 1996;45:103–18.
63. Nissen E, Gustavsson P, Widström AM, Uvnäs Moberg K. Oxytocin, prolactin, milk production and their relationship with personality traits in women after vaginal delivery or Cesarean section. J Psychosom Obstet Gynaecol. 1998;19:49–58.
64. Heinrichs M, Meinlschmidt G, Wippich W, Ehlert U, Hellhammer DH. Selective amnesic effects of oxytocin on human memory. Physiol Behav. 2004;83:31–8.
65. Waldenström U, Schytt E. A longitudinal study of women's memory of labour pain—from 2 months to 5 years after the birth. BJOG Int J Obstetr Gynaecol. 2009;116:577–83.
66. Li C, Wang X, Zhang G, Zhang Y, Xia F, Xu S, Shen X. Downregulation of microRNA 29c reduces pain after child delivery by activating the oxytocin GABA pathway. Mol Med Rep. 2020;22:1921–31.
67. Suzuki J, Nagase M, Sato N, Takahashi Y, Okamoto A, Kato F. Delivery-dependent shift in oxytocin-responsive cell population in the central amygdala of the female rat. Neuroendocrinology. 2023;113:48–63.
68. Buckley S, Uvnäs Moberg K, Pajalic Z, Luegmair K, Ekström-Bergström A, Dencker A, Massarotti C, Kotlowska A, Callaway L, Morano S, Olza I, Magistretti CM. Maternal and newborn plasma oxytocin levels in response to maternal synthetic oxytocin administration during labour, birth and postpartum—a systematic review with implications for the function of the oxytocinergic system. BMC Pregnancy Childbirth. 2023;23:137.
69. Marchini G, Lagercrantz H, Winberg J, Uvnäs Moberg K. Fetal and maternal plasma levels of gastrin, somatostatin and oxytocin after vaginal delivery and elective cesarean section. Early Hum Dev. 1988;18:73–9.
70. Widström AM, Ransjö-Arvidson AB, Christensson K, Matthiesen AS, Winberg J, Uvnäs Moberg K. Gastric suction in healthy newborn infants: effects on circulation and developing feeding behaviour. Acta Paediatr Scand. 1987;76:566–72.
71. Matthiesen AS, Ransjö-Arvidson AB, Nissen E, Uvnäs Moberg K. Postpartum maternal oxytocin release by newborns: effects of infant hand massage and sucking. Birth. 2001;28:13–9.
72. Vittner D, McGrath J, Robinson J, Lawhon G, Cusson R, Eisenfeld L, Walsh S, Young E, Cong X. Increase in oxytocin from skin-to-skin contact enhances development of parent-infant relationship. Biol Res Nurs. 2018;20:54–62.
73. Feldman R. The neurobiology of mammalian parenting and the biosocial context of human caregiving. Horm Behav. 2016;77:3–17.
74. Bystrova K, Matthiesen AS, Vorontsov I, Widström AM, Ransjö-Arvidson AB, Uvnäs Moberg K. Maternal axillar and breast temperature after giving birth: effects of delivery ward practices and relation to infant temperature. Birth. 2007;34:291–300.

75. Bystrova K, Matthiesen AS, Widström AM, Ransjö-Arvidson AB, Welles-Nyström B, Vorontsov I, Uvnäs Moberg K. The effect of Russian Maternity Home routines on breastfeeding and neonatal weight loss with special reference to swaddling. Early Hum Dev. 2007;83:29–39.
76. Bystrova K, Ivanova V, Edhborg M, Matthiesen AS, Ransjö-Arvidson AB, Mukhamedrakhimov R, Uvnäs Moberg K, Widström AM. Early contact versus separation: effects on mother-infant interaction one year later. Birth. 2009;36:97–109.
77. Kahalon R, Preis H, Benyamini Y. Mother-infant contact after birth can reduce postpartum post-traumatic stress symptoms through a reduction in birth-related fear and guilt. J Psychosom Res. 2022;154:110716.
78. Bigelow AE, Power M. Mother-infant skin-to-skin contact: short- and long-term effects for mothers and their children born full-term. Front Psychol. 2020;11:1921.
79. Kirca N, Adibelli D. Effects of mother-infant skin-to-skin contact on postpartum depression: a systematic review. Perspect Psychiatr Care. 2021;57:2014–23.
80. Westerfield KL, Koenig K, Oh R. Breastfeeding: common questions and answers. Am Fam Physician. 2018;98:368–73.
81. Bandoli G, Jelliffe-Pawlowski LL, Feuer SK, Liang L, Oltman SP, Paynter R, Ross KM, Schetter CD, Ryckman KK, Chambers CD. Second trimester serum cortisol and preterm birth: an analysis by timing and subtype. J Perinatol. 2018;38:973–81.
82. Christensson K, Cabrera T, Christensson E, Uvnäs Moberg K, Winberg J. Separation distress call in the human neonate in the absence of maternal body contact. Acta Paediatr. 1995;84:468–73.
83. Bergman NJ. Birth practices: maternal-neonate separation as a source of toxic stress. Birth Defects Res. 2019;111:1087–109.
84. Moore ER, Bergman N, Anderson GC, Medley N. Early skin-to-skin contact for mothers and their healthy newborn infants. Cochrane Database Syst Rev. 2016;11:CD003519.
85. Uvnäs Moberg K, Widström AM, Marchini G, Winberg J. Release of GI hormones in mother and infant by sensory stimulation. Acta Paediatr Scand. 1987;76:851–60.
86. Nolting IKL, Morina N, Hoppen TH, Tam KP, Kip A. A meta-analysis on gender differences in prevalence estimates of mental disorders following exposure to natural hazards. Eur J Psychotraumatol. 2025;16:2476809.
87. Hoirisch-Clapauch S, Brenner B, Nardi AE. Adverse obstetric and neonatal outcomes in women with mental disorders. Thromb Res. 2015;135:S60–3.
88. Carmassi C, Marazziti D, Mucci F, Della Vecchia A, Barberi FM, Baroni S, Giannaccini G, Palego L, Massimetti G, Dell'Osso L. Decreased plasma oxytocin levels in patients with PTSD. Front Psychol. 2021;12:612338.
89. Humble MB, Uvnäs Moberg K, Engström I, Bejerot S. Plasma oxytocin changes and anti-obsessive response during serotonin reuptake inhibitor treatment: a placebo controlled study. BMC Psychiatry. 2013;13:344.
90. Ellenbogen MA, Cardoso C, Serravalle L, Vadaga K, Joober R. The effects of intranasal oxytocin on the efficacy of psychotherapy for major depressive disorder: a pilot randomized controlled trial. Psychol Med. 2024;54:2122–32.
91. Lindley Baron-Cohen K, Feldman R, Fearon P, Fonagy P. Intranasal oxytocin administration improves mood in new mothers with moderate low mood but not in mothers with elevated symptoms of postnatal depression: a randomised controlled trial. J Affect Disord. 2022;300:358–65.
92. Carberg J. Statistics on postpartum depression, 2024. https://www.postpartumdepression.org/resources/statistics/. Accessed 6 April 2025.
93. Tambelli R, Tosto S, Favieri F. Psychiatric risk factors for postpartum depression: a systematic review. Behav Sci. 2025;15:173.
94. Arifunhera J, Mirunalini R. An update on the pharmacotherapy of postpartum depression. Int J Gynaecol Obstet. 2025;168:933–43.
95. Jobst A, Krause D, Maiwald C, Härtl K, Myint AM, Kästner R, Obermeier M, Padberg F, Brücklmeier B, Weidinger E, Kieper S, Schwarz M, Zill P, Müller N. Oxytocin course over

pregnancy and postpartum period and the association with postpartum depressive symptoms. Arch Womens Ment Health. 2016;19:571–9.

96. Figueiredo B, Dias CC, Brandão S, Canário C, Nunes-Costa R. Breastfeeding and postpartum depression: state of the art review. J Pediatr. 2013;89:332–8.
97. Zhu J, Jin J, Tang J. Oxytocin and women postpartum depression: a systematic review of randomized controlled trials. Neuropsychiatr Dis Treat. 2023;19:939–47.
98. Wei W, Feng X, Qin H, Yang X. Perception of traumatic childbirth of women, influencing factors and its relationship with post-traumatic stress disorder. Front Public Health. 2025;12:1485766.
99. Pfister HP, Muir JL. Psychological stress and administered oxytocin during pregnancy: effect corticosterone and prolactin response in lactating rats. Int J Neurosci. 1989;45:91–9.
100. Haim A, Albin-Brooks C, Brothers H, Breach M, Leuner B. Gestational stress disrupts dopamine and oxytocin signaling in the postpartum reward system of rats: implications for mood, motivation and mothering. Sci Rep. 2025;15:1450.
101. Buckley S, Uvnäs Moberg K, Dencker A, Kotlowska A, Massarotti C, Morano S, Olza I, Callaway L. Maternal and newborn plasma oxytocin levels in response to caesarean section—a systematic review with implications for the function of the oxytocinergic system. Under review with BMC Pregnancy and Childbirth, submitted 2024.
102. Velandia M. Parent-infant skin-to-skin contact studies. Stockholm: Department of Women's and Children's Health at Karolinska Institutet; 2012.
103. Özkan H, Aktaş EO, Işik HK. The effect of mode of delivery on postpartum comfort level and breastfeeding self-efficacy: a systematic review and meta-analysis. Maternal Health Neonatol Perinatol. 2024;10:17.
104. Wiberg-Itzel E, Uvnäs Moberg K. The correlation between synthetic oxytocin given during labor and women's personality traits according to the SSP (Swedish University Scales of Personality) survey: a pilot study. Open J Obstetr Gynecol. 2021;11:701–12.
105. Martínez-Hortelano JA, Saz-Lara A, González JLG, Cristóbal-Aguado S, Iglesias-Rus L, Martínez-Vizcaíno V, Garrido-Miguel M. Skin-to-skin contact and breastfeeding after caesarean section: a systematic review and meta-analysis of intervention studies. Int J Nurs Stud. 2025;166:105038.
106. Kennell JH, Trause MA, Klaus MH. Evidence for a sensitive period in the human mother. Ciba Found Symp. 1975;33:87–101.
107. WHO Immediate KMC Study Group. Impact of continuous Kangaroo Mother Care initiated immediately after birth (iKMC) on survival of newborns with birth weight between 1.0 to < 1.8 kg: study protocol for a randomized controlled trial. Trials. 2020;21:280.
108. Uvnäs Moberg K, Handlin L, Petersson M. Self-soothing behaviors with particular reference to oxytocin release induced by non-noxious sensory stimulation. Front Psychol. 2015;5:1529.
109. Moore SR, McEwen LM, Quirt J, Morin A, Mah SM, Barr RG, Boyce WT, Kobor MS. Epigenetic correlates of neonatal contact in humans. Dev Psychopathol. 2017;29:1517–38.
110. Unternaehrer E, Meyer AH, Burkhardt SC, Dempster E, Staehli S, Theill N, Lieb R, Meinlschmidt G. Childhood maternal care is associated with DNA methylation of the genes for brain-derived neurotrophic factor (BDNF) and oxytocin receptor (OXTR) in peripheral blood cells in adult men and women. Stress. 2015;18:451–61.
111. Uvnäs Moberg K, Gross MM, Agius A, Downe S, Calleja-Agius J. Are there epigenetic oxytocin-mediated effects on the mother and infant during physiological childbirth? Int J Mol Sci. 2020;21:9503.
112. Tschiderer L, Willeit P, Peters SAE. The cardiovascular benefits of breastfeeding to mothers. Expert Rev Cardiovasc Ther. 2022;20:589–92.
113. Binns C, Lee M, Low WY. The long-term public health benefits of breastfeeding. Asia Pac J Public Health. 2016;28:7–14.
114. Lara-Cinisomo S, McKenney K, Di Florio A, Meltzer-Brody S. Associations between postpartum depression, breastfeeding, and oxytocin levels in Latina mothers. Breastfeed Med. 2017;12:436–42.

115. Onozawa K, Glover V, Adams D, Modi N, Kumar RC. Infant massage improves mother-infant interaction for mothers with postnatal depression. J Affect Disord. 2001;63:201–7.
116. Glover V, Onozawa K, Hodgkinson A. Benefits of infant massage for mothers with postnatal depression. Semin Neonatol. 2002;7:495–500.
117. O'Higgins M, St James Roberts I, Glover V. Postnatal depression and mother and infant outcomes after infant massage. J Affect Disord. 2008;109:189–92.
118. Field T, Hernandez-Reif M, Diego M. Newborns of depressed mothers who received moderate versus light pressure massage during pregnancy. Infant Behav Dev. 2006;29:54–8.
119. Feijó L, Hernandez-Reif M, Field T, Burns W, Valley-Gray S, Simco E. Mothers' depressed mood and anxiety levels are reduced after massaging their preterm infants. Infant Behav Dev. 2006;29:476–80.
120. Field T, Diego M, Hernandez-Reif M. Depressed mothers' infants are less responsive to faces and voices. Infant Behav Dev. 2009;32:239–44.
121. Field T. Postpartum depression effects on early interactions, parenting, and safety practices: a review. Infant Behav Dev. 2010;33:1–6.
122. Stjernholm YV, Charvalho PDS, Bergdahl O, Vladic T, Petersson M. Continuous support promotes obstetric labor progress and vaginal delivery in Primiparous women—a randomized controlled study. Front Psychol. 2021;12:585823.
123. Hodnett ED, Gates S, Hofmeyr GJ, Sakala C. Continuous support for women during childbirth. Cochrane Database Syst Rev. 2003;3:CD003766.
124. Sobczak A, Taylor L, Solomon S, Ho J, Kemper S, Phillips B, Jacobson K, Castellano C, Ring A, Castellano B, Jacobs RJ. The effect of Doulas on maternal and birth outcomes: a scoping review. Cureus. 2023;15:e39451.
125. Bohren MA, Hofmeyr GJ, Sakala C, Fukuzawa RK, Cuthbert A. Continuous support for women during childbirth. The. Cochrane Database Syst Rev. 2017;7:CD003766.
126. Buerengen T, Bernitz S, Øian P, Dalbye R. Association between one-to-one midwifery care in the active phase of labour and use of pain relief and birth outcomes: a cohort of nulliparous women. Midwifery. 2022;110:103341.
127. Freak-Poli R, Ryan J, Neumann JT, Tonkin A, Reid CM, Woods RL, Nelson M, Stocks N, Berk M, McNeil JJ, Britt C, Owen AJ. Social isolation, social support and loneliness as predictors of cardiovascular disease incidence and mortality. BMC Geriatr. 2021;21:711.
128. Lindow SW, Hendricks MS, Thompson JW, van der Spuy ZM. The effect of emotional support on maternal oxytocin levels in labouring women. Eur J Obstet Gynecol Reprod Biol. 1998;79:127–9.
129. Sandall J, Soltani H, Gates S, Shennan A, Devane D. Midwife-led continuity models versus other models of care for childbearing women. The. Cochrane Database Syst Rev. 2016;4:CD004667.
130. Lisonkova S, Joseph KS. Why did preterm birth rates fall during the COVID-19 pandemic? Paediatr Perinat Epidemiol. 2023;37:113–6.
131. Shuman CJ, Peahl AF, Pareddy N, Morgan ME, Chiangong J, Veliz PT, Dalton VK. Postpartum depression and associated risk factors during the COVID-19 pandemic. BMC Res Notes. 2022;15:102.
132. Rodriguez ACI, Smith L, Harris R, Nephew BC, Santos HP Jr, Murgatroyd C. Oxytocin modulates sensitivity to acculturation and discrimination stress in pregnancy. Psychoneuroendocrinology. 2022;141:105769.

Partners' Stress Is Also a Source of Maternal Stress

12

Siti Khuzaiyah, Roseline Florence Gomes, Leila Nisya Ayuanda, Khadizah H. Abdul-Mumin, and Sarena H. Hashim

Abstract

Maternal stress is a global concern affecting both mothers and offspring adversely. There are several factors deemed to be significant risk factors for maternal stress, including partner stress. This chapter aims to examine partner stress as a contributor to maternal stress, encompassing the origins of partner stress, mechanisms of stress transmission between partners, psychological and physiological impacts of partner stress on maternal health, empirical evidence regarding partner stress and maternal well-being, strategies for mitigating partner-induced maternal stress, cultural and social viewpoints on partner stress and maternal health, and prospective avenues for research and intervention. Examining these elements is crucial for developing and designing an effective

S. Khuzaiyah (✉)
Midwifery Program, Faculty of Health Sciences, Universitas Muhammadiyah Pekajangan Pekalongan, Central Java, Indonesia

Nursing and Midwifery Program, PAPRSB Institute of Health Science, Universiti Brunei Darussalam, Gadong, Brunei
e-mail: 21h8722@ubd.edu.bn

R. F. Gomes
Department of Psychology, Jyoti Nivas College Autonomous, Bengaluru, India
e-mail: roselinegomes@jyotinivas.org

L. N. Ayuanda
Midwifery Program, Faculty of Health Sciences, Universitas Muhammadiyah Pekajangan Pekalongan, Central Java, Indonesia

K. H. Abdul-Mumin · S. H. Hashim
Nursing and Midwifery Program, PAPRSB Institute of Health Science, Universiti Brunei Darussalam, Gadong, Brunei

School of Nursing and Midwifery, La Trobe University, Melbourne, VIC, Australia
e-mail: khadizah.mumin@ubd.edu.bn; sarena.hashim@ubd.edu.bn

R. A. Caparros-Gonzalez (ed.), *Maternal Stress during Pregnancy and Postpartum*, https://doi.org/10.1007/978-3-032-09245-8_12

program to alleviate maternal stress caused by partner tension. The prior published studies were combined, presented, and analyzed thematically. The sources of partner stress included financial and work-related stress, anticipation of new roles and responsibilities, relationship adjustments, health concerns, and financial issues. The relationship between partner stress and maternal well-being is interconnected, and dyadic stress is essential in influencing mental well-being. The mechanism of partner stress affects maternal stress through three main routes, including emotional contagion, empathic distress, and behavioral responses. Partner-induced maternal stress affects maternal mental health, such as anxiety, depression, chronic maternal stress, reduced relationship quality, mirroring partner stressors, irritable action, and lack of motherhood adaptation. The physical health implications included hormonal transformation, higher cortisol, cardiovascular issues, reduced sleep quality, fatigue, weaker immune system, longer wound healing, and impaired breastfeeding process. The impact on pregnancy outcome and fetus includes organogenesis and placental growth problems, fetal growth restriction, fetus long-term metabolic problems, preterm labor, early labor onset, and reduced oxygen and nutrient flow. Management partner-induced maternal stress covers open communication, couples counseling and support programs, stress-education techniques for couples, parental leave for couples, and social and community support. Cultural norms establish the basis for maternal and partner experiences. Traditional gender roles significantly influence how partners manage stress during pregnancy. Economic disparities exacerbate these challenges, especially in marginalized or low-income communities. Addressing partner stress through inclusive, culturally informed, and systemic interventions provides a pathway to a more holistic and equitable maternal health framework, benefiting not only mothers but also entire families and communities. Future longitudinal study, especially in eastern countries with a diverse community, employing a family-centered policy approach and an intersectional framework to examine the influences of race, gender, socioeconomic status, and cultural norms on partner-induced maternal stress, is needed to gain a comprehensive understanding and robust recommendation.

Keywords

Partner stress · Maternal stress · Partner-induced maternal stress · Mental health

12.1 Background

Maternal stress becomes a global issue affecting mother and their children's well-being. The global prevalence of antenatal depression, postnatal depression, and antenatal-postnatal anxiety was 29%, 26%, and 31%, respectively [1]. A prospective study in Spain indicates that 23.1% of pregnant women experienced high levels of maternal stress at the end of pregnancy [2]. In low- and middle-income countries, one in five pregnant and postpartum women experience a generalized anxiety disorder, with 8.3% of women encountering post-traumatic stress disorder [3]. Another systematic review of studies conducted in 20 low- and middle-income countries (LMICs) revealed the prevalence of antepartum depression was 25.8%, and the prevalence of postnatal depression within 23 LMICs was 19.7% [4].For postnatal stress, a meta-analysis revealed that from 154 studies ($N = 54{,}711$), it found that the prevalence of birth-related post-traumatic stress disorder (PTSD) among mothers and fathers was 4.7% and 1.2%, respectively. In addition, the post-traumatic stress (PTSS) in correlation with childbirth traumatic events was 12.3% in mothers and 1.3% in fathers [5]. Around 4% of mothers and 1% of partners experience PTSD due to the childbirth process [5]. This indicates that both women and partners are at high risk of developing childbirth-related stress.

Maternal stress has been associated with adverse outcomes both in mothers and infants [6], negatively impacted health behavior, and increased morbidity [7]. In mothers, maternal prenatal stress is linked with spontaneous preterm birth, pre-eclampsia, neonatal morbidity, low birth weight, and predicted postpartum depression [6, 8]. While in children, maternal stress is linked to the development of a medical disease and psychiatric disorders, mainly on the development of autism spectrum disorder, obesity, and infantile colic [9]. Maternal stress is anticipated to impact neurodevelopment across various domains, including cognitive development, motor skills, behavior, temperament, memory, learning capabilities [10], and infant DNA methylation during their first year of life [11]. Moreover, a longitudinal study in Spain confirmed that prenatal stress increased blood cortisol levels and the caesarean section rate and decreased the APGAR score of babies in the first minute of life [7].

The factors associated with maternal stress and anxiety included age < 40 years, non-white ethnicity, and non-university studies [2]. For perinatal depression, the risk factors included lower educational attainment, low family income, mental health problems, domestic abuse, prenatal alcohol or tobacco use, and multiparity [12]. In LMICs, the risk factors of prenatal and postnatal depression were child abuse, adult abuse, low level of education, low economic status, low social support, and a history of mental issues [4].

Another source of maternal stress is partner stress and relationships. A study indicates that maternal emotional distress during pregnancy is significantly predicted by partner relationship dissatisfaction [13]. Not only does it increase child internalizing and externalizing behaviors [14] and buffer the correlation between mother's parental stress and children's behavioral issues [15], but paternal stress also has a reciprocal effect on the family relationship. While partner-relationship conflict and social support affect prenatal mental health [16], stress could harm intimate relationships and their longevity [17]. Support provided by the partner is essential to reduce prenatal and postnatal mental disorders [18]. Partner stress and conflicted relationships between women and partners might make it challenging to provide such support and eventually trigger more stressful conditions for women.

The mechanism of the relationship between partner stress and maternal stress seems complex, and understanding these issues is critical to providing a practical guide for managing partner and maternal stress. However, there is still limited literature discussing these essential issues. Thus, this chapter aims to examine the partner's stress as a source of maternal stress, including the source of partner stress, mechanisms of stress transmission between partners, psychological and physiological effects of partner's stress on maternal health, research evidence on partner's stress and maternal well-being, strategies for managing partner-induced maternal stress, cultural and social perspectives on partner's stress and maternal health, and future directions for research and intervention. Discussing these aspects is deemed to be essential to preparing and designing appropriate programs to mitigate maternal stress induced by partner stress.

12.2 Method

This chapter highlights the role of partner stress as the source of maternal stress. The format is based on earlier successful articles [19]. This chapter offers a thorough analysis of how the mechanism of partner stress as the source of maternal stress since there is a limited published study in this area of interest. Furthermore, it explores the physical and psychological impact of partner stress on maternal and strategies to mitigate partner-induced maternal stress. The authors end the chapter by synthesizing relevant recommendations and direction for health promotion programs and future research to maximize results despite facing partner stress. A synthesis of previous research findings obtained from reputable academic databases, including PubMed, Scopus, Science Direct, ProQuest, and Wiley, was used to form the empirical basis of this chapter. The available literature was also improved by utilizing Google Scholar to find comprehensive sources, especially those that were related to the following keywords: relationship of paternal stress and maternal stress, causes of paternal stress, impact or effect of partner stress on women, maternal stress management, paternal stress management, and intervention for maternal-paternal stress. Thematic analysis was used to comprehensively analyze, present, and discuss the findings.

12.3 Understanding the Sources of Partner's Stress

Various conditions trigger partner's stress, such as financial and work-related stress, new roles and responsibilities as new parents, relationship adjustment, mood swings, and other sources as described in this sub-theme.

12.3.1 Financial and Work-Related Stress

Globally, families have varying experiences with work and finances. Some families live with high levels of financial stress and pressure. On the other hand, some parents work but experience different challenges in managing the competing demands of work and family [20]. Economic problems and work demands can significantly increase stress in couples. This stress especially happens during the transition to parenthood since this transition requires increased responsibilities, including financial ones. Financial hardship and the occurrence of depression in the mother will put pressure on the parent-child relationship [21] since poverty harms family conditions such as difficulty in buying daily necessities, the poor mental health of parents, and conflict between parents (e.g., domestic violence).

There is a vicious cycle for women following childbirth related to economic disturbance. Economic difficulty exacerbates depression, while maternal depression concurrently heightens economic suffering. These reinforcing mechanisms exacerbate relational distress for both moms and fathers [21]. Another study concluded that there was a correlation between economic difficulties, parental depression, parenting, and internalizing and externalizing among adolescents [22]. Economic stress is also thought to directly and negatively impact the quality of the interparental relationship. Overall, economic pressure and stress to meet their families' daily material needs appear to be a trigger for fathers' mental health problems that then escalate into destructive interparental conflict. Family-strengthening policies and programs should examine whether families' material needs are adequately met and seek opportunities to address them to address parental mental health and strengthen the couple's relationship [23]. Providing paid leave policies might help to mitigate financial issues for new parents; for example, in developed countries such as Italy, new working mothers and fathers are entitled to 20 weeks of leave with 80% salary [24].

Another related partner stress source is work-related stress. Daily job stressors affect family interactions in the short term by influencing the employed individual's mood, thoughts, and coping behaviors [25]. The weeks following the birth of a child can be stressful for new mothers since maternal distress may increase when mothers are dissatisfied with their partner's instrumental support (e.g., division of childcare tasks and authority for family decision-making) [26]. The demands of work and family outside can increase stress in couples, resulting from conflicts in carrying out roles between husband and wife. However, the stress pattern is different between men and women. There is a spillover-crossover theory that refers to the process of stress transmission where stress at work is transferred to the family realm, and family-related stress is transferred to the workplace. Spillover is a process that occurs in individuals who perform their roles in two different domains. If there is a negative spillover, it can be called a conflict theory. Other domains are associated with various norms. If successful in one domain, sacrifices will likely be required in another domain, which means if they focus on using them in one area, they will not get benefits in other areas [27]. Certain spouse "cross-over" effects seem to reflect the adjustments made by the employed partner in response to stress. For example, a spouse may increase their social support and engagement with children, indicating dynamics beyond a straightforward transfer of stress from work to home [25].

12.3.2 Anticipation of New Roles and Responsibilities

The transition to parenthood can be a psychologically challenging experience for both mothers and fathers. Although often anticipated, the transition to parenthood can cause psychological distress for both mothers and fathers, with negative impacts on the infant. During the prenatal and postpartum periods, maternal and paternal emotional states were found to be significantly correlated, and parental mental health influenced self-efficacy and affected the quality of parent-infant interactions and parent-infant attachment [28]. It may also be detrimental to infants' early neurobehavioral and socio-emotional development. In addition to the general effects of reducing the quality of the couple's relationship, the transition to parenthood brings several life changes that may differ for new mothers and fathers. For example, the transition to parenthood often brings increased inequality in the division of household labor. Thus, detrimental effects on well-being may be more common for new mothers than new fathers [29].

Despite the detrimental effect of the transition period for women, men's mental health and well-being during this period remain under-researched, with new fathers' health needs often going unmet [30]. Differences in mental well-being between mothers and fathers are also reflected in the pressures in the environment. The primary issue of fathers was the increased pressure on new fathers to be the primary breadwinners at the expense of family time and increased demands for father involvement in childcare [31]. First-time fathers reported experiencing "high roller coasters" and challenges in their new identity and relationship dynamics. Men described a range of feelings associated with becoming a first-time father, with emotions ranging from happiness and joy to anxiety and stress in the antenatal period, with the baby not feeling "real" during their partner's pregnancy for many. However, men also described their experience of fatherhood as a sense of achievement and personal growth, enabling them to have a positive change that made them feel more secure and confident [32].

Some males felt that becoming a father made them "stronger" and "tougher" since they had to learn how to cope with the demands of fatherhood at a young age [33]. For example, fathers of premature infants in the NICU may experience emotional distress when supporting their partners, often hiding their own worries and negative emotions. Behind their idealized role as their partner's protector, they may hide the implementation of defense mechanisms that protect them from the reality of their inner experiences [28].

Despite their challenges facing the transition parenthood process, fathers described a lack of appropriate support and information for new fathers. Fathers could only access information through antenatal classes more tailored to women, but this was not enough. Some struggled to get an appointment with a GP for their own mental health needs. Yet many were unaware of any specific mental health support available to fathers [33]. Social support plays a key role in alleviating psychological distress for both parents, with support from friends being beneficial for mothers and family support being helpful for fathers [29]. Improving a father's mental well-being is essential to support mothers' well-being since emotional conditions in fathers can positively influence the support given to their partners and their involvement with the baby.

12.3.3 Relationship Adjustments

Parenthood is a potentially stressful transition, which can negatively impact both partners' individual and relational well-being [34]. Pregnancy and the transition to parenthood are significant life events that increase exposure to psychological stress and the likelihood of developing psychiatric disorders, most commonly depression, in both parents [35]. During pregnancy, there are significant physiological changes that support a healthy fetus. Parasympathetic activity typically decreases during pregnancy [36], and psychological stress can lead to further decreases in heart rate variability (HRV) [37].

The pregnancy and postpartum period can significantly impact the emotional well-being of both partners. Women often experience higher levels of depression and anxiety during pregnancy and postpartum compared to men. Pregnancy and postpartum can lead to increased emotional and psychopathological symptoms in women compared to men, potentially putting a strain on the couple dynamic [38].

Couples may also be at increased risk for depression and anxiety, especially those who report poor sexual satisfaction, unemployment, or financial difficulties. Negative partner relationship quality during pregnancy is associated with lower heart rate variability and more severe depressive symptoms in the postpartum period [35].

One study found that most new fathers described their relationships with their partners as having become stronger since the birth of their baby. However, another study found a decline in the relationship between couples after birth. These two conditions differed, perhaps because they reflected different populations in the research settings. It is clear that those who described their relationships as having become more potent because they worked together to fulfill the tasks of achieving the parenting role early in the process [36].

Thus, in prenatal classes, it is necessary to promote the involvement of both partners in household tasks. Anticipating a fair division of household tasks can enable couples to prepare for childbirth and limit stress for both partners, thereby reducing parenting stress and improving parental well-being [39].

12.3.4 Other Sources

Research on postpartum depression and parental stress in partners suggests that similar mood swings impact both mothers and fathers during the transition to parenthood and that their mental health has a significant impact on child development and family health [43].

Parents face a variety of stressors, including family-related issues, work challenges, health concerns, and financial pressures. These issues are triggered by several factors, namely, gender, marital status, education level, physical health conditions, and economic pressures [40].

Many mothers view childcare as their responsibility and display a range of distressing emotions, including sadness, anger, guilt, feeling overwhelmed, anxiety, loneliness, and feeling like they are shouldering the entire responsibility for the family [41]. The involvement and support of partners or other family members will reduce parenting stress. So, it is essential to understand the two-way relationship between joint parenting and marital function. The more mothers perceive their partners to be involved in childcare responsibilities, the less they experience symptoms of depression and stress related to their parenting responsibilities [42].

Regarding the partners anxiety, experiences in pregnancy and childbirth problems in mothers will contribute to postpartum depression and anxiety. These problems will also impact fathers' psychological well-being, affecting partner relationships. From the father's perspective, some circumstances that trigger stress are usually external factors such as work, the economy, compensation for not working when caring for a baby, or restrictions in childcare. The stress experienced is typically related to the dual role of carrying out the role of parents and the demands of work life. Meanwhile, mothers express pressure as parents about internal demands such as childcare dynamics, family, and household situations. They describe their well-being as decreasing drastically by feeling burdened by the responsibility of caring for the family [43].

Other stress sources, such as the fertility rate of a couple, the number of children they have, and the spacing between them, will increase the stress of parenting for mothers and fathers [44].

12.4 Partner's Stress and Maternal Well-Being

The relationship between partner stress and maternal well-being is well documented in several studies. Dyadic stress is a stressful event or interaction that invariably pertains to both partners, either directly when both are faced with the same stressor or when the stress originates within the couple, or indirectly when one partner's stress permeates the relationship, impacting both individuals. Many academics and theorists concur that stress in couples is inherently a dyadic event that affects both spouses somehow [17]. It means that partner stress can significantly influence women's psychological well-being.

Studies indicate that poor partner relationships are correlated with mother depression and anxiety symptoms. In contrast, lower relationship quality has been associated with heightened parental stress and predicts greater maternal general anxiety disorder [45]. From a psychological viewpoint, a partner's mental health, such as stress, anxiety, or depression, can significantly influence maternal well-being. A study indicates that depression among partners has a moderate positive correlation with maternal depression [30]. When the partners suffer from depression, they can't provide sufficient help for women to tackle their problems during maternal perinatal. Furthermore, once women are abused by their partner, they are vulnerable to anxiety, depression, and post-traumatic stress [46].

12.5 Mechanisms of Stress Transmission Between Partners

The mechanism of stress transmission between women and partners will be explained through emotional contagion, empathic distress, and behavioral response mechanism.

12.5.1 Emotional Contagion

Emotional contagion is reflected as a vicious cycle that acts as a contagious indicator within intimate relationships among partners. There has also been the presence of empathy and the processes of shared experiences that impact these relationships. This emotional contagion has been viewed from the lens of intimate interpersonal relationships, which shows that the intensity of intimacy empowers affective contagion among partners [47].

Apart from the emotional paradigm, partner-related stress can also erupt from clinical signs like negative affective states. It was found that depressive symptomatic patterns during the perinatal pregnancy have been observed if the partners have witnessed an insecure partner attachment pattern in their initial year of parenthood [48]. Thus, it was recommended that clinicians need to develop their awareness regarding vulnerable fathers during the time of childbirth to tailor-make further interventions and treatment methodologies that address the needs of these partners.

Historically, it was recognized that the partner's stressors or outcomes are transmitted during stressful situations, strengthening the emotional contagion [49]. Therefore, how partners intersect effectively affects their empathetic response to emotional regulation that develops as automatic and self-controlled [50].

Empathy and shared experiences among partners can outcome this mechanism of emotional contagion. This empathy is a socio-emotional experiential construct that is an integral part of partners [51]. The presence of these attributes denotes the interplay of psychosocial stress. This type of stress is acute and adaptive and impacts the neurobiological systems [52]. It also reflected and implicated the outcome of chronic empathetic stressful experiences.

12.5.2 Empathic Distress

Pregnancy is a progressive, challenging period of physiological transformations and mental health concerns. Hence, it is necessary to understand that this period is the epitome of multilevel risk factors that require resilience [41]. Thus, community institutions need to work toward need-based interventions that understand and combat empathetic distress and guide partners with the family. The process of witnessing a partner's stress can transition into additional stressful experiences for the other partner, especially in pregnancy when the emotional sensitivity is heightened. These can contain emotional distress, fear, and apprehensions, ubiquitous attributes of experiences [53].

Partners of pregnant women experience empathetic distress that heightens their emotional sensitivity. Similarly, Vallian et al. found that these partners witnessed more significant fears, apprehensions, and stress accompanied by feelings of helplessness as an outcome of nurturing women for childbirth [54]. Johanson et al. found that these partners are generally overwhelmed by these experiences that resulting in physiological concerns [55]. These fathers perceived childbirth as a dynamic experience that needed a sense of preparedness. Some of these developmental ages experienced social pressures. There were feelings of worry and shock, resulting in behavioral responses [56].

12.5.3 Behavioral Responses

These behavioral responses among partners depict aspects of irritability, anxiety, overwhelmed feelings, social withdrawal, etc., which may have a negative influence on maternal emotional health. Women, during their pregnancy, go through an array of affective concerns. They show distinct behaviors in challenging times [57]. Research findings showed that in this apprehensive context, it was difficult for women to identify distress among their partners.

Paternal factors are also indicators that impact the maternal affective state. Contemporary findings highlighted that fatherhood in times of the perinatal stage has been demanding as an outcome of environmental stressors [58]. These factors include unfavorable factors regarding the pregnancy processes, fears related to childbirth, and feelings of incompetency related to nurturance that can further contribute to clinical mental health concerns, behavioral distress, and fatigue.

There is also the presence of neuroticism, a lack of social networking that increases social withdrawal, and dissatisfaction related to environmental events [59]. Kowlessar et al. [60] found that there is an interplay of affective, psychological, and behavioral distress among expectant fathers during the period of pregnancy. These behavioral distressing factors include irritability and indicators of hostility, where the stressors manifest through conflicts that can emotionally drain pregnant women by aggravating their anxiety [61]. This may further reduce coping skills during the times of pregnancy or the postpartum phase.

The aspect of emotional withdrawal and unavailability is also considered as other causal factors where partners who have experienced stress may withdraw physiologically and emotionally, which may deplete their capacity for engagement. This unavailability can transition attributes of social isolation, loneliness, and mental health challenges among to-be mothers [62, 63]. Thus, stress can impair behavioral responses where the partners cannot initiate a consistent support pattern, which can develop maternal stressors [64]. Hence, these behavioral responses strengthen overwhelmed feelings that can empower frustration, bitterness, and stress among mothers [65].

There are some instances where partners excessively rely on pregnant partners for affective or logistic support that compounds into stress instead of alleviation the stressors [61]. Thus, stress within close relationships, like among partners, is considered "contagious" whenever they share everyday experiences and affective states through the empathetic paradigm. This proposed phenomenon is known as affective contagion, which occurs whenever a partner experiences stress and gets amplified onto the other partner, especially during pregnancy, when there is greater affective sensitivity. Thus, witnessing the partner's psychosocial distress may fuel empathic concerns by intensifying the emotional strain, which further can create a sensitive feedback-driven loop of the partner's mutual stress experiences.

This dyadic dynamic cycle can further strain affective health and relationships [61]. Behavioral stress-related responses like irritability, social withdrawal, or affective unavailability can further alleviate the issues. This irritability can result in conflicts by also reducing affective support and leaving pregnant women overwhelmed. These actions, coupled with neglect and lack of support, can exacerbate maternal-related stressors. Therefore, recognizing these present patterns while initiating open communication and more excellent mutual supportive frameworks can be critical to the dissolution of the stress-based contagion [62, 63].

12.6 Effects of Partner's Stress on Maternal Mental Health, Physical Health, and Pregnancy Outcome

12.6.1 Impact on Maternal Mental Health

There is a need to recognize maternal affective distress during pregnancy and identify risk-related factors as the causal factors of the distress that can be considered of clinical and community importance [13]. This mental health of the pregnant mother is relevant both for the individual and the partner. There are instances when the partner's levels of stress impact the mental health of pregnant women, which can aggregate the stress and result in anxiety and depression. Stressors within the environment of couples are common and are associated with depression [66].

Partners' stressors are mostly underestimated and affect women's distress [67]. The partners' levels of stressors significantly influence maternal mental concerns that are observed during times of pregnancy. Thus whenever partners witness greater stress levels, their affective and behavioral outcomes exacerbate maternal apprehensions, depression, and stress. Findings show that maternal-related mental health is intricately associated with the quality of partner relationships and mutual stressors that are shared. For example, partners who reflect stress-related actions like irritability, emotional withdrawal, or hostility leave pregnant women unsupported with heightened affective distress [61]. This emotional unavailability increases vulnerability among mothers, which fuels anxiety and depression within the context of pregnancy that are marked by hormonal transformations, which further amplify affective sensitivity [64].

Empirical findings reveal the work of stress contagion among intimate associations. This affective contagion occurs when one partner's stress influences the other through shared affective experiences. Empathic distress during pregnancy guides the absorption and mirroring of a partner's stressors. Mohler et al. found that pregnant mothers, along with their stressed partners, exhibited higher cortisol, which is a biomarker of stressors connected to adverse results like complications in pregnancy and postpartum depression [62]. These action-oriented patterns as an outcome of partner stress can directly relate to maternal mental health concerns.

The withdrawal and negation of parental roles and responsibilities force mothers to carry the burdens of caregiving, which develops stress and dissolves self-care opportunities. The consistent and systematic exposure to the other partners' vulnerability and negative mindset undermines the maternal affective well-being, thereby fostering helplessness [65]. In addition, the interplay of relational mechanisms deteriorates coping patterns in mothers by increasing levels of susceptibility to episodes of depression [63].

The stressful associations also affect the physical stress patterns among women who are pregnant. Shishido [61] emphasized that these elevated forms of partner-related stressors can further dysregulate the hypothalamic-pituitary-adrenal (HPA) axis among mothers, leading to chronically stressed states. Thus this dynamic dysregulation can be associated with the development of anxiety, irritable actions, and a lowered capacity to adapt to the complexities of motherhood. Over time, these stressors impact maternal health and pose risks for the development of the fetus, leading to longitudinal complexities [64].

To mitigate these adverse outcomes, addressing the stressors within couples is integral. Evidence-based relationship-driven interventions, like mindfulness or couple therapy, can guide partners in developing healthy communication methodologies and mutual coping skills [63]. Thus, an extension of support to maternal mental health concerns requires the provision of an ecosystem backed by mutual understanding and affective availability to dissolve the unfavorable impact of partner-related stress.

12.6.2 Physical Health Implications

The levels of stress during the preliminary phases of pregnancy can outcome in significant physiological health-related concerns for emerging mothers, with a heightened cascading influence on both maternal and fetal well-being. These longitudinal mechanisms revolving near stress further activate the hypothalamic-pituitary-adrenal (HPA) axis, increasing the cortisol levels that can cause hypertension. Thus, these can precede hypertensive disorders like preeclampsia that can have greater challenges associated with maternal stress and increased risks of maternal cardiovascular concern [68, 69]. These chronic stressors further disrupt the quality of sleep, which was also highlighted in a study that depicted 81% of pregnant women, who experienced exacerbated fatigue, had weaker immune functioning and were susceptible to environmental infections [69].

Stress-embedded inflammation is another risk factor, as are inflammatory indicators like the rise of interleukin-6 (IL-6) with stressors. This can lead to poor placental health, leading to complications like fetal growth restriction [70]. Additionally, the presence of gestational diabetes has also been influenced by cortisol dysregulation, which poses risks to the mother and the fetus, thereby affecting long-term metabolic health [71]. Therefore, these postpartum stressor-related physiological conditions like delayed healing of wounds, excessive fatigue, and disturbances in sleep quality hinder recovery.

Tremendous stress also impairs the process of breastfeeding as it interferes with hormonal interference and milk production [68]. Thus, stress reduction methods that include mindfulness-based interventions are greatly recommended to combat these physical risks and handhold maternal health during and after pregnancy.

12.6.3 Impact on Pregnancy and Birth Outcomes

Maternal stress as an outcome of the partner's stress has been associated with adverse pregnancy and birth causal outcomes like preterm labor and also low birth weight. These chronic stressors thus activate the hypothalamic-pituitary-adrenal (HPA) axis, resulting in elevated cortisol, which deteriorates the placental functioning. Scientific findings have consistently reflected that maternal stressors increase the risk of preterm birth. Lobel et al. [72] also found that mothers exposed to more tremendous stress due to their strained partner relationships were at significantly greater risk of preterm labor. Stress-induced inflammation assessed by elevated cytokines also contributed to uterine contractions and early labor onset [70].

Low birth weight is the outcome of preterm birth of restricted fetal development, which is again another significant outcome associated with maternal stress. Findings have indicated that maternal stress has been instrumental in reducing uteroplacental blood flow, thereby limiting the flow of nutrients and oxygen into the fetus. Dunkel Schetter and Tanner [71] stressed that higher maternal stressors are often exacerbated through unsupportive partner dynamics and were strongly associated with fetal growth restriction and lower birth weights.

Stress also influences the maternal immune system, increasing the risk of infections like bacterial vaginosis, a risk factor for preterm labor [73]. These psychosocial stressors caused by withdrawal from the partner or conflict are damaging during the critical periods of fetal growth. Lederman et al. [74] highlighted that stressors during this second trimester, whenever organogenesis and placental growth levels increase, lead to the most profound effects on birth outcomes. Additionally, lowered affective or financial assistance from partners intensifies maternal stressors, thereby compounding its influence on the outcomes of pregnancy. Thus, intervention findings underscore the mitigating aspects of partner-induced stress to improve birth outcomes. It's necessary to apply mindfulness techniques and couple therapy in dissolving maternal stressors and lowering the adverse risks.

12.7 Strategies for Managing Partner-Induced Maternal Stress

Several strategies could be considered to manage partner stress and partner-induced maternal stress, including open communication, couples counseling, stress reduction techniques for couples, parental leave, and social and community support.

12.7.1 Open Communication

Research emphasizes the importance of communication between couples in dealing with stressors and providing emotional support. Explicit stress communication facilitates perceived responsiveness in dyadic coping, contributing to relationship satisfaction [75]. Couples' shared responses to stressors can buffer the relationship from the strain of daily stress, increase intimacy, and strengthen the relationship [76]. Intimate relationships are a principal source of emotional support, which fosters recipients' health and well-being. Yet, being able to provide support can be stressful, particularly if people are burdened with their emotional difficulties, and such stress may interfere with people's ability to behave in emotionally supportive ways. Open communication and mutual support are needed to maintain relationship quality and manage stressors. Developing communication skills and fostering supportive behaviors can help couples navigate challenges and strengthen their emotional bonds [77].

Key elements of the communication process include one partner disclosing relevant information about the event, the stress and negative emotions they are feeling, and the other partner responding to this disclosure [78]. Once the partners have engaged in such a communication sequence, the partner who initiated the sequence understands, interprets, and evaluates their partner's reactions, being sensitive to how the partner responds to their concerns and needs. Perceptions of responsiveness are part of the dyadic coping process with stress. However, it is not uncommon for partners to fail to respond to expressions of stress. This response is due to a lack of motivation or skills. Therefore, explicit and unambiguous stress communication strategies can protect couples from maladaptive coping dynamics, increase couple responsiveness in the dyadic coping process, enhance adaptation to stressors, and strengthen the relationship [75].

In addition, concerning parent-child communication, open communication between parents and children facing health challenges is also essential to improving psychosocial well-being and reducing stress. Studies have shown that open communication is associated with positive illness attitudes, better self-perceptions, higher quality of life for children, and more positive responses to illness for parents [79].

12.7.2 Couples Counseling and Support Programs

Psychological distress before and after childbirth is common in both parents. Depression in one parent poses significant coping challenges for their partner and increases their own risk of depression. Preventive interventions that target both parents' distress and improve quality of life will also likely benefit the couple's relationship and their child's emotional and social adjustment [80].

One educational program for couples is the Family Hope Program, which provides an integrative program model for new and expectant parents that includes couple/relationship education and parenting elements. It is a 12-week, face-to-face, group-based program for expectant or new parents designed to provide couples with information and skills to help during this transition, including topics related to newborn care, stress management, co-parenting, and the role of partners [81]. The program effects were moderated by socioeconomic factors, such that socioeconomically disadvantaged individuals showed increased communication and relationship stability benefits. A study investigating changes in couple, parenting, and individual functioning following family expectations program participation showed short-term changes, mainly reduced psychological distress. The effects were stronger for married than unmarried participants [82].

In addition to the Family Hope Program, there is the Baby Steps Well-Being program. This is a free, self-guided web program optimized for various devices. It aims to prevent stress and improve the well-being of new parents. The program contains four modules with practical tips on preparing for a baby and dealing with issues related to feeding, sleeping, and soothing (baby care). The complete Baby Steps Well-Being program has four additional modules that provide information and interactive problem-solving on self-care, relationships, interacting with the baby, and adjusting to a new role, as well as a module focused explicitly on fathers discussing ways to support their partners and share parenting duties [83].

12.7.3 Stress Reduction Techniques for Couples

Another stress management technique for couples is stress reduction techniques. Numerous studies examine various stress releases to address a couple of types of stress, such as mindfulness, meditation, and relaxation exercises. Stress management programs such as mindfulness exercises, cognitive-behavioral intervention, exercise, and relaxation techniques affect neurobiological, psychological, and physiological processes, decreasing stress and improving well-being [84]. Regarding mindfulness, Cambridge Dictionary defines mindful as "deliberately aware of your body, mind, and feelings in the present moment, in order to create a feeling of calm" [85]. The Merriam-Webster Dictionary defines mindfulness as "the practice of maintaining a nonjudgmental state of heightened or complete awareness of one's thoughts, emotions, or experiences on a moment-to-moment basis" [86]. In the context of family therapy, ultimately, mindfulness refers to the present, an attribute that may be cultivated to perceive oneself and others with diminished judgment and increased love [87].

When people act mindfully, they will keep calm when reacting to the thoughts or emotions that come to their mind. The fundamental idea of practicing mindfulness is that it enables individuals to modify their interaction with traumatic or distressing thoughts and feelings. Mindfulness-based stress reduction (MBSR) is a training and practice designed for those experiencing psychological and emotional distress due to life events, physical problems, or pain, aimed at alleviating stress and anxiety symptoms, mitigating negative emotions, and enhancing overall mental health and functioning [88].

One mindfulness intervention relevant for women and partners is mindfulness-based relationship enhancement (MBRE). MBRE refers to a set of methods used for couples who agree with each other to enhance their coping ability related to relational stress [89]. There are four specific areas of MBRE: mindfulness, acceptance, relaxation, and self-broadening through techniques such as partner-centered loving-kindness meditation, learning to be mindful of daily happy situations, and enhancing closeness through mindful touch and eyecontact [89].

A study conducted by Winter et al. [90] indicates that mindfulness-based programs for women and their partners can potentially increase the perceived relationship between couples and the individual burden. The improved relationship quality will eventually reduce the risk of maternal stress. Several types of mindfulness therapies and their outcomes are available in Table 12.1.

Mindfulness, which can strengthen relationship quality between couples, is an effective technique to reduce partner and maternal stress since stress can be mitigated by co-regulation and adaptive self-regulation in a close relationship [21, 91]. Mindfulness couple and family therapy can improve mindfulness in both spouses and foster their autonomy and acceptance [92]. Furthermore, mindfulness focusing on family relationships has been connected to broad positive results, including empathy, resolving conflict skills, emotion regulation, and partnership satisfaction [87].

Another management to reduce stress is meditation. Mindfulness meditation is a broad word that refers to several methods empirically shown to enhance clinically significant cognitive and health benefits [93]. A study on mindfulness meditation in 15 healthy individuals showed significantly lower pain receiving brief four-session

Table 12.1 The type of mindfulness intervention and the outcomes [90]

Type of intervention	Effects on dyadic outcomes	Effects on individual outcomes
Mindfulness-based stress reduction (MBSR) and mindfulness-based relationship enhancement (MBRE) Psychoeducation Loving-kindness meditation Compassion exercises Group-based interventions offline and online	Relationship satisfaction	Mindfulness Increase self-compassion Decrease symptom burden Increase well-being Improvements in psychological stress parameters

therapy. Participants, instructed to concentrate on breath sensations and release feelings without judgment, exhibited a 40% reduction in pain intensity and a 57% drop in painful unpleasantness when exposed to noxious heat. Functional MRI revealed increased activation in brain areas such as the subgenual anterior cingulate cortex, orbitofrontal cortex, and right anterior insula, which is associated with pain regulation and sensory modification in conjunction with bilateral thalamic inactivation. The findings indicate that mindfulness alleviates pain via many brain pathways that engage top-down regulation. The study lacked a control group; however, later research rectified this deficiency [93]. If the couple uses this method, it can bring both women and partners the dyad effect. A study among patients with metastatic brain tumors indicates that online couple-based meditation intervention using videoconferencing was feasible; participants and partners mentioned the intervention as beneficial. This method also increased patients' cognitive and general disease symptoms, interference from symptoms, depressive manifestations, relationship well-being, and compassion [94].

Regarding relaxation exercise, the National Center for Complementary and Integrative Health acknowledges that relaxation methods may be beneficial in managing several stress-related health events, such as anxiety associated with progressive health issues and in people experiencing medical treatment [95]. The relaxation sample includes progressive muscle relaxation, deep breathing, and guided imagery, significantly increasing psychological relaxation and improving coping with stress and well-being [96]. In the diaphragmatic breathing condition, a study indicated that when a substantial interaction effect of group by time on sustained attention was observed, sustained attention markedly improved post-training, accompanied by a notable reduction in cortisol levels following the training [97]. By relaxing together, women and partners can release stress and improve their well-being.

Since stress reduction can significantly reduce stress and improve a couple's well-being, the maternity healthcare professional and related stakeholders can facilitate or support women and partners in stress reduction techniques. Programs such as mindfulness-based relationship enhancement (MBRE), mindfulness couple and family therapy, couple-based meditation intervention, or couple relaxation classes implementing progressive muscle relaxation, deep breathing, and guided imagery can also be implemented in primary health services from pregnancy until postpartum.

12.7.4 Parental Leave for Women and Partners

Being a parent is not an easy process; it takes a challenging adaptation stage. New parenthood can be difficult for couples since a newborn brings changes and stress that might lower the relationship's happiness and partner's social support [98]. These challenges were exacerbated by exhaustion and sleep deprivation, social seclusion and feelings of loneliness, and the challenge of managing work, education, and family obligations [99]. Positive emotions may help adapt healthy relationships to severely stressful situations that risk intimate partnerships, such as when adapting to becoming parents [98]. Interventions targeting parental emotional and psychological interventions, mainly for fathers, benefit the transition to parenthood [100]. In addition, work allocation, parental leave distribution, and the gendered aspects of maternity enable parents to be aware of the parenthood transition [99].

Regarding leave distribution, providing leave enables new parents to have adequate time to take care of the baby. New parents face burdens that trigger stressful conditions without proper time available. Thus, parental leave is essential to support them in becoming parents, as it gives parents more time and serves newborn babies with the best service they can provide. When both mothers and fathers have parental leave together, it allows them to build intimacy. A balanced relationship's intimacy will enhance mothers' mental and physical health [18]. In addition, paid leave for new parents positively impacts children's health and development, and paid paternity significantly impacts gender equality, family well-being, and financial returns [101].

Partner parental leave also benefits maternal health and well-being by enhancing partner support availability and sharing domestic job responsibilities. Partners felt that taking paternal leave can help mothers in the early phase of motherhood [102]. Moreover, parental leave supports the subversion of maternal ideals and transformations in domestic gender roles, liberating mothers from some household responsibilities, allowing them to engage in self-care, and prioritizing their wellness. The prevalence of paternal depression in those who used paternal leave was lower compared to those who did not use paternity leave [103]. For mothers, a longer duration of leave was correlated with a decreased risk of poor maternal mental health, such as the symptoms of depression, psychological distress, and burnout. It reduced mental healthcare utilization [104]. Specifically, for first-time mothers, more generous maternity leave decreases 0.38 point Euro-D depression indicator grade in old age [105].

Since paid maternity leave provides benefits for not only maternal mental well-being but also the whole family members, facilitating paid maternity leave of at least 14 weeks should be encouraged per the Maternity Protection Convention, 2000, The General Conference of the International Labor Organization [106]. However, a report from the World Policy Analysis Center highlights that as of 2023, there are 186 nations globally providing only some maternal paid leave, 120 nations offer at least 14 weeks, and only 55 nations guarantee 6 months or more maternal leave. For paternal leave, 108 nations provide some form of paternal paid leave, several countries such as Australia, Japan, New Zealand, and the Republic of Korea provide 14 weeks or more paternal paid leave, and unfortunately, Indonesia only guarantees 2–5 days paternal paid leave [107, 108]. Thus, issuing a global policy to push countries to implement at least 14 weeks of paternal leave is urgent, ensuring fathers have adequate time to assist mothers in caring for newborn babies and preventing maternal and paternal stress.

Regarding maternal and paternal paid leave, the Organization for Economic Co-operation and Development (OECD) reported that in April 2022, OECD countries offered nationwide paid maternity and paternity leave around delivery, but duration, payment, and uptake vary widely [109]. Paid maternity leave ranges from

43 weeks in Greece to none in the USA (though some US states give it). The OECD averages 18.5 weeks. Most OECD nations offer paid paternity leave; however, it averages 2.3 weeks. Spain leads with 16 weeks, three times longer than Portugal. Four countries offer only 1 week of paid paternity leave, while nine do not [109]. In addition to maternity and paternity leave, all but 11 OECD nations offer paid parental and/or homecare leave. Finland provides the most prolonged parental and homecare leave until the child's third birthday, while the OECD average is 39 weeks [109].

12.7.5 Social and Community Support

New parents may feel lonely and isolated while taking care of newborn babies. Social support is essential at this period, encompassing emotional support, companionship, knowledge and resources, and practical assistance such as meal preparation or errands [110]. Social support is valuable when people who are being supported feel cared for and valued and have a sense of belonging to a broader network by partners, family members, friends, peers, colleagues, and others from the broader community [102].

Social support is not only essential for mothers but also critical for fathers as they are the primary support for mothers. Fathers may experience heightened stress and loneliness, which the availability of social support can mitigate [111]. Feeling loneliness of fathers is due to perceived exclusion from maternity care services and low information access in the healthcare system. Thus, promoting social support from experienced fathers, friends, family, and partners would be prudent to mitigate paternal postnatal sadness [111].

Social support received by the father has a dyadic correlation with maternal stress. Higher quality support received by father's correlates with reduced maternal pregnancy stress, mitigating impairments in mother-infant bonding. Similarly, higher-quality support provided to mothers mitigated paternal pregnancy stress and subsequent impairments in father-infant bonding [112]. For mothers, inadequate support from partners, friends, and family correlates with an increased risk of depressive and anxiety symptoms. Distance-delivered programs, utilizing Internet or telephone modalities, have been shown to reduce levels of depression and anxiety [113–115]. For adolescent parents, social support will also increase their parenting competence mediated by parental depression [116]. Providing support using WhatsApp groups might benefit adolescents living in a country that utilizes WhatsApp as main communication media since it is considered a feasible and efficient consultation method [117].

12.8 Cultural and Social Perspectives on Partner's Stress and Maternal Health

As highlighted in the earlier section of this chapter, partners' stress can significantly contribute to maternal stress, reflecting the interconnected nature of shared emotional and social dynamics within a relationship. This interplay highlights the importance of addressing both partners' well-being, as unresolved stress in one partner may amplify maternal stress, potentially impacting maternal health and overall family functioning. Additionally, maternal health is not an isolated phenomenon but a deeply interconnected experience, influenced by the social context and the cultural norms, within which there are relational dynamics [118, 119]. A partner's stress, while often underexplored in scholarly discourse, plays a critical role in shaping maternal health outcomes. The intricate relationship between these factors necessitates a deeper examination of the cultural expectations, gender roles, and systemic structures that frame the maternal experience and the psychosocial pressures partners endure during this transformative period.

Cultural norms form the foundation upon which maternal and partner experiences are constructed. In collectivist societies, such as those prevalent in Southeast Asia, sub-Saharan Africa, and parts of the Middle East, the partner's role is often laden with expectations to fulfill familial and societal obligations [120]. This may include economic provision, deference to elder family members' decisions, and adherence to traditional gender roles [118, 121]. Moreover, the pressure to meet these cultural benchmarks often manifests as heightened stress, with adverse consequences for maternal well-being [122]. Stress, even when not directly expressed, can influence maternal psychological states, creating an environment where anxiety and emotional strain are mutually amplified. Stress also triggered mothers to be less likely to adopt a healthy lifestyle [123].

In contrast, individualistic cultures, which focus on nuclear family autonomy, offer different challenges. The emphasis on self-sufficiency and limited reliance on extended family networks often isolates partners from external support [124]. In such contexts, partners may experience heightened anxiety related to managing parental responsibilities alone. This isolation, coupled with occupational demands, creates an environment where stress is internalized, further complicating maternal health dynamics.

12.8.1 Gender Roles, Socioeconomic Structure, and Emotional Dynamics

The perpetuation of traditional gender roles significantly shapes how partners cope with stress during pregnancy. Societal constructions of masculinity often discourage men from articulating their emotional struggles, fostering a culture of silence that indirectly burdens maternal health [122]. A partner's unaddressed stress can intensify relational tensions, leading to diminished emotional support for the expectant mother. Studies in psychosocial health suggest that maternal stress is intricately linked to adverse pregnancy outcomes, such as preterm labor and reduced fetal growth, emphasizing the relational impact of a partner's mental state on maternal health [119, 120].

In societies where egalitarian ideals are embraced, partners are increasingly expected to share caregiving roles. However, the transition toward such models is not without challenges. Partners may feel unprepared for these expanded responsibilities, primarily when societal structures do not provide adequate support or resources to facilitate this shift. This underscores the importance of fostering educational and institutional interventions that equip partners to navigate their roles effectively without exacerbating stress levels [125].

The availability and accessibility of social support systems, both informal and institutional, serve as critical buffers against stress for partners and, by extension, for maternal health [126, 127]. In nations with progressive parental leave policies, universal healthcare, and robust community-based support, partners are better positioned to provide consistent emotional and physical support during pregnancy [128–130]. Conversely, partners often face compounded stress from economic and occupational pressures in societies with minimal state intervention or inadequate healthcare infrastructure. This stress invariably seeps into the maternal experience, further complicating health outcomes for both mother and child.

Economic disparities deepen these challenges, particularly in marginalized or low-income communities. For these groups, the strain of securing necessities often supersedes emotional well-being, creating an environment of chronic stress [125]. This is especially pronounced in contexts where structural inequities, such as systemic racism, limited healthcare access, or cultural stigmatization, in turn, amplified existing vulnerabilities [127]. Addressing these disparities requires material support and culturally informed policies that recognize the nuanced interplay between systemic inequity and individual health outcomes.

12.8.2 Sociocultural Approach to Addressing Paternal Stress

Cultures influence positive or negative attitudes toward health practice and belief [131]. To meaningfully address the relationship between partner stress and maternal health, it is imperative to adopt an intersectional and culturally sensitive approach. This involves recognizing the interplay between cultural identity, socioeconomic status, gender dynamics, and systemic inequalities [127]. For example, within Indigenous or diasporic communities, unique historical and cultural contexts often shape health behaviors and perceptions of care [132]. Any intervention that disregards these dimensions risks perpetuating inequities and failing to address the root causes of stress.

Parallel to the above, healthcare systems and policymakers must prioritize the inclusion of partners in maternal health initiatives. Prenatal and postnatal care programs that actively involve partners have shown promise in reducing stress and improving maternal outcomes [133]. Educational campaigns that challenge restrictive gender norms and equip partners with strategies for managing stress and providing emotional support are essential for fostering equitable caregiving roles [118, 120, 134]. For adolescent pregnancy, where typically they have less ANC and a high risk of stress, facilitating friendly and easy access to psychological healthcare might improve quality and appropriate care for adolescent mothers [135, 136]. Moreover, community-based initiatives that bridge cultural traditions with contemporary healthcare practices can further enhance relational and maternal well-being.

The intricate relationship between partner stress and maternal health underscores the profound influence of cultural and social structures on health outcomes. Scholars and practitioners can better understand the multifaceted nature of maternal care by critically examining the cultural constructs, gendered expectations, and systemic inequities that frame this relationship. Addressing partner stress through inclusive, culturally informed, and systemic interventions offers a pathway toward a more holistic and equitable maternal health framework that ultimately benefits not only mothers but entire families and communities.

12.9 Future Directions for Research and Intervention

Partner stress is a crucial but underexplored determinant of maternal well-being during the perinatal period. Despite a growing body of evidence demonstrating the profound impact of relational stress on maternal health outcomes, significant gaps remain in the literature, and opportunities for targeted interventions have yet to be fully realized. This section highlights these gaps, outlines potential areas for research, and proposes interventions emphasizing family-centered prenatal care to mitigate partner-induced maternal stress.

Gaps in the Current Literature

Several methodological and conceptual constraints still limit research on partner stress and maternal health. Longitudinal studies that track partner stress across pregnancy and postpartum are scarce, leaving a gap in understanding how cumulative stress affects maternal mental health, pregnancy outcomes, and postpartum recovery [137]. Moreover, much of the existing research is conducted in Western settings, failing to account for the diverse cultural and socioeconomic contexts that influence partner and maternal stress. For instance, in collectivist societies, extended family involvement and community expectations may amplify partner stress, which in turn exacerbates maternal stress [138].

The mechanisms linking partner stress to maternal outcomes also remain underexplored. While emotional contagion, empathic distress, and behavioral responses have been identified as potential pathways, further investigation is needed to elucidate how these mechanisms interact and how they can be mitigated [139]. Additionally, most studies focus on heteronormative, nuclear family structures, neglecting the experiences of single parents, LGBTQ+ families, and families with non-marital partners, thus limiting the generalizability of findings [140]. Expanding research to encompass these diverse family dynamics is critical for developing inclusive interventions.

Potential Areas for Intervention

Addressing partner-induced maternal stress requires a multifaceted approach that integrates evidence-based strategies into prenatal care frameworks. One promising avenue is the development of couple-based stress reduction programs, including cognitive-behavioral therapy (CBT), mindfulness practices, and problem-solving techniques tailored to expectant parents. These programs could be incorporated into routine antenatal care, with modules addressing shared stress management and emotional support [141]. Family-centered prenatal care models represent another area of innovation. Involving partners in antenatal consultations, educational workshops, and decision-making processes can foster mutual understanding and reduce relational stress.

At the policy level, interventions to reduce external stressors, such as financial and work-related pressures, are essential. Policies promoting parental leave, flexible work arrangements, and affordable childcare can alleviate partner stress, indirectly benefiting maternal health. For example, countries with a more generous paid leave policy help improve family well-being [142]. Parental leave policies might impact parent mental health [104, 143].

Culturally tailored community-based interventions are crucial in addressing the unique stressors faced by families in non-Western contexts. Community health workers or peer support groups could deliver culturally relevant stress management programs, incorporating traditional practices alongside evidence-based techniques [144]. In Western countries such as the United States, most community-based programmes and interventions for perinatal mental health are delivered in home or community settings by individuals regarded as community change agents, including doulas, nurses, midwives, and community health workers [145]. Similarly, digital health tools like mobile applications offering stress management resources, virtual counseling, and psychoeducation for couples can provide scalable solutions, particularly for families in underserved areas [146–148].

Future Research Directions

Future studies should adopt an intersectional framework to examine how race, gender, socioeconomic status, and cultural norms intersect to influence partner-induced maternal stress. Additionally, research on biomarkers such as cortisol levels in both partners could provide insights into the physiological pathways linking stress to maternal and fetal outcomes [139]. Investigating the intergenerational effects of partner-induced maternal stress on child development, including neurodevelopmental and behavioral outcomes, is another critical area for exploration. For future qualitative studies involving mothers with young babies, it is challenging for mothers to participate in an interview when their babies are unsettled, hungry, or sleepy [149]. Thus, it is essential to discuss with mothers the effective time for interviewing starting the interview process.

12.10 Conclusions

Partner stress is correlated with maternal stress through mechanism such as emotional contagion, empathic distress, and behavioral responses. The causes of partner stress include financial and work-related stress, anticipation of new roles and responsibilities, relationship adjustments, health concerns, and financial issues. The partner stress brings a dyadic effect, leading to maternal stress. The impact of partner-induced maternal stress on maternal mental health includes anxiety, depression, chronic maternal stress, lower relationship quality, mirroring partner stressors, irritable action, and motherhood adaptation issues. The impacts of paternal-induced maternal stress were hormonal alteration, increased cortisol, cardiovascular problems, lower sleep quality, fatigue, decreased immune system, longer wound healing, and breastfeeding-related issues.

Furthermore, the effect of partner-induced maternal stress on pregnancy and fetus includes organogenesis and placental growth issues, fetal growth retardation, fetus long-term metabolic problems, preterm labor, early labor onset, and lower oxygen and nutrient flow. To manage partner-induced maternal stress, several programs benefit, such as building open communication, providing counseling and support programs for couples, giving stress-education intervention for couples, facilitating sufficient parental leave for couples, and enhancing social and community support. Since cultural norms establish the basis for maternal and partner experiences, it is crucial to address paternal stress by using inclusive, culturally informed, and systemic programs with a more holistic and equitable maternal health framework to gain favorable outcomes not only for women and partners but also for the communities. Further longitudinal studies, mainly in eastern countries and with a diverse population, employing a family-centered policy approach and an intersectional framework to analyze the correlation of race, gender, socioeconomic status, and cultural beliefs on partner-induced maternal stress can fill the gap to reach more holistic understanding and provide a stronger recommendation.

12.11 Clinical and Research Implications

This chapter highlights the correlation between partner and maternal stress. Since partner stress is deemed to significantly affect maternal stress, early screening and intervention are needed to ensure partner stress can be assessed in the early stage, thus, preventing the worst impact on mothers. In addition, maternity healthcare professionals must provide comprehensive interventions to prevent and manage couple stress.

References

1. Caffieri A, Gómez-Gómez I, Barquero-Jimenez C, De-Juan-Iglesias P, Margherita G, Motrico E. Global prevalence of perinatal depression and anxiety during the COVID -19 pandemic: an umbrella review and meta-analytic synthesis [Internet]. 2024 [cited 2025 Jan 6]. Available from: https://obgyn.onlinelibrary.wiley.com/doi/full/10.1111/aogs.14740.
2. Pascal R, Casas I, Genero M, Nakaki A, Youssef L, Larroya M, et al. Maternal stress, anxiety, well-being, and sleep quality in pregnant women throughout gestation [Internet]. 2023 [cited 2025 Jan 6]. Available from: https://pmc.ncbi.nlm.nih.gov/articles/PMC10707410/.
3. Mitchell AR, Gordon H, Atkinson J, Lindquist A, Walker SP, Middleton A, et al. Prevalence of perinatal anxiety and related disorders in low- and middle-income countries: a systematic review and meta-analysis [Internet]. 2023 [cited 2025 Jan 6]. Available from: https://pmc.ncbi.nlm.nih.gov/articles/PMC10656650/.
4. Gelaye B, Rondon MB, Araya R, Williams MA. Epidemiology of maternal depression, risk factors, and child outcomes in low-income and middle-income countries. Lancet Psychiatry. 2016;3(10):973–82. https://doi.org/10.1016/S2215-0366(16)30284-X.
5. Heyne C-S, Kazmierczak M, Souday R, Horesh D, Lambregtse-van den Berg M, Weigl T, Horsch A, Oosterman M, Dikmen-Yildiz P, Garthus-Niegel S. Prevalence and risk factors of birth-related posttraumatic stress among parents: a comparative systematic review and meta-analysis. Clin Psychol Rev. 2022;94(94):102157. https://doi.org/10.1016/j.cpr.2022.102157.
6. Cheng CY, Chou YH, Chang CH, Liou SR. Trends of perinatal stress, anxiety, and depression and their prediction on postpartum depression. Int J Environ Res Public Health. 2021;18(17):9307. https://doi.org/10.3390/ijerph18179307.
7. Palomo-Gómez R, Rúger-Navarrete A, Antúnez-Calvente I, Vázquez-Lara JM, Rodríguez-Díaz L, Gómez-Salgado J, et al. Prenatal stress as a risk factor for maternal–foetal morbidity: a longitudinal study. Healthcare [Internet]. 2024;12(3):312. Available from: https://www.ncbi.nlm.nih.gov/pmc/articles/PMC10855075/. https://doi.org/10.3390/healthcare12030312.
8. Traylor CS, Johnson JD, Kimmel MC, Manuck TA. Effects of psychological stress on adverse pregnancy outcomes and nonpharmacologic approaches for reduction: an expert review. Am J Obstetr Gynecol MFM [Internet]. 2020;2(4):100229. Available from: https://www.ncbi.nlm.nih.gov/pmc/articles/PMC7513755/.
9. Caparros-Gonzalez RA, de la Torre-Luque A, Romero-Gonzalez B, Quesada-Soto JM, Alderdice F, Peralta-Ramírez MI. Stress during pregnancy and the development of diseases in the offspring: a systematic-review and meta-analysis. Midwifery. 2021;97:102939. https://doi.org/10.1016/j.midw.2021.102939. https://www.sciencedirect.com/science/article/abs/pii/S0266613821000188.
10. Matas-Blanco C, Caparros-Gonzalez RA. Influence of maternal stress during pregnancy on child's neurodevelopment. Psych. 2020;2(4):186–97. https://doi.org/10.3390/psych2040016.
11. Abrishamcar S, Zhuang BC, Thomas M, Gladish N, MacIsaac JL, Jones MJ, et al. Association between maternal perinatal stress and depression and infant DNA methylation in the first year of life. Transl Psychiatry [Internet]. 2024;14(1) Available from: https://www.nature.com/articles/s41398-024-03148-8.
12. Yang K, Wu J, Chen X. Risk factors of perinatal depression in women: a systematic review and meta-analysis. BMC Psychiatry [Internet]. 2022;22(1) Available from: https://bmcpsychiatry.biomedcentral.com/articles/10.1186/s12888-021-03684-3.
13. Røsand GMB, Slinning K, Eberhard-Gran M, Røysamb E, Tambs K. Partner relationship satisfaction and maternal emotional distress in early pregnancy. BMC Public Health. 2011;11(1) http://www.biomedcentral.com/1471-2458/11/161
14. Fisher SD. Paternal mental health: why is it relevant? Am J Lifestyle Med [Internet]. 2016;11(3):200–11. Available from: https://www.ncbi.nlm.nih.gov/pmc/articles/PMC6125083/. https://doi.org/10.1177/1559827616629895.

15. Trumello C, Babore A, Cofini M, Baiocco R, Chirumbolo A, Morelli M. The buffering role of paternal parenting stress in the relationship between maternal parenting stress and children's problematic behaviour. Int J Psychol. 2021; https://doi.org/10.1002/ijop.12758.
16. Daugherty JC, Bueso-Izquierdo N, Lara-Cinisomo S, Lozano-Ruiz A, Caparros-Gonzalez RA. Partner relationship quality, social support and maternal stress during pregnancy and the first COVID-19 lockdown. J Psychosom Obstet Gynecol. 2022;43(4):563–73. https://doi.org/10.1080/0167482X.2022.2101446.
17. Randall AK, Bodenmann G. The role of stress on close relationships and marital satisfaction. Clin Psychol Rev [Internet]. 2009;29(2):105–15. Available from: https://www.sciencedirect.com/science/article/pii/S0272735808001402.
18. Antoniou E, Tzanoulinou MD, Stamoulou P, Orovou E. The important role of partner support in women's mental disorders during the perinatal period. Liter Rev Mædica [Internet]. 2022;17(1):194–200. Available from: https://www.ncbi.nlm.nih.gov/pmc/articles/PMC9168558/.
19. Nixon N, Lin Y, Snow L. Catalyzing equity in STEM teams: harnessing generative AI for inclusion and diversity. Policy Insights Behav Brain Sci. 2024; https://doi.org/10.1177/23727322231220356.
20. Haslam DM, Burke K. Work, poverty, and financial stress. In: Handbook of parenting and child development across the lifespan; 2018. p. 495–510. https://doi.org/10.1007/978-3-319-94598-9_21.
21. Williams DT, Cheadle JE. Economic hardship, parents' depression, and relationship distress among couples with young children. Soc Mental Health. 2015;6(2):73–89. https://doi.org/10.1177/2156869315616258.
22. Zietz S, Lansford JE, Liu Q, Long Q, Oburu P, Pastorelli C, et al. A longitudinal examination of the family stress model of economic hardship in seven countries. Child Youth Serv Rev. 2022;143:106661. https://doi.org/10.1016/j.childyouth.2022.106661.
23. Lee JY, Lee SJ, Volling BL, Grogan-Kaylor AC. Examining mechanisms linking economic insecurity to interparental conflict among couples with low income. Fam Relat. 2022; https://doi.org/10.1111/fare.12698.
24. Candelori C, Trumello C, Babore A, Keren M, Romanelli R. The experience of premature birth for fathers: the application of the Clinical Interview for Parents of High-Risk Infants (CLIP) to an Italian sample. Front Psychol. 2015:6. https://doi.org/10.3389/FPSYG.2015.01444/BIBTEX.
25. Repetti R, Wang SW, Karantzas G, Mccabe M, Simpson J. ScienceDirect Spillover as a short-term process. Effects of job stress on family relationships [Internet]. 2017.; Available from: http://shuwen.haverford.edu/wp-content/uploads/2016/04/RepettiWang2017-job-stress-and-families-Curr-Opinion.pdf https://doi.org/10.1016/j.copsyc.2016.03.010.
26. Thorp SR, Krause ED, Cukrowicz KC, Lynch TR. Postpartum partner support, demand-withdraw communication, and maternal stress. Psychol Women Q. 2004;28(4):362–9. https://doi.org/10.1111/j.1471-6402.2004.00153.x.
27. Smoktunowicz E, Cieślak R. How job and family demands impact change in perceived stress: a dyadic study. Int J Occup Med Environ Health. 2017; https://doi.org/10.13075/IJOMEH.1896.01134.
28. Stefana A, Biban P, Padovani EM, Lavelli M. Fathers' experiences of supporting their partners during their preterm infant's stay in the neonatal intensive care unit: a multi-method study. J Perinatol. 2021; https://doi.org/10.1038/S41372-021-01195-3.
29. Hughes C, Devine TR, Foley S, Ribner DA, Mesman J, Blair C. Couples becoming parents: trajectories for psychological distress and buffering effects of social support. J Affect Disord. 2020;265:372–80. https://doi.org/10.1016/J.JAD.2020.01.133.
30. Paulson JF, Bazemore SD. Prenatal and postpartum depression in fathers and its association with maternal depression. JAMA [Internet]. 2010;303(19):1961. Available from: https://pubmed.ncbi.nlm.nih.gov/20483973/. https://doi.org/10.1001/JAMA.2010.605.

31. Raley S, Bianchi SM, Wang W. When do fathers care? Mothers' economic contribution and fathers' involvement in child care. Am J Sociol. 2012;117(5):1422–59. https://doi.org/10.1086/663354.
32. Shorey S, Chan V. Paternal mental health during the perinatal period: a qualitative systematic review. J Adv Nurs. 2020;76(6):1307–19. https://doi.org/10.1111/JAN.14325.
33. Baldwin S, Malone M, Sandall J, Bick D. A qualitative exploratory study of UK first-time fathers' experiences, mental health and wellbeing needs during their transition to fatherhood. BMJ Open [Internet]. 2019;9(9):e030792. Available from: https://bmjopen.bmj.com/content/9/9/e030792. https://doi.org/10.1136/BMJOPEN-2019-030792.
34. Molgora S, Acquati C, Saita E. The role of dyadic coping for the individual and relational well-being of couples during the transition to parenthood. J Fam Issues. 2021:0192513X2110223. https://doi.org/10.1177/0192513X211022394.
35. Finnbogadóttir H, Persson E. Risk for partners' depression and anxiety during pregnancy and up to one year postpartum: a longitudinal cohort study. Eur J Midwifery. 2022;6(June):1–12. https://doi.org/10.18332/EJM/148162.
36. Baldwin S, Malone M, Sandall J, Bick D. Mental health and wellbeing during the transition to fatherhood. JBI Database Syst Rev Implement Rep [Internet]. 2018;16(11):2118–91. Available from: https://journals.lww.com/jbisrir/pages/articleviewer.aspx?year=2018&issue=11000&article=00010&type=Fulltext. https://doi.org/10.11124/JBISRIR-2017-003773.
37. Brown RL, Fagundes CP, Thayer JF, Christian LM. Longitudinal changes in HRV across pregnancy and postpartum: effect of negative partner relationship qualities. Psychoneuroendocrinology. 2021;129:105216. https://doi.org/10.1016/J.PSYNEUEN.2021.105216.
38. Forte Camarneiro AP, de Miranda Justo JMR. Emotional states and psychopathological symptoms in couples during pregnancy and post-partum. J Reprod Infant Psychol. 2020:1–15. https://doi.org/10.1080/02646838.2020.1814226.
39. Smorti M, Ponti L, Prino LE, Rollè L. Maternal perception of couple relationship before and after the birth of first and second child and twins. Fam Relat. 2021; https://doi.org/10.1111/FARE.12610.
40. Alonzi S, Park J Eun PA, Saulsman C, Silverstein MW. An examination of COVID-19-related stressors among parents. Eur J Investig Health Psychol Educ [Internet]. 2021 [cited 2021 Aug 23];11(3):838–48. Available from: https://www.mdpi.com/2254-9625/11/3/61. https://doi.org/10.3390/EJIHPE11030061.
41. Davis K, Lu L, Gomez-Roas M, Leziak K, Jackson JL, Williams BR, et al. Psychosocial stressors of parenting and the postpartum period during COVID-19. Am J Obstet Gynecol. 2022;226(1):S208. https://doi.org/10.1016/J.AJOG.2021.11.356.
42. deMontigny F, Gervais C, Pierce T, Lavigne G. Perceived paternal involvement, relationship satisfaction, mothers' mental health and parenting stress: a multi-sample path analysis. Front Psychiatry. 2020:11. https://doi.org/10.3389/FPSYT.2020.578682/PDF.
43. Johansson M, Benderix Y, Svensson I. Mothers' and fathers' lived experiences of postpartum depression and parental stress after childbirth: a qualitative study. Int J Qual Stud Health Well Being. 2020;15(1):1722564. https://doi.org/10.1080/17482631.2020.1722564.
44. Tach L, Mincy R, Edin K. Parenting as a "Package Deal": relationships, fertility, and nonresident father involvement among unmarried parents. Demography [Internet]. 2010;47(1):181–204. Available from: https://www.jstor.org/stable/25651496.
45. Daundasekara SS, Schuler BR, Beauchamp JES, Hernandez DC. The mediating effect of parenting stress and couple relationship quality on the association between material hardship trajectories and maternal mental health status. J Affect Disord. 2021;290:31–9. https://doi.org/10.1016/j.jad.2021.04.058.
46. Aeri R, Farhoud F. Intimate Partner Violence during pregnancy: impact on women and children: a review. J Soc Behav Commun Health. 2024; https://doi.org/10.18502/jsbch.v8i1.15676.

47. Kimura M, Daibo I, Yogo M. The study of emotional contagion from the perspective of interpersonal relationships. Soc Behav Personal Int J [Internet]. 2008;36(1):27–42. https://psycnet.apa.org/doi/10.2224/sbp.2008.36.1.27.
48. Simpson JA, Rholes WS, Campbell L, Tran S, Wilson CL. Adult attachment, the transition to parenthood, and depressive symptoms. J Pers Soc Psychol. 2003;84(6):1172. https://doi.org/10.1037/0022-3514.84.6.1172.
49. Hompson A, Bolger N. Emotional transmission in couples under stress. J Marriage Fam. 1999;61(1):38. https://psycnet.apa.org/doi/10.2307/353881.
50. Mazzuca S, Kafetsios K, Livi S, Presaghi F. Emotion regulation and satisfaction in long-term marital relationships: the role of emotional contagion. J Soc Pers Relat. 2018;36(9):2880–95. https://psycnet.apa.org/doi/10.1177/0265407518804452.
51. Nitschke JP, Bartz JA. The association between acute stress & empathy: a systematic literature review. Neurosci Biobehav Rev. 2023;144:105003. https://doi.org/10.1016/j.neubiorev.2022.105003.
52. Engert V, Linz R, Grant JA. Embodied stress: the physiological resonance of psychosocial stress. Psychoneuroendocrinology. 2018; https://doi.org/10.1016/j.psyneuen.2018.12.221.
53. Greene JO, Burleson BR, editors. Handbook of communication and social interaction skills. Routledge; 2003. https://doi.org/10.4324/9781410607133.
54. Alio AP, Lewis CA, Scarborough K, Harris K, Fiscella K. A community perspective on the role of fathers during pregnancy: a qualitative study. BMC Pregnancy Childbirth. 2013;13:1. https://doi.org/10.1186/1471-2393-13-60.
55. McCarthy M, Houghton C, Matvienko-Sikar K. Women's experiences and perceptions of anxiety and stress during the perinatal period: a systematic review and qualitative evidence synthesis. BMC Pregnancy Childbirth. 2021;21:1–2. https://doi.org/10.1186/s12884-021-04271-w.
56. Poh HL, Koh SSL, Seow HCL, He HG. First-time fathers' experiences and needs during pregnancy and childbirth: a descriptive qualitative study. Midwifery. 2014;30(6):779–87. https://doi.org/10.1016/j.midw.2013.10.002.
57. Beck LA, Pietromonaco PR, DeBuse CJ, Powers SI, Sayer AG. Spouses' attachment pairings predict neuroendocrine, behavioral, and psychological responses to marital conflict. J Pers Soc Psychol. 2013;105(3):388–424. https://doi.org/10.1037/a0033056.
58. Philpott LF, Leahy-Warren P, FitzGerald S, Savage E. Stress in fathers in the perinatal period: a systematic review. Midwifery. 2017;55:113–27. https://doi.org/10.1016/j.midw.2017.09.016.
59. Boyce P, Condon J, Barton J, Corkindale C. First-time fathers' study: psychological distress in expectant fathers during pregnancy. Aust NZ J Psychiatry. 2007;41(9):718–25. https://doi.org/10.1080/00048670701517959.
60. Kowlessar O, Fox JR, Wittkowski A. The pregnant male: a metasynthesis of first-time fathers' experiences of pregnancy. J Reprod Infant Psychol. 2014;33(2):106–27. https://doi.org/10.1080/02646838.2014.970153.
61. Shishido Y, Latzman RD. Mother–son discrepant reporting on parenting practices: the contribution of temperament and depression. J Fam Psychol. 2017;31(4):398–408. https://doi.org/10.1037/fam0000284.
62. Witcher PM, Harvey CJ. Modifying labor routines for the woman with cardiac disease. J Perinat Neonatal Nurs. 2006;20(4):303–10. https://doi.org/10.1097/00005237-200610000-00008.
63. Antenatal depression programs cortisol stress reactivity in offspring through increased maternal inflammation and cortisol in pregnancy: the Psychiatry Research and Motherhood—Depression (PRAM-D) study. Psychoneuroendocrinology [Internet]. 2018;98:211–21. Available from: https://www.sciencedirect.com/science/article/pii/S0306453017316311. https://doi.org/10.1016/j.psyneuen.2018.06.017.
64. Van den Bergh BRH, Beijers R, Jaddoe VWV, Rijlaarsdam J. Emotional stress during pregnancy and its long-term impact on maternal and child development. Dev Rev. 2017;47:17–30. https://doi.org/10.1016/j.dr.2017.01.002.
65. Graignic-Philippe R, Dayan J, Chokron S, Jacquet A-Y, Tordjman S. Effects of prenatal stress on fetal and child development: a critical literature review. Neurosci Biobehav Rev [Internet].

2014;43(43):137–62. Available from: https://www.ncbi.nlm.nih.gov/pubmed/24747487. https://doi.org/10.1016/j.neubiorev.2014.03.022.
66. Divney AA, Sipsma H, Gordon D, Niccolai L, Magriples U, Kershaw T. Depression during pregnancy among young couples: the effect of personal and partner experiences of stressors and the buffering effects of social relationships. J Pediatr Adolesc Gynecol. 2012;25(3):201–7. https://doi.org/10.1016/j.jpag.2012.02.003.
67. Chapman HA, Hobfoll SE, Ritter C. Partners' stress underestimations lead to women's distress: a study of pregnant inner-city women. J Pers Soc Psychol. 1997;73(2):418–25. https://psycnet.apa.org/doi/10.1037/0022-3514.73.2.418.
68. Saur AM, Dos Santos MA. Risk factors associated with stress symptoms during pregnancy and postpartum: integrative literature review. Women Health. 2021;61(7):651–67. https://doi.org/10.1080/03630242.2021.1954132.
69. Pascal R, Casas I, Genero M, Nakaki A, Youssef L, Larroya M, Benitez L, Gomez Y, Martinez-Aran A, Morilla I, Oller-Guzmán TM. Maternal stress, anxiety, well-being, and sleep quality in pregnant women throughout gestation. J Clin Med. 2023;12(23):7333. https://doi.org/10.3390/jcm12237333.
70. Christian LM. Psychoneuroimmunology in pregnancy: immune pathways linking stress with maternal health, adverse birth outcomes, and fetal development. Neurosci Biobehav Rev. 2012;36(1):350–61. https://doi.org/10.1016/j.neubiorev.2011.07.005.
71. DunkelSchetter C, Tanner L. Anxiety, depression and stress in pregnancy: implications for mothers, children, research, and practice. Curr Opin Psychiatry [Internet]. 2012;25(2):141–8. Available from: https://www.ncbi.nlm.nih.gov/pmc/articles/PMC4447112/. https://doi.org/10.1097/yco.0b013e3283503680.
72. Lobel M, Cannella DL, Graham JE, DeVincent C, Schneider J, Meyer BA. Pregnancy-specific stress, prenatal health behaviors, and birth outcomes. Health Psychol. 2008;27(5):604–15. Available from: https://pubmed.ncbi.nlm.nih.gov/18823187/. https://doi.org/10.1037/a0013242.
73. Grote NK, Bridge JA, Gavin AR, Melville JL, Iyengar S, Katon WJ. A meta-analysis of depression during pregnancy and the risk of preterm birth, low birth weight, and intrauterine growth restriction. Arch General Psychiatry [Internet]. 2010;67(10):1012. https://doi.org/10.1001/archgenpsychiatry.2010.111.
74. Lederman RP, Weis KL, Lederman RP, Weis KL. Psychosocial anxiety, stress, and adaptation in pregnancy: assessment of seven dimensions of maternal development. Springer International Publishing; 2020. https://doi.org/10.1007/978-3-030-45738-9_1.
75. Pagani AF, Donato S, Parise M, Bertoni A, Iafrate R, Schoebi D. Explicit stress communication facilitates perceived responsiveness in Dyadic Coping. Front Psychol. 2019:10. https://doi.org/10.3389/FPSYG.2019.00401/PDF.
76. Milek A, Butler EA, Bodenmann G. The interplay of couple's shared time, women's intimacy, and intradyadic stress. 2015;29(6):831–42. https://doi.org/10.1037/FAM0000133.
77. Jayamaha SD, Overall NC, Girme YU, Hammond MD, Fletcher GJO. Depressive symptoms, stress, and poorer emotional support when needed by intimate partners. Emotion. 2021; https://doi.org/10.1037/EMO0001000.
78. Reis HT, Gable SL. Responsiveness. Curr Opin Psychol [Internet]. 2015;1:67–71. https://doi.org/10.1016/J.COPSYC.2015.01.001.
79. O'Toole S, Gallagher P, Benson A, Shahwan A, Austin JK, Lambert V. Exploring the relationship between parent–child communication about epilepsy and psychosocial well-being. J Health Psychol [Internet]. 2019;26(8):135910531987164. https://doi.org/10.1177/1359105319871642.
80. Nishimura A, Fujita Y, Katsuta M, Ishihara A, Ohashi K. Paternal postnatal depression in Japan: an investigation of correlated factors including relationship with a partner. BMC Pregnancy Childbirth. 2015;15(1):1–8. https://doi.org/10.1186/S12884-015-0552-X/TABLES/3.

81. Ritchie LL, Stanley SM, Allen MOT, Rhoades GK. Impact evaluation of the family expectations program and moderation by sociodemographic disadvantage. Fam Process. 2022; https://doi.org/10.1111/FAMP.12762.
82. Barton AW, Gong Q, Stanley SM, Rhoades GK. Changes in couple, parenting, and individual functioning following family expectations program participation. J Marital Fam Ther. 2022; https://doi.org/10.1111/JMFT.12613.
83. Kavanagh DJ, Connolly J, Fisher J, Halford WK, Hamilton K, Hides L, et al. The baby steps web program for the well-being of new parents: randomized controlled trial. J Med Internet Res. 2021;23(11):e23659. https://doi.org/10.2196/23659.
84. Geetanjali G, Wahane AS, Sharma A. Exploring effective strategies for stress management: enhancingmental well-being through mindfulness, CBT, exercise, and relaxation techniques. Bullet Environ Pharmacol Life Sci [Internet]. 2023;12(5):345–8. Available from: https://www.researchgate.net/publication/374290227_Exploring_Effective_Strategies_for_Stress_Management_Enhancing_Mental_Well-being_through_Mindfulness_CBT_Exercise_and_Relaxation_Techniques.
85. MINDFUL | meaning in the Cambridge English Dictionary [Internet]. dictionary.cambridge.org. Available from: https://dictionary.cambridge.org/dictionary/english/mindful.
86. Merriam-Webster. Definition of MINDFULNESS [Internet]. Merriam-webster.com. 2019. Available from: https://www.merriam-webster.com/dictionary/mindfulness.
87. Gambrel L. Mindfulness in marriage and family therapy [Internet]. Wiley Online LIbrary. American Association for Marriage and Family Therapy; [cited 2025 Jan 8]. Available from: https://onlinelibrary.wiley.com/page/journal/17520606/homepage/mindfulness_in_marriage_and_family_therapy.
88. Raj A, Kumar P. Efficacy of mindfulness based stress reduction (MBSR):a brief overiew. J Disabil Manag Rehabil [Internet]. 2018 [cited];4(1). Available from: https://www.researchgate.net/publication/328540330_Efficacy_of_Mindfulness_Based_Stress_Reduction_MBSR_A_Brief_Overiew.
89. Cuncic, Arlin. How mindfulness-based relationship enhancement can benefit you [Internet]. Verywell Mind, 2023. Available from: https://www.verywellmind.com/understanding-mindfulness-based-relationship-enhancement-4685242.
90. Winter F, Steffan A, Warth M, Ditzen B, Aguilar-Raab C. Mindfulness-based couple interventions: a systematic literature review. Fam Process. 2021;60(3) https://doi.org/10.1111/famp.12683.
91. Zaki J. Integrating empathy and interpersonal emotion regulation. Annu Rev Psychol. 2020;71:517–40. https://doi.org/10.1146/annurev-psych-010419-050830.
92. Gemescu M. Mindfulness-based couples and family therapy: a literature review. J Exp Psychother [Internet]. 2019;22(3) Available from: https://www.researchgate.net/publication/344666070_Mindfulness-Based_Couples_and_Family_Therapy_a_Literature_Review.
93. Zeidan F, Vago DR. Mindfulness meditation-based pain relief: a mechanistic account. Ann New York Acad Sci [Internet]. 2016;1373(1):114–27. Available from: https://www.ncbi.nlm.nih.gov/pmc/articles/PMC4941786/. https://doi.org/10.1111/nyas.13153.
94. Milbury K, Weathers SP, Durrani S, Li Y, Whisenant M, Li J, et al. Online couple-based meditation intervention for patients with primary or metastatic brain tumors and their partners: results of a pilot randomized controlled trial. J Pain Sympt Manag [Internet]. 2020 [cited 2022 Oct 11];59(6):1260–7. Available from: https://pubmed.ncbi.nlm.nih.gov/32061834/.
95. NIH. Mind and body approaches for stress and anxiety: what the science says [Internet]. NCCIH. 2024. Available from: https://www.nccih.nih.gov/health/providers/digest/mind-and-body-approaches-for-stress-science.
96. Toussaint L, Nguyen QA, Roettger C, Dixon K, Offenbächer M, Kohls N, et al. Effectiveness of progressive muscle relaxation, deep breathing, and guided imagery in promoting psychological and physiological states of relaxation. Taylor-Piliae R, editor. Evid Based Complement Alternat Med. 2021;2021(1):1–8. https://doi.org/10.1155/2021/5924040.

97. Ma X, Yue ZQ, Gong ZQ, Zhang H, Duan NY, Shi YT, et al. The effect of diaphragmatic breathing on attention, negative affect and stress in healthy adults. Front Psychol. 2017;8(874):1–12. https://doi.org/10.3389/fpsyg.2017.00874.
98. Don BP, Eller J, Simpson JA, Fredrickson BL, Algoe SB, Rholes WS, et al. New parental positivity: the role of positive emotions in promoting relational adjustment during the transition to parenthood. J Pers Soc Psychol. 2021; https://doi.org/10.1037/pspi0000371.
99. Lévesque S, Bisson V, Charton L, Fernet M. Parenting and relational well-being during the transition to parenthood: challenges for first-time parents. J Child Family Stud [Internet]. 2020;29(7):1938–56. Available from: https://link.springer.com/article/10.1007/s10826-020-01727-z.
100. Refaeli LB, Rodrigues M, Neaman A, Bertele N, Ziv Y, Talmon A, et al. Supporting the transition to parenthood: a systematic review of empirical studies on emotional and psychological interventions for first-time parents. Patient Educ Couns. 2023;120:108090. https://doi.org/10.1016/j.pec.2023.108090.
101. Herbert Smith Freehills. Indonesia: New law on maternity and paternity leave [Internet]. Herbert Smith Freehills | Global law firm. 2024. Available from: https://www.herbertsmithfreehills.com/notes/employment/2024-posts/indonesia-new-law-on-maternity-and-paternity-leave-.
102. Nisbet L. Partner support in the postnatal period: the impact of partner parental leave on maternal health and wellbeing in New Zealand [Internet] [Thesis]. [Te Herenga Waka, Victoria University of Wellington]; 2023 [cited 2025 Jan 8]. Available from: https://openaccess.wgtn.ac.nz/articles/thesis/Partner_Support_In_The_Postnatal_Period_the_Impact_of_Partner_Parental_Leave_on_Maternal_Health_and_Wellbeing_in_New_Zealand/23906265?file=41912946.
103. Barry KM, Gomajee R, Benarous X, Dufourg MN, Courtin E, Melchior M. Paternity leave uptake and parental post-partum depression: findings from the ELFE cohort study. Lancet Public Health. 2023;8(1):e15–27. https://doi.org/10.1016/s2468-2667(22)00288-2.
104. Heshmati A, Honkaniemi H, Juárez SP. The effect of parental leave on parents' mental health: a systematic review. Lancet Public Health [Internet]. 2023;8(1):e57–75. https://doi.org/10.1016/S2468-2667(22)00311-5.
105. Avendano M, Berkman LF, Brugiavini A, Pasini G. The long-run effect of maternity leave benefits on mental health: evidence from European countries. Soc Sci Med. 2015;132(132):45–53. https://doi.org/10.1016/j.socscimed.2015.02.037.
106. International Labour Organization, C183—Maternity Protection Convention, 2000 (No. 183), 2000. https://www.ilo.org/dyn/normlex/en/f?p=NORMLEXPUB:12100:0::NO::P12100_ILO_CODE:C183, Accessed 8 Jan 2025.
107. World Policy Analysis Centre. Extending Paid Maternal And Paternal Leave: Feasible Options For Indonesia Paid Parental Leave Indonesia in Context . November 2023. [Internet]. [cited 2025 Jan 9]. Available from: https://www.worldpolicycenter.org/sites/default/files/2024-04/Paid%20parental%20Leave%20Indonesia_WORLD%20Policy%20Analysis%20Center.pdf.
108. Republic of Indonesia. Undang-undang (UU) Nomor 4 Tahun 2024 tentang Kesejahteraan Ibu danAnak pada Fase Seribu Hari Pertama Kehidupan. Database Peraturan | JDIH BPK, 2024. Available from: https://peraturan.bpk.go.id/Details/289997/uu-no-4-tahun-2024.
109. Oecdstatistics. Paid parental leave: Big differences for mothers and fathers [Internet]. oecdstatistics.blog, 2023. Available from: https://oecdstatistics.blog/2023/01/12/paid-parental-leave-big-differences-for-mothers-and-fathers/.
110. MMHLA. Maternal mental health overview, 2023. https://www.mmhla.org/fact-sheets.
111. Cunningham SM, Power JM, Hyland P, Casey AM. Support for the supporter: paternal postpartum loneliness and social support during the COVID-19 pandemic. Am J Mens Health. 2024;18(3) https://doi.org/10.1177/15579883241249921.
112. Martin RCB, Brock RL. The importance of high-quality partner support for reducing stress during pregnancy and postpartum bonding impairments. Arch Womens Ment Health. 2023;26(2):201–9. https://doi.org/10.1007/s00737-023-01299-z.

113. Sufredini F, Catling C, Zugai J, Chang S. The effects of social support on depression and anxiety in the perinatal period: a mixed-methods systematic review. J Affect Disord. 2022;319:119–41. https://doi.org/10.1016/j.jad.2022.09.005.
114. MacMillan KK, Lewis AJ, Watson SJ, Bourke D, Galbally M. Maternal social support, maternal depression and emotional availability in early mother-infant interaction: findings from a pregnancy cohort. J Affect Disord. 2021; https://doi.org/10.1016/j.jad.2021.05.048.
115. Khuzaiyah S, Adnani QES, Chabibah N, Khanifah M, Lee KY. A qualitative study on mothers' experiences attending an online infant massage class: "It is funny! I feel close to my baby!". BMC Nurs. 2022;21(1) https://doi.org/10.1186/s12912-022-00952-9.
116. Angley M, Divney A, Magriples U, Kershaw T. Social support, family functioning and parenting competence in adolescent parents. Maternal Child Health J [Internet]. 2014;19(1):67–73. Available from: https://www.ncbi.nlm.nih.gov/pmc/articles/PMC4233010/
117. Khuzaiyah S, Adnani QES, Muthoharoh A, Chabibah N, Widyastuti W, Susiatmi SA, et al. Indonesian COVID-19 lesson: a mixed-methods study on adolescent health status and health services during pandemic. J Child Adolesc Psychiatr Nurs. 2024;37(2) https://doi.org/10.1111/jcap.12457.
118. Vasilevski V, Sweet L, Bradfield Z, Wilson AN, Hauck Y, Kuliukas L, Homer CSE, Szabo RA, Wynter K. Receiving maternity care during the COVID-19 pandemic: experiences of women's partners and support persons. Women Birth. 2022;35:298–306.
119. Finlayson K, Sacks E, Brizuela V, et al. Factors that influence the uptake of postnatal care from the perspective of fathers, partners and other family members: a qualitative evidence synthesis. BMJ Glob Health. 2023;8:e011086.
120. Abie A, Belay G, Asmare E, Ayalew N, Feyisa W, Kassie N. Male partner involvement in postnatal care service utilization and associated factors: a community-based cross-sectional study in Motta district, Northwest Ethiopia. PLoS One. 2023;18:e0276477.
121. Zhong Q, Xu Y. Dyadic coping mediates between parenting stress and marital adjustment among parents of 0–6 years old children. J Child Fam Stud. 2024;33:2337–47.
122. Nambile Cumber S, Williams A, Elden H, Bogren M. Fathers' involvement in pregnancy and childbirth in Africa: an integrative systematic review. Glob Health Action. 2024; https://doi.org/10.1080/16549716.2024.2372906.
123. Maulina R, Kuo SC, Liu CY, Lu YY, Khuzaiyah S, Caparros-Gonzalez RA. Does attachment and prenatal depression affect maternal health-promoting lifestyle during pregnancy? A cross-sectional study. Clin Epidemiol Glob Health. 2025;31:101904. https://doi.org/10.1016/j.cegh.2024.101904.
124. Lambermon F, Vandenbussche F, Dedding C, van Duijnhoven N. Maternal self-care in the early postpartum period: an integrative review. Midwifery. 2020;90:102799.
125. Oladeji O, Elmi Farah A, Oladeji B, Mohamed J. Male involvement in pregnancy and childbirth: a qualitative study in rural population in Awbare District of Somali region of Ethiopia. J Womens Health Dev. 2022; https://doi.org/10.26502/fjwhd.2644-28840074.
126. Hodnett ED, Gates S, Hofmeyr GJ, Sakala C. Continuous support for women during childbirth. Cochrane Database Syst Rev. 2013; https://doi.org/10.1002/14651858.CD003766.pub5.
127. Kashaija DK, Mselle LT, Mkoka DA. Husbands' experience and perception of supporting their wives during childbirth in Tanzania. BMC Pregnancy Childbirth. 2020;20:85.
128. Pizarro J, Gartzia L. Paternity leave: a systematic review and directions for research. Hum Resour Manag Rev. 2024;34:101001.
129. Saime SH, Abdul-Mumin KH, Hashim S. Admission to delivery suites: the importance of antenatal education. Br J Midwifery. 2022;30(4):215–21. https://doi.org/10.12968/bjom.2022.30.4.215.
130. Latiff HSB, Saime NS, Idris DR, Mohamad SM, Husaini A, Matassan NS, et al. Providing care to couples experiencing pregnancy loss. Br J Midwifery. 2023;31(3):172–6. https://doi.org/10.12968/bjom.2023.31.3.172.
131. Yıldız M, Gomes RF, Felix EO, Ademiju O, Tayyeb M, Noibi TO, et al. Attitudes of different religions towards breast milk bank: analysis of 17 countries with data mining. Women's Stud Int Forum. 2023;101:102840. https://doi.org/10.1016/j.wsif.2023.102840.

132. Navarro-Prado S, Sánchez-Ojeda MA, Plaza del Pino FJ, Vázquez-Sánchez MÁ, Tovar-Gálvez MI, Azirar-Mohamed N. Coping strategies during childbirth related to cultural identity: companionship, choice of analgesia and maternal satisfaction. Healthcare. 2023;11:1714.
133. McKinlay AR, Fancourt D, Burton A. Factors affecting the mental health of pregnant women using UK maternity services during the COVID-19 pandemic: a qualitative interview study. BMC Pregnancy Childbirth. 2022; https://doi.org/10.1186/s12884-022-04602-5.
134. Saime NS, Hashim SH, Mohamad SM, Sharbini SH, McKenna L, Abdul-Mumin KH. Initial care during miscarriage in the emergency department: a discussion of international context. 2023;31(11):646–51. https://doi.org/10.12968/bjom.2023.31.11.646.
135. Khuzaiyah S, Mumin KHA, McKenna L, Hashim SH. Health-seeking behaviours of pregnant adolescents: a scoping review. Br J Midwifery [Internet]. 2023;31(7):408–17. https://doi.org/10.12968/bjom.2023.31.7.408.
136. Khuziayah S, Hashim SH. Mental health problems among adolescents during pregnancy and postpartum. In: Unveiling shadows: nurturing maternal mental health. Jejak Publisher; 2023. https://www.researchgate.net/publication/374447224_MENTAL_HEALTH_PROBLEMS_AMONG_ADOLESCENTS_DURING_PREGNANCY_AND_POSTPARTUM.
137. Kingston D, Tough S, Whitfield H. Prenatal and postpartum maternal psychological distress and infant development: a systematic review. Child Psychiatry Hum Dev. 2012;43(5):683–714. https://doi.org/10.1007/s10578-012-0291-4.
138. Yim IS, Tanner Stapleton LR. The psychological and physiological sequelae of prenatal stress. Curr Psychiatry Rep. 2019;21(12):115.
139. Field T. Prenatal depression effects on early development: a review. Infant Behav Dev [Internet]. 2011;34(1):1–14. https://doi.org/10.1016/j.infbeh.2010.09.008.
140. Reblin M, Uchino BN. Social and emotional support and its implication for health. Curr Opin Psychiatry [Internet]. 2018;21(2):201–5. Available from: https://www.ncbi.nlm.nih.gov/pmc/articles/PMC2729718/. https://doi.org/10.1097/yco.0b013e3282f3ad89.
141. Feinberg ME, Kan ML. Establishing family foundations: intervention effects on coparenting, parent/infant well-being, and parent-child relations. J Fam Psychol. 2008;22(2):253–63. https://doi.org/10.1037/0893-3200.22.2.253.
142. Nandi A, Jahagirdar D, Dimitris MC, Labrecque JA, Strumpf EC, Kaufman JS, et al. The impact of parental and medical leave policies on socioeconomic and health outcomes in OECD countries: a systematic review of the empirical literature. Milbank Q. 2018;96(3):434–71. https://doi.org/10.1111/1468-0009.12340.
143. Jefferson EEY. Will it ever change? Lack of parental leave and its detrimental effects on maternal well-being. Lancet Region Health Am [Internet]. 2023;25:100572. https://doi.org/10.1016/j.lana.2023.100572.
144. Ramadani S, Sutrisno B, Zainal R. Community-based maternal mental health programs: lessons from Indonesia. Matern Child Health J. 2020;24(5):621–8.
145. Scroggins JK, Harkins SE, Brown S, Clair VS, LeBron GK, Barcelona V. A systematic review of community-based interventions to address perinatal mental health. Semin Perinatol. 2024:151945. https://doi.org/10.1016/j.semperi.2024.151945.
146. Chua JYX, Shorey S. Effectiveness of mobile application-based perinatal interventions in improving parenting outcomes: a systematic review. Midwifery. 2022;114:103457. https://doi.org/10.1016/j.midw.2022.103457.
147. Spadaro B, Martin-Key NA, Funnell E, Bahn S. m-Health solutions for perinatal mental health: a scoping review and appraisal following the MIND framework (preprint). JMIR Mhealth Uhealth. 2021; https://doi.org/10.2196/30724.
148. Hussain-Shamsy N, Shah A, Vigod SN, Zaheer J, Seto E. Mobile health for perinatal depression and anxiety: scoping review. J Med Internet Res. 2020;22(4):e17011. https://doi.org/10.2196/17011.
149. Khuzaiyah S, Abdul-Mumin KH, McKenna L, Hashim SH. The importance of reflexivity in data collection methods for qualitative midwifery research. Br J Midwifery. 2023;31(12):701–5. https://doi.org/10.12968/bjom.2023.31.12.701.

Fetal Programming: An Explanation on How Maternal Stress Impacts Future Generations

13

Jorge Lopez-Tello, Álvaro Llorente-Berzal, Silvia M. Arribas, and David Ramiro-Cortijo

Abstract

The prevalence of stress in society is dramatically increasing and has been linked to several medical complications, including cardiovascular disease, metabolic disorders, and immune dysfunction. This issue is particularly critical for pregnant women, one of the most vulnerable groups in our society. Maternal stress during pregnancy can negatively impact pregnancy outcomes and, in severe cases, may even lead to pregnancy loss. Moreover, stress during pregnancy not only affects maternal health but also disrupts placental growth and function, which in turn can impair fetal development. As a result, fetal growth and organ maturation may be compromised, increasing the risk of late-onset diseases in adulthood due to stress-induced fetal programming. This chapter presents compelling epidemiological and experimental evidence demonstrating how maternal

J. Lopez-Tello
Department of Physiology, Faculty of Medicine, Universidad Autónoma de Madrid, Madrid, Spain

Á. Llorente-Berzal
Department of Physiology, Faculty of Medicine, Universidad Autónoma de Madrid, Madrid, Spain

Food, Oxidative Stress and Cardiovascular Health (FOSCH), Instituto de Investigación Sanitaria, Hospital Universitario La Paz (IdiPAZ), Madrid, Spain

S. M. Arribas · D. Ramiro-Cortijo (✉)
Department of Physiology, Faculty of Medicine, Universidad Autónoma de Madrid, Madrid, Spain

Food, Oxidative Stress and Cardiovascular Health (FOSCH), Instituto de Investigación Sanitaria, Hospital Universitario La Paz (IdiPAZ), Madrid, Spain

Instituto Universitario de Estudios de la Mujer (IUEM), Universidad Autónoma de Madrid, Madrid, Spain
e-mail: david.ramiro@uam.es

R. A. Caparros-Gonzalez (ed.), *Maternal Stress during Pregnancy and Postpartum*, https://doi.org/10.1007/978-3-032-09245-8_13

stress influences offspring health and its effects on fetal organ development. Specifically, it describes how prenatal stress increases the risk of adult-onset conditions, including cardiometabolic disorders, neurological diseases, alterations in reproductive health, and even certain types of cancer. Additionally, it discusses emerging interventions aimed at mitigating the adverse effects of prenatal stress on both maternal well-being and fetal programming.

Keywords

Fetal programming · Cortisol · Maternal stress · Prenatal exposure delayed effects · Developmental origins of health and disease

13.1 Introduction

For many women, pregnancy is a cause for celebration. However, in other cases, it can be a vulnerable period marked by high levels of stress, depression, and anxiety [1]. Maternal stress refers to the physiological and psychological responses triggered when a pregnant woman faces significant psychosocial challenges that may exceed her ability to cope if left unaddressed. Studies have pointed out that around 15–20% of pregnant women experience mental health issues during gestation [2, 3]. Common social stressors include financial strain or poverty, community disasters, violence, partner abuse or mistreatment, divorce, loss of a family member, and social isolation. Additional stressors may include environmental factors, such as limited access to healthy food, pollution, workplace stress, and disruptions in the sleeping patterns [4, 5]. Alongside these external stressors, the maternal physical changes required to support fetal growth and prepare for childbirth and lactation can also impact maternal mental health [6]. Indeed, physical changes like weight gain can lead to negative self-image, altered eating patterns, and added stress [7] (Fig. 13.1).

In addition to the environmental, social, and psychological stressors, maternal stress can be exacerbated by preexisting medical conditions such as asthma or autoimmune disorders, as well as pregnancy-related complications like preeclampsia or gestational diabetes. Another source of stress is assisted reproduction, which has been associated with greater pregnancy-specific anxiety and poorer quality of life [8] (Fig. 13.1). These factors are especially concerning because maternal stress has been linked to an increased risk of adverse pregnancy outcomes, including preeclampsia, premature rupture of membranes, and, in severe cases, miscarriage [9]. Moreover, maternal stress can impair placental growth and function, which may result in a lower capacity of the placenta to transport oxygen and nutrients to the developing fetus [10]. These alterations in placental function, known as placental insufficiency, can disrupt fetal growth trajectory and interfere with the proper development and maturation of key fetal organs such as the brain, the heart, and the kidneys [11].

Fetal programming, or Developmental Origins of Health and Disease (DOHaD), refers to the process by which adverse conditions during critical periods of

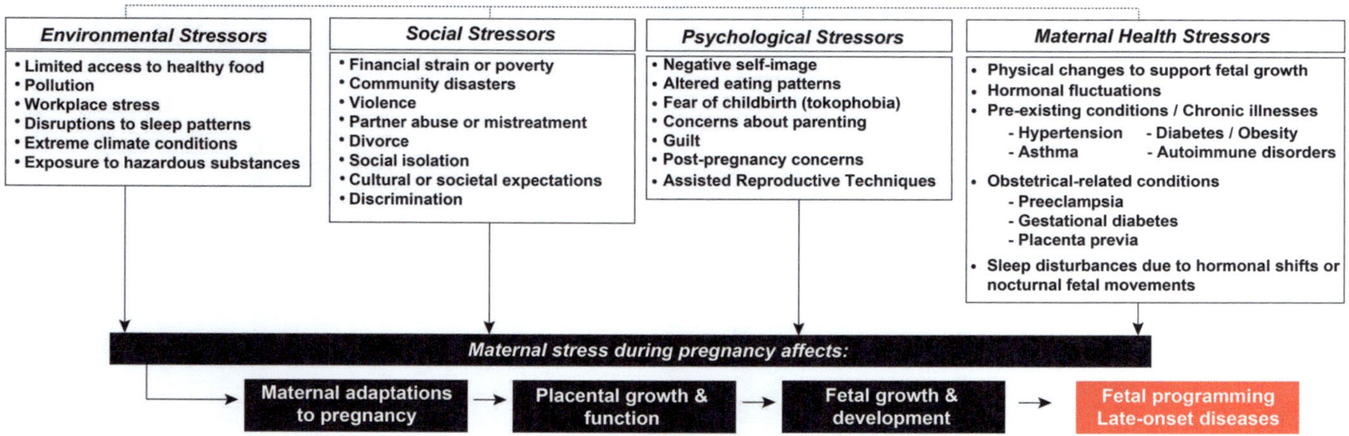

Fig. 13.1 Summary illustration shows how the different stressors are interconnected and contribute to maternal stress, affecting maternal adaptations to pregnancy, placental growth and function, and ultimately fetal growth. Exposure to intrauterine stress can impair fetal growth, leading to fetal programming, which can increase the risk of developing late-onset diseases in adulthood. Note that these stressors can act independently or synergistically, amplifying their effects

development cause permanent changes in organ structure and function, increasing the offspring's vulnerability to diseases later in life. As we will describe in the following sections of this chapter, among the various factors contributing to fetal programming, maternal stress plays a significant role by directly influencing the development and maturation of fetal organs. As a result, the negative effects of maternal stress can persist beyond birth. Newborns exposed to intrauterine stress are not only at greater risk of adverse outcomes but also have an increased likelihood of developing chronic diseases in adulthood, including schizophrenia, obesity, and hypertension. These long-term outcomes are attributed to stress-induced disruptions in the maturation of fetal organs [12].

Given the high prevalence of stress in the population and its association with increased obstetric complications and long-term effects on offspring health, this chapter aims to review: (1) the physiological responses of mother, placenta, and fetus in response to stress and (2) present findings from human studies and experimental animal models to provide a comprehensive view of how maternal stress affects fetoplacental development and its potential lifelong consequences for the health of the infants.

13.2 Changes in Maternal Physiology in Response to a Situation of Stress

During gestation, the body undergoes profound physiological changes to support fetal growth and development. These adaptations involve a wide range of organs and systems, including cardiovascular, metabolism, and endocrine systems, as reviewed elsewhere [6, 13–15].

One critical adaptation during a normal pregnancy occurs in the maternal hypothalamic–pituitary–adrenal (HPA) axis, which regulates the stress response via glucocorticoids. During gestation, the HPA axis becomes less sensitive to glucocorticoid feedback suppression, while the adrenal glands show enhanced responsiveness to adrenocorticotrophic hormone (ACTH) [16]. This is reflected in elevated levels of HPA axis hormones. In fact, maternal cortisol levels rise progressively throughout gestation, reaching approximately three times the levels observed in non-pregnant women by the third trimester [17, 18]. In addition, ACTH, corticosteroid-binding globulin, and corticotropin-releasing hormone (CRH) levels also rise in response to gestation [19, 20]. While these increments in the circulating levels of hormones regulating the HPA axis and the stress responses are considered normal and necessary for the course of pregnancy, excessive levels of cortisol may impact on the progression of the pregnancy. In fact, studies have found that high levels of maternal CRH at mid-gestation are associated with spontaneous preterm birth [21]. Moreover, maternal stress during the first trimester results in high glucocorticoid levels, which can also result in miscarriage [22].

Cortisol plays a crucial role in regulating immune responses. The maternal immune system undergoes extensive remodeling to balance immune tolerance toward the fetus with the need for protection against pathogens. This delicate balance requires profound modifications to the maternal immune tolerance capacity [23]. The first trimester of pregnancy is characterized by a controlled pro-inflammatory environment, predominantly driven by uterine innate immune cells. Notably, there is an increased abundance of noncytotoxic uterine natural killer (uNK) cells, which play a critical role in promoting angiogenesis and facilitating trophoblast invasion [24]. Additionally, macrophages are present in higher abundance to support trophoblast migration [25]. These immune cells are particularly important in regulating inflammation and are also prone to modulation by maternal stress. Thus, under adverse stimuli or stressful conditions, uNK may adopt cytolytic mechanisms that can negatively affect fetal implantation [26].

By the second trimester, when maternal cortisol levels continue rising as part of the normal physiological changes [19], an anti-inflammatory profile predominates to support the rapid growth of the fetus. By the end of gestation, the maternal immune system shifts back to a pro-inflammatory state to aid in the labor process. It has been observed that concurrent stress during pregnancy is associated with elevated pro-inflammatory gene expression in the maternal circulation [27]. Moreover, prenatal maternal stress alters offspring cytokine profiles at birth, increasing pro-inflammatory cytokines (IL-1β, IL-6, IL-8) and T helper lymphocytes [28, 29]. Taking together, adequate maternal adaptations, particularly in the HPA axis and the maternal immune system, are necessary for the success of pregnancy, and maternal stress during pregnancy may disrupt these systems, affecting fetal growth and the immune system of the developing offspring.

13.3 Changes in Placental Function in Response to Maternal Stress

The placenta is a transient organ responsible for multiple functions, including the transport of nutrients and the production of endocrine factors required for adapting maternal physiology in response to pregnancy [30]. The placenta, as a potent endocrine organ [6], plays a crucial role in regulating maternal stress responses. In fact, the placenta is a major producer of CRH and ACTH [31, 32]. CRH is released into maternal and fetal circulations, although the CRH levels are 20- to 30-fold lower in the umbilical cord plasma compared to the levels in the maternal circulation [32]. Therefore, during pregnancy, the placenta can also modulate the HPA axis.

Cortisol can cross the placenta, playing a role in fetal development, particularly in the maturation of the lungs in late pregnancy, when its levels rise [33]. However, continuous exposure to elevated levels of this hormone can be detrimental to fetal development (which will be discussed in the following sections) [34, 35]. To protect the fetus against excessive maternal cortisol levels, the placenta has several biological mechanisms to control the metabolism and transport of cortisol, primarily via enzymatic regulation. In fact, maternal endogenous cortisol concentrations are five to ten times higher than those in the fetus, with this gradient being maintained by a placental enzymatic barrier [33]. The maternal decidua and chorionic villi layers produce the glucocorticoid-inactivating enzyme 11β-hydroxysteroid dehydrogenase type 2 (11β-HSD2), an important unidirectional enzyme that converts biologically active cortisol into inactive cortisone [36–38]. In addition, the placenta also has a bidirectional glucocorticoid-regenerating enzyme called 11β-HSD1. This enzyme, located in decidual cells (stromal and epithelial cells) and fetal endothelial cells in the villous core, is involved in prostaglandin biosynthesis [39] and can convert biologically inactive cortisone into active cortisol [36].

Maternal stress can reduce this physiological cortisol barrier and also alter placental structure and function. It is known that placentas from mothers experiencing stress during pregnancy are larger and thicker [40]. Functionally, studies conducted in pregnant women with dysregulation of the HPA axis had reduced placental 11β-HSD2 expression along with higher placental 11β-HSD2 methylation levels, an epigenetic mechanism controlling gene expression [41]. In addition, there is evidence for an association between prenatal maternal stress and downregulation of placental 11β-HSD2 [42, 43]. This is worrying as decreasing placental 11β-HSD2 levels can elevate maternal cortisol levels reaching the fetus and cause fetal growth restriction [44, 45], a pathological condition associated with placental insufficiency [46]. Excess access to cortisol could also disrupt the fetal HPA axis with long-term consequences in neurobehavior and metabolism [41]. Moreover, experimental animal models have also observed that maternal stress and low food intake during gestation can reduce placental *Hsd11b2* gene expression resulting in low birth weight and programming changes in the HPA axis and the cardiovascular system of the offspring [47, 48]. However, human and animal studies evidence that acute stress has a differential influence on enzyme expression, inducing an upregulation, possibly as a mechanism to counteract a sudden surge in maternal cortisol, while chronic stress reduces the capacity of the placenta to upregulate 11β-HSD2 activity [41, 49]. Taken together, it can be concluded that the placenta, as a protective organ, plays a crucial role in the metabolism of cortisol and glucocorticoids, thus preventing fetal exposure to elevated cortisol levels but also modulating hormonal milieu according to the period of gestation.

13.4 Fetal Adaptive Changes in Response to Maternal Stress

Professor David Barker was the first to establish a link between poor intrauterine development, infant birth weight and the risk of adult-onset diseases, setting the so-called Barker Hypothesis [50, 51]. In his work, he proposed that adverse environmental factors, particularly maternal nutrition, are key determinants in shaping fetal growth and development. Since then, many other environmental and maternal stressors such as pollutants [52], microplastics [53, 54], or chronic maternal stress [55] have been identified in the pathogenesis of fetal programming.

The mechanisms by which adverse intrauterine environments affect the lifelong health of the offspring are complex and are thought to be mediated through epigenetic processes, including DNA methylation and covalent posttranslational histone modifications [56]. These processes influence the formation, structure, and function of offspring organs and tissues. As will be discussed in the following sections, the timing and duration of exposure to these aberrant intrauterine conditions play a critical role in shaping fetal development and long-term health. For example, stress during late gestation can negatively impact offspring motor development, while stress during early gestation can adversely affect cognitive function [57]. Additionally, the fetal sex can also modulate the effect, being male sex, and its placenta, more susceptible to maternal stress [58], concluding that male and female fetuses may use different strategies when adapting to maternal adversity [59]. These differences may be linked to the capacity of the fetus to adapt to the intrauterine stressor but are also likely associated with cellular events occurring during specific developmental windows, particularly during organogenesis.

It has been proposed that under adverse intrauterine conditions, the fetus may prioritize the growth of vital organs, such as the brain, at the expense of others, like the kidneys or the liver. This "survival strategy," known as brain sparing, allows the fetus to preserve the growth of essential organs in response to an adverse intrauterine environment [60]. However, while this may be beneficial for survival, it may not be advantageous postnatally, when the external environment differs from that predicted during early development, but the structural and functional development of organs has already been altered. Therefore, understanding the mechanisms underlying fetal programming is essential for improving lifelong health outcomes.

13.5 What Are the Long-Term Effects of Maternal Stress on Offspring Health?

13.5.1 Maternal Stress and Fetal Programming of Cardiovascular Health in the Offspring

Cardiovascular diseases (CVD), a leading cause of death worldwide [61], include disorders that directly affect the heart and blood vessels, such as coronary artery disease, heart failure, stroke, and peripheral arterial disease. These conditions are commonly associated with risk factors like hypertension and represent structural or functional abnormalities of the cardiovascular system that can lead to both acute events (e.g., heart attacks, strokes) and chronic conditions (e.g., chronic heart failure, arrhythmia, peripheral artery disease) [62]. While smoking and metabolic diseases, such as diabetes and dyslipidemia, are well-established contributors to the development of CVD [63–65], additional risk factors such as low birth weight can also predispose individuals to cardiovascular disease later in life. This link between low birth weight and CVD was identified by Professor Barker, whose epidemiological studies conducted in Hertfordshire, England, revealed that men born with low birth weight had the highest mortality rates from ischemic heart disease [51]. Years later, Professor Barker discovered the connection between intrauterine conditions and the risk of CVD, particularly through the placenta. Professor Barker and colleagues found that individuals who were born small but had large placentas tended to have elevation of blood pressure, placing them at greater risk of developing hypertension later in life. The authors hypothesized that the redistribution of fetal cardiac output to maintain brain perfusion (fetal brain sparing), could explain this association. They suggested that reduced blood flow to other organs, such as the trunk, might alter arterial structure, thus programming the offspring for cardiovascular dysfunction in adulthood [66].

Since Professor Barker formulated the DOHaD hypothesis, numerous research groups and human epidemiological studies have built upon it, providing further mechanistic evidence linking adverse intrauterine environments to the development of CVD. Interestingly, the Raine Study, a longitudinal study conducted in Australia that assessed the health outcomes of offspring from 2900 pregnant women, found a negative correlation between birth weight and blood pressure at the age of five. Additionally, the study revealed a negative association between offspring blood pressure and antenatal femur length [67], suggesting the relationship with birth size. Similarly, research conducted at Helsinki University Central Hospital, which analyzed the child welfare records of over 5000 men, found that both low birth weight and rapid postnatal weight gain were linked to an increased risk of coronary heart disease [68]. Collectively, these studies emphasize that both intrauterine and immediate postnatal events can program offspring for CVD. Moreover, these studies suggest that the placenta—and potentially the maternal environment—may play key roles in influencing these fetal changes. Considering this, *what is the contribution of maternal stress in programming offspring for CVD?*

Maternal bereavement, a term referring to the emotional and psychological distress that a mother can experience after losing a family member, is considered an important source of stress. A study conducted with 6.8 million participants from Denmark and Sweden found no overall association between maternal bereavement and offspring susceptibility to ischemic heart disease or stroke. However, a more detailed analysis revealed that fetuses exposed to intrauterine stress due to maternal bereavement during the third trimester were at higher risk of developing ischemic heart disease later in life [69]. Another study conducted on pregnant women observed that children born to bereaved mothers tended to be born preterm and with lower birth weight. However, as the authors noted, these bereaved mothers were older and had higher parity, factors that may influence the observed outcomes in their offspring. Interestingly, the study also identified a modestly increased risk of CVD in children who were prenatally exposed to maternal stress following the death of a close relative [70].

Building on the connection between maternal stress and offspring health, a study conducted in China with over 2000 women found that the risk of congenital heart diseases in offspring increased by 62% among pregnant women who experienced negative stress events compared to those who experienced positive events [71]. Similarly, an observational study from Germany reported that maternal emotional state influences the fetal and infant autonomic nervous system by modulating heart rate variability [72]. However, the researchers did not find a significant association between maternal metabolic factors such as cortisol levels, inflammatory markers, or prepregnancy adiposity and these cardiovascular outcomes.

Given the ethical limitations inherent in conducting experimental research on humans, animal models have been instrumental in advancing our understanding of the molecular mechanisms underlying fetal programming and its link to CVD. In a rat model of maternal stress induced by repeated restraint, both male and female offspring of stressed mothers exhibited increased blood pressure and elevated atrial diastolic dimensions [73]. Interestingly, the American Society of Echocardiography has highlighted that an increase in atrial diastolic dimension during adolescence can contribute to higher left atrial pressure in adulthood, potentially predisposing individuals to cardiovascular complications later in life [74]. Mechanistically, researchers observed that adult rat male offspring of stressed mothers displayed elevated tropomyosin-related kinase receptor B (TrkB) signaling in the left ventricle, a pathway implicated in the regulation of cardiac contraction force and calcium signaling [75]. Notably, a sex-specific effect was observed, with male offspring exhibiting greater left ventricular diastolic dimensions compared to females, underscoring a potential sexual dimorphism in the cardiovascular responses to maternal stress [74]. In sheep, widely recognized as one of the most suitable animal models for fetal programming due to their similarities in fetal growth rates to humans, researchers observed significant cardiac transcriptomic changes following exogenous exposure to maternal cortisol. Specifically, 260 genes in the left ventricle were altered by cortisol exposure [76]. Additionally, cortisol was found to influence gene expression in the interventricular septum and epicardial adipose tissue. Pathway analysis of the dysregulated genes revealed that cortisol primarily impacts mitochondrial function and ubiquitin-mediated proteolysis [76].

Collectively, findings from human epidemiological studies and work conducted in animal models underscore that maternal stress, as well as stress-related hormones like cortisol, can induce both structural and functional alterations in the heart of the offspring, highlighting the critical influence of the intrauterine environment on cardiovascular health.

13.5.2 Maternal Stress on Fetal Programming of Metabolic Health of the Offspring

Professor Barker's observations extended beyond the link between the intrauterine environment and CVD in adulthood. He and his team also investigated the associations between adverse intrauterine conditions and metabolic diseases. Professor Barker found that men who experienced restricted growth early in life were more susceptible to impaired glucose tolerance and β-cell dysfunction [77]. Years later, this observation was also confirmed in women [78]. Furthermore, like the cardiovascular phenotype, the authors identified a connection between impaired glucose tolerance or non-insulin-dependent diabetes mellitus and the placenta. Individuals with programmed metabolic dysfunction had a higher ratio of placental weight to birth weight, suggesting anomalies in placental function that could contribute to these long-term metabolic outcomes [78].

Regarding the topic of maternal bereavement and maternal depression, a study found that children born to mothers who experienced stress due to the loss of a family member had an increased body mass index (BMI) and a higher prevalence of overweight status by the age of ten. Moreover, the authors found this association to be stronger when the stress exposure occurred in the months just before conception [79], suggesting that maternal stress may have a greater impact on the embryo than on the fetus. However, other studies have not identified significant correlations between BMI and intrauterine stress resulting from maternal bereavement. In a study conducted in Copenhagen, Denmark, researchers evaluated the BMI of 492 children who experienced parental bereavement during the first 6 years of life. They found no significant changes in BMI between the ages of 7 and 13 [80]. Project Viva, a prospective cohort study of pregnant women conducted in the areas of Boston (Massachusetts, USA), evaluated how maternal depression during the mid-pregnancy affects anthropometric data for children at the age of three. After controlling potential confounder factors, the authors found that children exposed to antenatal depression had more central adiposity even though they weighed less [81].

The Amsterdam Born Children and their Development study is a longitudinal birth cohort study in which maternal prenatal psychosocial stress and offspring metabolic health were evaluated at the age of 5–6 years. The authors did not find any association between depressive symptoms, state of anxiety, pregnancy-related anxiety, parenting daily hassles, job strain, or cumulative stress with circulating levels of glucose, C-peptide, or insulin resistance in their offspring. Moreover, the results were the same when the authors assessed a potential sexual dimorphism response between males and females [82]. However, another study found that prenatal psychosocial stress can program glucose metabolism and C-peptide levels [83]. Several factors may explain these differences, including the intensity of maternal stress and the age of the offspring studied. Indeed, the first study focused on children, while the second examined young adults. Together, these findings suggest that the severity of in utero stress exposure and the aging process are key factors influencing the development of metabolic diseases.

Because maternal bereavement, depression, and anxiety can broadly impact various aspects of a pregnant woman's health and well-being, including physical activity, diet, and sleep patterns, animal models have been valuable in isolating these confounding factors. In this regard, pregnant mice treated with corticosterone (the primary glucocorticoid produced in rodents) showed that the capacity of the placenta to transport amino acids was affected by exposure to this hormone. Moreover, these fetuses were growth-restricted, and placental expression of *Hsd11b2*, the enzyme responsible for regulating feto-placental glucocorticoid bioavailability, was also altered [84]. In rats, offspring from mothers exposed to undernutrition during pregnancy had lower weight and higher plasma corticosterone, particularly in male. In addition, placenta of male dams showed lower vascularization and reduced glucocorticoid barrier, indicating poorer adaptation to undernutrition with nutrient deficiency likely influencing developmental programming [85]. In baboons, exposure to exogenous doses of dexamethasone (a steroid hormone that mimics the action of cortisol) affected placental thickness in a dose-dependent manner, although it did not alter birth weight. However, consistent with the previous results from human studies, antenatal dexamethasone attenuated growth (weight and length) and increased subcutaneous fat thickness. At 12–14 months of age, baboons exposed to glucocorticoids had heavier pituitary glands compared to control animals, along with reduced pancreatic β-cell mass. Examination of the liver revealed that exposure to this steroid hormone reduced the activity of the gluconeogenic enzyme phosphoenolpyruvate carboxykinase. These findings obtained in a nonhuman primate model indicate that dexamethasone can induce structural changes in the organs of offspring. Metabolically, these offspring exhibited higher fasting plasma insulin levels and reduced glucose clearance, indicative of early-stage insulin resistance and glucose intolerance [86].

In summary, adverse intrauterine conditions, including malnutrition and stress, increase the risk of metabolic diseases by affecting fetal growth, placental function, and glucose metabolism. Maternal stress, especially before conception, is linked to higher BMI in children. Animal studies confirm that glucocorticoid exposure disrupts placental function, fetal development, and metabolic regulation, leading to long-term health risks like insulin resistance and glucose intolerance.

13.5.3 Maternal Stress on Fetal Programming of the Neurological Health of the Offspring

The brain is not an exception to the Barker hypothesis. Several reports have shown impaired development of the offspring's brain under maternal stress. It is important to identify not only the intensity and the nature of maternal stress but also the timing. Brain development starts in the third week after conception and grows progressively during gestation [87]. However, the developmental timeline of each brain region varies, and stress at specific time points may disrupt the normal neurodevelopment of one or more regions. Prenatal stress has been related to changes in the volume of the brain of 6- to 9-year-old infants [88] and decreased cortical gray matter in young adults [89]. Moreover, these changes in neurodevelopment induce organizational alterations in brain structure, functional connectivity, metabolism, and neurotransmission systems that, in the long-term, might have adverse behavioral outcomes in the adult, such as social-emotional difficulties, language, memory deficits, and neuropsychiatric disorders [90].

As stated above, maternal stress may generate neurological alterations and mental illness in the adult offspring. However, it is unclear the mechanisms by which antenatal stress can induce these effects. The developing brain is highly sensitive to the effects of cortisol, and disruptions in the HPA axis are believed to have harmful effects on the development of the central nervous system. A rat model showed that maternal stress induces on male offspring alterations in the corticosterone levels (like cortisol in humans), decreasing hippocampal expression of glucocorticoid and mineralocorticoid receptors. These results suggest maternal stress-induced molecular pathway dysregulation [91]. Since glucocorticoid receptor (GR) induces alterations in cell's transcription upon activation and neuron expresses GRs early during development, elevated cortisol levels may alter normal gene expression in human fetal brain [92]. Connected with this, in pregnant women with anxiety, a downregulation of placental *Hsd11b2* can be observed [42]. This downregulation could imply higher levels of maternal cortisol transmitted into the fetus, which consequently may increase the activation of brain's GRs and alterations in fetal brain development. For instance, in pregnant rats exposed to carbenoxolone, inhibitor of 11β-HSD2, higher corticosterone levels were observed as well as altered GRs in the hypothalamus and amygdala of the offspring. Moreover, the increased maternal corticosterone crossing the placenta induced anxiety-like behaviors in the offspring under stressful situations [93].

In recent years, a new maternal stress-mediated factor has been put in the spotlight, i.e., epigenetic alterations. Epigenetics refers to changes in gene expression that are not related to changes in DNA. The best epigenetic alterations studied are the DNA methylation at cytosine level [94]. This transformation is catalyzed by DNA methyltransferases (DNMTs). The results of DNMTs activity are the shutdown of genes [95]. These DNA marks are dynamic and responsive to environmental cues, prenatal development being the most vulnerable period for epigenetic disruption. The epigenome resets to get naïve pluripotency and reprograms to induce cellular differentiation during prenatal stage [94, 96]. During neurogenesis, neural precursors express specific factors that promote the transcription of neuronal genes and silence those genes that are typically expressed by glial cells [97]. Maternal stress alters physiological epigenetic programming of the brain offspring. Moreover, maternal anxiety and depression have been linked to higher methylation of the gene *Nc3r1*, responsible for the synthesis of GR [98, 99], and the placental gene *Hsd11b2* [100, 101]. This may imply that maternal psychological distress during pregnancy influences the regulation of the HPA axis due to epigenetic alterations. However, maternal stress does not only cause changes in the methylation related to the HPA axis. It has been observed that prenatal stress induces epigenetic modifications that affect schizophrenia-related glutamatergic and GABAergic pathway [102, 103] and increase DNA methylation of the *Bdnf* gene (responsible for synthesis of brain-derived neurotrophic factor; BDNF) in the hippocampus and prefrontal cortex of rodents [102, 104]. Interestingly, it has been suggested that an increased blood DNA methylation of promoter for *Bdnf* can be used as a diagnostic biomarker for major depression [105]. It was shown that maternal stress in mice induced anxiety- and depressive-like behaviors which were accompanied by low hippocampus BDNF levels induced by a high methylation of the *Bdnf*. Authors also reported an increase in DNMT1 in the hippocampus [106]. To sum up, prenatal stress induces epigenetic alterations during neurodevelopment affecting the expression of genes related to developing mood and neuropsychiatric disorders in adult life.

Anxiety and depression have been connected to brain modification patterns during prenatal stages induced by gestational maternal stress. For instance, prenatal maternal stress was associated with less cortical thickness in frontal and temporal regions and child cortical thickness correlated with depressive symptoms during adolescence [107]. In addition, prenatal stress increased cortical gyrification index in the temporal region, being associated with adult mood disorders [108, 109].

Women's psychological well-being can also influence the development of psychopathologies such as schizophrenia, attention deficit hyperactivity disorder (ADHD), and autism spectrum disorder (ASD). All these disorders have in common an early brain developmental alteration, influenced by maternal stress mixed with the activation of susceptibility genes [110]. Most epidemiological studies have reported that maternal exposure to natural disasters, wars, terrorist attacks, and famines increase the prevalence of schizophrenia [111]. Likewise, death of a close relative during the first trimester also increases schizophrenia in the offspring [110]. Unfortunately, these studies are not able to extract information about mechanisms involved in maternal stress-related neurodevelopmental alterations. From animal models, some hypotheses have been extracted from DNA methylation of *Bdnf* promoters during brain development [112].

Maternal stress also increases ADHD and ASD [113]. One study analyzed the rates of ASD in Louisiana (USA) associated with the storms occurring between 1980 and 1995. It was observed that there was a higher prevalence of ASD in children whose mother was exposed to a severe storm during pregnancy. Interestingly, they also observed that the increase of the prevalence of ASD was dependent on two main factors: (1) the severity of the storm and (2) the vulnerability of the parish to the storm effects [114]. In addition, mother's exposure to loss of a first-degree relative increased the risk of ADHD and ASD when the loss happened in the third trimester of gestation [115]. Like schizophrenia, the mechanisms by which these early neurodevelopmental insults induce ADHD and ASD are unclear, although it has been, again, suggested the implication of epigenetic changes [116, 117].

It is important to highlight that all mechanisms and behavioral outcomes induced by maternal stress are often sex-specific. This is not surprising since brain's HPA axis, epigenome, and epigenetic pathway are sex-dependent. It could explain, at least in part, the different prevalence and severity observed in mood disorders and neurodevelopmental psychiatric disorders. In view of this, it is essential that future studies focus their efforts on including in their analysis of both sexes.

To sum up, maternal stress during pregnancy disrupts fetal brain development through hormonal and epigenetic changes, increasing the risk of neuropsychiatric disorders like anxiety, depression, or schizophrenia. Timing and intensity of stress are key, as different brain regions develop at different stages. The HPA axis plays a central role, with excess cortisol altering gene expression and brain structure. Animal models confirm sex-specific differences.

13.5.4 Maternal Stress on Fetal Programming of Offspring Reproductive Organs

Compared to cardiovascular, metabolic, and neurological outcomes, less is known about the intrauterine effects of maternal stress on the development and function of reproductive organs in offspring. Indeed, most of the findings regarding the effects of fetal programming on the reproductive capacity of female offspring have been obtained from animal models, as reviewed elsewhere [118]. However, both human and experimental animal models highlight that prenatal maternal stress can affect the HPA and hypothalamic-pituitary-gonadal (HPG) axes [118, 119].

In the Raine Study, scientists evaluated the programming effects of maternal stress on female offspring aged 14–16 years. Interestingly, the authors found that intrauterine exposure to maternal stress in late, but not early, gestation increased the offspring's uterine volume by 13% and resulted in an 18% increase in ovarian antral follicle count [120]. Moreover, prenatal stress was associated with an earlier onset of puberty in female offspring, independently of their BMI. Specifically, the authors observed a 3.5-month advancement in menarche when the female offspring was exposed in utero to only one stressful life event and a 1.7-month advancement with exposure to two or more stressful life events. The authors suggested that the potential cause for the early onset of the menarche could be due to programming effects in the HPA axis of the offspring [121] as it is known that the HPA axis regulates the onset of puberty [122] and several studies conducted in humans have observed that the HPA axis can be programmed by maternal stress [123–125].

Evidence regarding the effects of maternal stress on the human male offspring's reproductive system remains relatively scarce. A human study examining the impact of prenatal stress associated with the Chernobyl disaster on circulating reproductive hormones found that testosterone levels were significantly higher in female, but not male offspring exposed to maternal stress from the second trimester onward compared to the control population [126], suggesting a sexually dimorphic response to stress on circulating levels of sex steroids. In the Raine Study, scientists found that maternal stress during early gestation negatively affected total sperm count, progressive motile sperm count, and serum testosterone levels in male offspring. Interestingly, these programming effects were not observed when mothers experienced stress in late gestation, suggesting that the timing of exposure can differentially program the fetus [127]. Additionally, men exposed to prenatal stress due to maternal bereavement during the first trimester of pregnancy showed an increased risk of cryptorchidism and hypospadias [128]. However, the fertility of these men was not affected by maternal stress [128].

Taken together, there is evidence suggesting that maternal stress can affect both male and female offspring, although the intensity of maternal stress, the sex of the offspring, and the timing of exposure seem to be critical determinants of reproductive outcomes in the offspring.

13.5.5 Maternal Stress on Cancer Risk in the Offspring

The interplay between prenatal stress, the maternal hormonal milieu, and epigenetic modifications in the developing fetus has raised questions about long-term health consequences for offspring, including the risk of cancer. Emerging evidence highlights the critical importance of understanding how maternal stressors may shape the future oncological landscape of children [129]. A cohort study found that children born to mothers who experienced stress during pregnancy had an increased incidence of neuroblastoma [130, 131]. Similarly, it was reported that maternal stress due to bereavement in pregnancy was associated with a higher risk of pediatric cancers [130]. In male offspring, this prenatal stressor at first trimester was associated with a high risk of testicular cancer [128]. The offspring of women who experienced parental death during pregnancy were affected by cancer within 22 years of follow-up, particularly important for leukemia and Hodgkin's lymphomas [132]. However, these studies also underscore the multifactorial nature of cancer risk, which includes genetic predisposition, environmental exposures, and lifestyle factors.

Elevated cortisol levels can cross the placenta, exposing the fetus to heightened glucocorticoid concentrations. This exposure can disrupt physiological cellular programming and lead to epigenetic changes in key tumor-suppressor genes and oncogenes [129]. Additionally, maternal stress may reduce nutrient and oxygen delivery to the fetus. Such conditions have been associated with intrauterine growth restriction, a factor linked to increased susceptibility to pediatric cancers, including leukemia and neuroblastoma [133]. Studies suggest that stress-induced epigenetic alterations can be transmitted across generations, potentially influencing cancer risk in subsequent progeny [134]. This transgenerational transmission underscores the broader implications of maternal stress for public health and cancer prevention strategies. The potential impact of maternal stress during pregnancy on offspring cancer risk represents a critical area of research with significant public health implications. However, research is necessary to disentangle the direct effects of prenatal stress from these confounding variables, and longitudinal studies with large cohorts and precise stress quantification are essential to establish causality.

In summary, maternal stress can influence offspring cancer risk through hormonal changes, epigenetic modifications, and impaired fetal development. Elevated maternal cortisol levels and disrupted placental function are key mechanisms linking prenatal stress to increased susceptibility to pediatric cancers. Furthermore, epigenetic changes may have transgenerational effects, highlighting the importance of maternal well-being for long-term child health.

13.5.6 Effects of Maternal Stress on Fetal Programming on Offspring Microbiota

Microbial colonization of the gut is essential for the natural maturation of both the intestine and the immune system. The infant gut microbiome is highly sensitive to environmental exposures, and it has been shown that early life imbalances in the gut microbiota composition increase the risk of chronic immune-related conditions such as allergy and type 1 diabetes mellitus [135–138].

During normal pregnancy, the maternal gut microbiota differs substantially from the non-gravid microbiota [139]. Additionally, chronic psychological stress can elevate cortisol levels, leading to alterations in the gut microbiome [140]. Nevertheless the impact of microbiota on fetal development, particularly its role in placental growth and function, is still debated, with some researchers suggesting the presence of a "placental microbiome" and others opposing it [141–143]. Because studying the contribution of the maternal gut microbiota to fetoplacental growth is challenging in humans, studies in germ-free mice have provided valuable insights.

These studies have shown that maternal gut microbiota plays a critical role in feto-placental growth [144]. Specifically, the absence of maternal gut microbiota results in smaller placentas with reduced fetal capillary formation. These alterations in placental vascular development caused fetal growth restriction and fetal hypoglycemia [144]. Moreover, fetuses from mothers lacking gut microbiota exhibited smaller fetal liver size, further suggesting that the maternal microbiome can influence offspring growth even in utero [144]. Furthermore, it has been suggested that prenatal stress can even unbalance offspring's gut microbiota during the fetal stage, resulting in alterations in the offspring behavior and cognition in adult life [145].

Regarding the postnatal effects and the interplay between maternal stress and gut microbiome composition, studies in infants whose mothers had high levels of stress have shown that these infants exhibited lower gut microbiome beta diversity. Specifically, the levels of *Lactobacillus gasseri* and *Bifidobacterium pseudocatenulatum*, which are considered beneficial bacteria, were reduced [146]. In another study, scientists compared the development of the intestinal microbiota and health of infants from stressed mothers and concluded that maternal stress and salivary cortisol concentrations during late pregnancy were associated with significant shifts in the infant microbiota [147]. Another example of how maternal stress induced by natural disasters can affect offspring's gut microbiota is the human HOLA study. This study showed that infants exposed in utero to Hurricane Maria in Puerto Rico, USA, had reduced diversity in their gut microbiome compared to control infants. Specifically, *Clostridium innocuum*, *Clostridium neonatale*, *Bacteroides vulgatus*, and *Bifidobacterium pseudocatenulatum* were depleted in the exposed group [148].

Taken together, findings from both human and experimental animal models highlight that maternal gut composition during and after pregnancy can influence offspring growth and gut microbiome diversity. These conditions may increase offspring susceptibility to metabolic diseases later in life, although further research in this area is needed.

13.6 What Do Historical Famines and Wars Reveal About Fetal Programming?

In war times women are exposed to life-endangering conditions and traumatic events, being frequently the target of physically violence such as rape and trafficking [149]. Thus, the burden of both physical and psychological trauma also compromises pregnancy. In fact, evaluation of the impact of armed conflicts in 53 developing countries in the last decade gave the result that exposure of the women to war-related stress conditions, particularly in the first trimester, is unambiguously associated with a low infant birth weight [149].

The impact of war on fetal programming is influenced by diverse factors, being the best studied nutrient deprivation. Studies in populations from different ethnic origins who suffered starvation derived from wars and famines over the past decades have provided compelling evidence about DOHaD hypothesis. The most extensively assessed has been the Dutch famine cohort, with over 250 studies [150]. This famine took place in the German-occupied Netherlands during the harsh winter of 1944–1945, near the end of World War II. It was found that individuals exposed to undernutrition in early, but not in middle or late gestation, had higher rates of coronary heart disease associated with low birth weight [151]. This has also been documented in descendants from pregnant women during the Spanish Civil war (1936–1939) [152]. Population exposed to the Dutch famine also evidenced increased risk of cancer [153], pulmonary obstructive disease [154], metabolic diseases, obesity [155], altered lipid profiles [156], and type 2 diabetes [150]. Although the Dutch famine did not affect reproductive performance, it advanced menopause, suggesting that early life stress also has negative effects at ovarian level [157]. Another World War II population evaluated was the descendants from women pregnant during the Leningrad Siege (Russia), the longest siege of history (1941–1944). In this population it has been found evidence of endothelial dysfunction [158, 159], reduced kidney filtration [160], and telomere shortening, a marker of accelerated aging [161]. However, studies conducted in this cohort did not find a disbalance in glucose and lipids homeostasis, or cardiovascular diseases in adulthood. The larger effect of fetal starvation on Dutch compared to Russian cohorts may be related to postnatal living conditions during early childhood. Firstly, in the studies of the Leningrad siege, the populations compared (during and after the siege) had differences in caloric intake in the fetal period but equally experienced famine during infancy, which may have influenced the results [162]. Besides, the improved living conditions during childhood after the war in the Dutch cohort may have been detrimental, leading to a rapid postnatal growth, known to increased susceptibility to noncommunicable diseases development in adult life [163].

Increased risk of disease development after famines has also been demonstrated in offspring from populations of other ethnic origins, being the most studied the Great Chinese famine (1959–1961). Descendants from this cohort had increased BMI and blood pressure [164]. The incidence of type 2 diabetes was also higher in this population, identical to the Dutch famine [150]. In addition, studies in the Chinese famine evidenced high risk of cancer [165, 166] and advanced aging, largely influenced by the severity of the famine [167]. Interestingly, the adverse outcome is not restricted to the exposed descendants, and obesity and hypertension have been also found in the second generation [164, 168]. Sub-Saharan Africa is facing increasing prevalences of hypertension, obesity, and diabetes, which may have roots in undernutrition caused by wars and famines in the last part of the twentieth century. The descendants of women who suffered the Biafran War (1967–1970) exhibit increased rates of obesity and hypertension [169, 170]. Adults who had prenatal exposure to the Great Ethiopian Famine (1984–1985) are more likely to develop metabolic syndrome [171], showing also higher risk of chronic kidney disease and hypertension [172].

Besides nutrient deprivation, psychological factors are a key determinant of fetal programming associated with war times and other stressful situations, particularly if pregnant women were exposed during the first trimester or to a high intensity stressor. A systematic review showed that the severity of the exposure is the major predictor of mental health issues among pregnant women and the factor that most strongly influence child development [173]. As examples, reduced pregnancy length and birth weight have been documented in relation to terrorist attacks, such as the September 9, 2001, in New York City (USA), the March 11, 2004, train bombings in Madrid (Spain) [174, 175], the July 7, 2005, attacks in London (UK) [176], and sustained Spanish national terrorism during the 1980–2003 period [177]. Descendants from pregnant women who suffered economic crisis, such as the Great depression in the 1930s, also had low birth weight associated with later obesity development, particularly for women, and signs of accelerated aging [178]. Exposure to natural disasters during gestation also has negative consequences for the offspring. Descendants from women pregnant during the 1998 ice storm in Quebec (Canada) had insulin resistance and worse cognitive and language development [179], and those exposed to floods in 2011 in Queensland (Australia) had children with poorer fine motor development [180]. The aftermaths of the 1918 influenza pandemic have also been documented, evidencing a transgenerational effect increasing the risk of hypertension [181]. In view of this, it is foreseen that the recent COVID-19 pandemic (2020–2023) will also have negative consequences for future generations, not only directly related to the virus, but also to the traumatic consequences of isolation, death, and economical loss [182]. In fact, a systematic review evidenced that COVID-19 was associated with increased risks of preeclampsia and preterm birth [183], which are known factors compromising the future health of the descendants.

Taken together, there is compelling evidence from around the world on historical wars, famines and natural disasters, showing that maternal stress, alone or in combination with other factors such as malnutrition, have an enormous impact on gestational health and results in intergenerational negative outcomes for the offspring, being the impact larger during the first trimester and directly proportional to the level of stressor (Table 13.1).

Table 13.1 Summary of global evidence linking maternal stress during pregnancy and adverse intergenerational health outcomes

Event	Stressor	Place	Date	Health consequences in the offspring
Spanish Civil War	Undernutrition	Spain	1936–1939	Cardiovascular disease
The Leningrad siege	Undernutrition	Russia	1941–1944	Reduced kidney filtration, endothelial dysfunction, telomere length shortening
The Dutch Famine	Undernutrition	The Netherlands	1944–1945	Cardiovascular disease, type 2 diabetes, obesity, advanced menopause, mental disorders, cancer, respiratory disorders, accelerated aging
Korean War	Undernutrition	South Korea	1950–1953	Obesity, metabolic syndrome, dyslipidemia
The Great Chinese Famine	Undernutrition	China	1959–1961	Type 2 diabetes, hypertension, obesity, cancer, advanced aging

(continued)

Table 13.1 (continued)

Event	Stressor	Place	Date	Health consequences in the offspring
Biafra War	Undernutrition	Nigeria	1967–1970	Hypertension, obesity
Ethiopian famine	Undernutrition	Ethiopia	1984–1985	Hypertension, metabolic syndrome, reduced kidney filtration
The Flue pandemic	Psychological	World	1918	Hypertension
The Great Depression	Psychological	Iceland	1929–1933	Obesity
The Great Depression	Psychological	USA	1929–1933	Accelerated aging
Quebec ice storm	Psychological	Canada	1998	Poorer cognitive and language development
Queensland floods	Psychological	Australia	2011	Poorer fine motor development

13.7 Clinical and Research Implications

As mentioned before, the DOHaD theory explains how negative events occurring during early life, such as maternal stress, influence the risk of chronic diseases from childhood to adulthood. However, in some cases, the effects of fetal programming can be modulated, or even reversed, through various intervention strategies. Psychological maternal interventions for mood control and activation regulation, such as mindfulness or yoga, can effectively manage stress during pregnancy, reducing risks to fetal programming [184]. These practices have been shown to lower anxiety, depression, and stress levels in pregnant individuals, thus potentially preventing negative fetal outcomes caused by daily stressors. Thus, government public health policies should focus on lifestyle strategies for women to alleviate the impact of fetal programming in maternally stressful pregnancies. Among others, physical activity in combination with adequate nutrition, such as the Mediterranean diet that promotes beneficial microbiota, and reduction of maternal cortisol levels during pregnancy have been proposed [185].

Immediate postnatal stages also play a critical role in the perpetuation or mitigation of fetal programming, with breastfeeding consistently identified as a protective factor across studies [186, 187]. For infants, the benefits of breast milk (BM) feeding are well established, including protection against respiratory and gastrointestinal tract infection, overweight, diabetes, allergy, and inflammatory bowel disease [188]. BM not only supplies optimal infant nutrition but also provides protective and immunomodulatory components, which can block infection, promote antigen tolerance, stimulate mucosal immunity, induce regulatory T-cell production, select for the beneficial bacteria in the gut, and provide passive immunity [189, 190]. Thus, nutritional programming can be seen as a sequence of events through which nutrition—particularly breastfeeding in neonates—can help counteract the adverse effects of fetal programming. However, if maternal stress progresses during postnatal life, it can have a negative effect on BM. It has been shown that the mother's mood during breastfeeding alters the bacterial diversity of their BM without altering its macronutrient composition, affecting also the neonatal intestinal microbiota and mental health [191, 192]. Furthermore, postnatal environmental mismatches, such as shifts from stress-adaptive fetal programming in utero to a non-stressful postnatal setting, may exacerbate the risk of overweight or obesity, hypertension, or diabetes in the offspring. These effects are influenced by epigenetic modifications and nutrient acquisition during breastfeeding, which are critical for long-term metabolic health outcomes [193, 194].

It is important to consider that the prenatal stress effects are modulated by the individual's own lifestyle. Factors such as a sedentary lifestyle, smoking, and nutritional imbalance in adulthood can lead the individual to have similar risks of getting sick [195] even if their pregnancy has been free of stressful events. In contrast, maintaining a healthy lifestyle can protect against, or at least mitigate or delay, the onset of noncommunicable diseases in adulthood, even if the fetal stage has been significantly influenced by maternal stress [196].

13.8 Conclusions

Exposure to stress factors during pregnancy has deleterious effects on the woman and programs the offspring, inducing structural and functional changes across multiple systems, with a large impact on future health. In this process, the maternal and fetal HPA axis seems to be crucial, being the placenta, a central element regulating maternal stress hormones, and fetal responses to stress (Fig. 13.2). The underlying mechanisms and the influence of some factors, such as fetal sex, are gradually being revealed. However, further research is needed to identify the cellular targets to prevent and mitigate the adverse effects of fetal programming, as well as to design effective strategies to alleviate maternal stress before, during, and after gestation. These interventions will improve the health of both pregnant women and future generations.

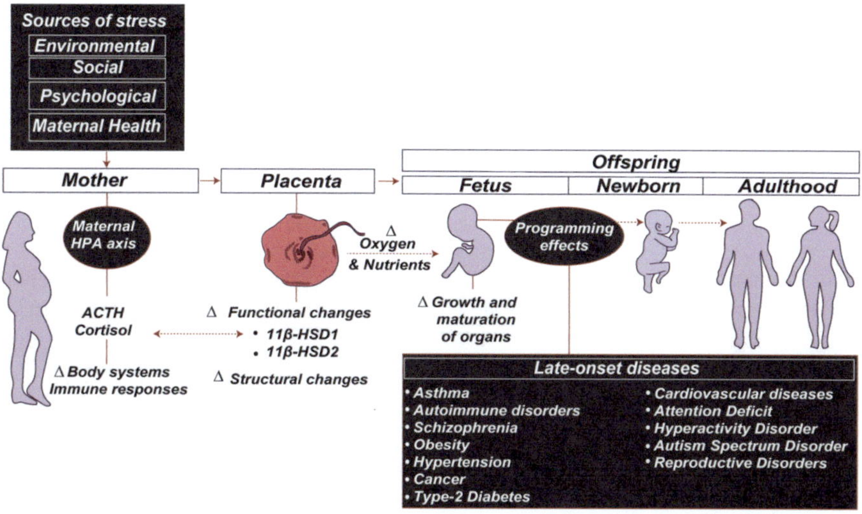

Fig. 13.2 Maternal stress during pregnancy can affect maternal physiology. Activation of the maternal HPA axis leads to increased levels of stress-related hormones, such as adrenocorticotropic hormone (ACTH) and cortisol, in maternal circulation. These changes (displayed as Δ) can alter maternal adaptations to pregnancy, including immune system function. In response to maternal stress, the placenta can modify the expression of enzymes that regulate stress hormones (e.g., 11β-HSD1 and 11β-HSD2), potentially affecting placental structure. If maternal stress remains uncontrolled and placental defenses become overwhelmed, placental function may be compromised, impairing the transport of oxygen and nutrients to the developing fetus. This disruption can impact fetal growth and organ maturation. As a result of this intrauterine environment, offspring may be more susceptible to developing late-onset diseases in adulthood (the list of pathologies presented in the figure is based on the references provided in the text)

Acknowledgments David Ramiro-Cortijo received the "Dr. Luis Álvarez" 2024 grant from the Mentor-2025 program of IdiPAZ (Spain; Grant No. PI-6493). Jorge López-Tello is supported by the Attraction of Talent Grant from the Community of Madrid (Spain; Grant No. 2023-T1/SAL-GL-28960, CESAR NOMBELA Fellowship).

References

1. Coussons-Read ME. Effects of prenatal stress on pregnancy and human development: mechanisms and pathways. Obstet Med. 2013;6:52–7.
2. Wu Y, De Asis-Cruz J, Limperopoulos C. Brain structural and functional outcomes in the offspring of women experiencing psychological distress during pregnancy. Mol Psychiatry. 2024;29:2223–40.
3. Dahlerup BR, Egsmose EL, Siersma V, Mortensen EL, Hedegaard M, Knudsen LE, Mathiesen L. Maternal stress and placental function, a study using questionnaires and biomarkers at birth. PLoS One. 2018;13:e0207184.
4. Woods SM, Melville JL, Guo Y, Fan M-Y, Gavin A. Psychosocial stress during pregnancy. Am J Obstet Gynecol. 2010;202:61.e1–7.

5. Miller GE, Chen E, Parker KJ. Psychological stress in childhood and susceptibility to the chronic diseases of aging: moving toward a model of behavioral and biological mechanisms. Psychol Bull. 2011;137:959–97.
6. Napso T, Yong HEJ, Lopez-Tello J, Sferruzzi-Perri AN. The role of placental hormones in mediating maternal adaptations to support pregnancy and lactation. Front Physiol. 2018;9:1091.
7. Grajek M, Krupa-Kotara K, Grot M, Kujawińska M, Helisz P, Gwioździk W, Białek-Dratwa A, Staśkiewicz W, Kobza J. Perception of the body image in women after childbirth and the specific determinants of their eating behavior: cross-sectional study (Silesia, Poland). Int J Environ Res Public Health. 2022;19:10137. https://doi.org/10.3390/ijerph191610137.
8. Gourounti K. Psychological stress and adjustment in pregnancy following assisted reproductive technology and spontaneous conception: a systematic review. Women Health. 2016;56:98–118.
9. Dunkel Schetter C, Tanner L. Anxiety, depression and stress in pregnancy: implications for mothers, children, research, and practice. Curr Opin Psychiatry. 2012;25:141–8.
10. Cowell W, Deyssenroth M, Chen J, Wright RJ. Maternal stress in relation to sex-specific expression of placental genes involved in nutrient transport, oxygen tension, immune response, and the glucocorticoid barrier. Placenta. 2020;96:19–26.
11. Gagnon R. Placental insufficiency and its consequences. Eur J Obstet Gynecol Reprod Biol. 2003;110(Suppl 1):S99–107.
12. Entringer S, Buss C, Wadhwa PD. Prenatal stress, development, health and disease risk: a psychobiological perspective-2015 Curt Richter Award Paper. Psychoneuroendocrinology. 2015;62:366–75.
13. Sferruzzi-Perri AN, Lopez-Tello J, Napso T, Yong HEJ. Exploring the causes and consequences of maternal metabolic maladaptations during pregnancy: lessons from animal models. Placenta. 2020;98:43–51.
14. Rizi SS, Wiens E, Hunt J, Ducas R. Cardiac physiology and pathophysiology in pregnancy. Can J Physiol Pharmacol. 2024;102:552–71.
15. Soma-Pillay P, Nelson-Piercy C, Tolppanen H, Mebazaa A. Physiological changes in pregnancy. Cardiovasc J Afr. 2016;27:89–94.
16. Green D, Dineen R, O'Reilly MW, Sherlock M. Fertility and pregnancy in adrenal insufficiency. Endocr Connect. 2024;13:e230088. https://doi.org/10.1530/EC-23-0088.
17. Duthie L, Reynolds RM. Changes in the maternal hypothalamic-pituitary-adrenal axis in pregnancy and postpartum: influences on maternal and fetal outcomes. Neuroendocrinology. 2013;98:106–15.
18. Jung C, Ho JT, Torpy DJ, Rogers A, Doogue M, Lewis JG, Czajko RJ, Inder WJ. A longitudinal study of plasma and urinary cortisol in pregnancy and postpartum. J Clin Endocrinol Metab. 2011;96:1533–40.
19. Gardella B, Gritti A, Scatigno AL, Gallotti AMC, Perotti F, Dominoni M. Adrenal crisis during pregnancy: case report and obstetric perspective. Front Med (Lausanne). 2022;9:891101.
20. Lebbe M, Arlt W. What is the best diagnostic and therapeutic management strategy for an Addison patient during pregnancy? Clin Endocrinol. 2013;78:497–502.
21. Hobel CJ, Dunkel-Schetter C, Roesch SC, Castro LC, Arora CP. Maternal plasma corticotropin-releasing hormone associated with stress at 20 weeks' gestation in pregnancies ending in preterm delivery. Am J Obstet Gynecol. 1999;180:S257–63.
22. Nepomnaschy PA, Welch KB, McConnell DS, Low BS, Strassmann BI, England BG. Cortisol levels and very early pregnancy loss in humans. Proc Natl Acad Sci USA. 2006;103:3938–42.
23. Guleria I, Sayegh MH. Maternal acceptance of the fetus: true human tolerance. J Immunol. 2007;178:3345–51.
24. Hanna J, Goldman-Wohl D, Hamani Y, et al. Decidual NK cells regulate key developmental processes at the human fetal-maternal interface. Nat Med. 2006;12:1065–74.
25. Moser G, Windsperger K, Pollheimer J, de Sousa Lopes SC, Huppertz B. Human trophoblast invasion: new and unexpected routes and functions. Histochem Cell Biol. 2018;150:361–70.

26. Kalkunte S, Chichester CO, Gotsch F, Sentman CL, Romero R, Sharma S. Evolution of non-cytotoxic uterine natural killer cells. Am J Reprod Immunol. 2008;59:425–32.
27. Ross KM, Carroll JE, Dunkel Schetter C, Hobel C, Cole SW. Pro-inflammatory immune cell gene expression during the third trimester of pregnancy is associated with shorter gestational length and lower birthweight. Am J Reprod Immunol. 2019;82:e13190.
28. Andersson NW, Li Q, Mills CW, Ly J, Nomura Y, Chen J. Influence of prenatal maternal stress on umbilical cord blood cytokine levels. Arch Womens Ment Health. 2016;19:761–7.
29. Wright RJ, Visness CM, Calatroni A, et al. Prenatal maternal stress and cord blood innate and adaptive cytokine responses in an inner-city cohort. Am J Respir Crit Care Med. 2010;182:25–33.
30. Lopez-Tello J, Yong HEJ, Sandovici I, et al. Fetal manipulation of maternal metabolism is a critical function of the imprinted Igf2 gene. Cell Metab. 2023;35:1195–1208.e6.
31. Petraglia F, Sawchenko PE, Rivier J, Vale W. Evidence for local stimulation of ACTH secretion by corticotropin-releasing factor in human placenta. Nature. 1987;328:717–9.
32. Florio P, Petraglia F. Human placental corticotropin-releasing factor (CRF) in the adaptive response to pregnancy. Stress. 2001;4:247–61.
33. Zhao C, He L, Li L, Deng F, Zhang M, Wang C, Qiu J, Gao Q. Prenatal glucocorticoids exposure and adverse cardiovascular effects in offspring. Front Endocrinol (Lausanne). 2024;15:1430334.
34. Migeon C, Bertrand J, Gemzell C. The transplacental passage of various steroid hormones in mid-pregnancy. Recent Prog Horm Res. 1961;17:207–48.
35. Reynolds RM. Glucocorticoid excess and the developmental origins of disease: two decades of testing the hypothesis—2012 Curt Richter Award Winner. Psychoneuroendocrinology. 2013;38:1–11.
36. Zhu P, Wang W, Zuo R, Sun K. Mechanisms for establishment of the placental glucocorticoid barrier, a guard for life. Cell Mol Life Sci. 2019;76:13–26.
37. Murphy BE, Clark SJ, Donald IR, Pinsky M, Vedady D. Conversion of maternal cortisol to cortisone during placental transfer to the human fetus. Am J Obstet Gynecol. 1974;118:538–41.
38. Beitins IZ, Bayard F, Ances IG, Kowarski A, Migeon CJ. The metabolic clearance rate, blood production, interconversion and transplacental passage of cortisol and cortisone in pregnancy near term. Pediatr Res. 1973;7:509–19.
39. Patel FA, Sun K, Challis JR. Local modulation by 11beta-hydroxysteroid dehydrogenase of glucocorticoid effects on the activity of 15-hydroxyprostaglandin dehydrogenase in human chorion and placental trophoblast cells. J Clin Endocrinol Metab. 1999;84:395–400.
40. Saeed H, Lu Y-C, Andescavage N, et al. Influence of maternal psychological distress during COVID-19 pandemic on placental morphometry and texture. Sci Rep. 2023;13:7374.
41. Jahnke JR, Terán E, Murgueitio F, Cabrera H, Thompson AL. Maternal stress, placental 11β-hydroxysteroid dehydrogenase type 2, and infant HPA axis development in humans: psychosocial and physiological pathways. Placenta. 2021;104:179–87.
42. O'Donnell KJ, Bugge Jensen A, Freeman L, Khalife N, O'Connor TG, Glover V. Maternal prenatal anxiety and downregulation of placental 11β-HSD2. Psychoneuroendocrinology. 2012;37:818–26.
43. Tartour AI, Chivese T, Eltayeb S, Elamin FM, Fthenou E, Seed Ahmed M, Babu GR. Prenatal psychological distress and 11β-HSD2 gene expression in human placentas: systematic review and meta-analysis. Psychoneuroendocrinology. 2024;166:107060.
44. McTernan CL, Draper N, Nicholson H, Chalder SM, Driver P, Hewison M, Kilby MD, Stewart PM. Reduced placental 11β-hydroxysteroid dehydrogenase type 2 mRNA levels in human pregnancies complicated by intrauterine growth restriction: an analysis of possible mechanisms. J Clin Endocrinol Metab. 2001;86:4979–83.
45. Shams M, Kilby MD, Somerset DA, Howie AJ, Gupta A, Wood PJ, Afnan M, Stewart PM. 11Beta-hydroxysteroid dehydrogenase type 2 in human pregnancy and reduced expression in intrauterine growth restriction. Hum Reprod. 1998;13:799–804.

46. Nardozza LMM, Caetano ACR, Zamarian ACP, Mazzola JB, Silva CP, Marçal VMG, Lobo TF, Peixoto AB, Araujo Júnior E. Fetal growth restriction: current knowledge. Arch Gynecol Obstet. 2017;295:1061–77.
47. Lesage J, Blondeau B, Grino M, Bréant B, Dupouy JP. Maternal undernutrition during late gestation induces fetal overexposure to glucocorticoids and intrauterine growth retardation, and disturbs the hypothalamo-pituitary adrenal axis in the newborn rat. Endocrinology. 2001;142:1692–702.
48. de Oliveira JC, Gomes RM, Miranda RA, et al. Protein restriction during the last third of pregnancy Malprograms the neuroendocrine axes to induce metabolic syndrome in adult male rat offspring. Endocrinology. 2016;157:1799–812.
49. Welberg LAM, Thrivikraman KV, Plotsky PM. Chronic maternal stress inhibits the capacity to up-regulate placental 11beta-hydroxysteroid dehydrogenase type 2 activity. J Endocrinol. 2005;186:R7–R12.
50. Barker DJ, Osmond C. Infant mortality, childhood nutrition, and ischaemic heart disease in England and Wales. Lancet. 1986;1:1077–81.
51. Barker DJ, Winter PD, Osmond C, Margetts B, Simmonds SJ. Weight in infancy and death from ischaemic heart disease. Lancet. 1989;2:577–80.
52. Koshko L, Scofield S, Mor G, Sadagurski M. Prenatal pollutant exposures and hypothalamic development: early life disruption of metabolic programming. Front Endocrinol (Lausanne). 2022;13:938094.
53. Zurub RE, Cariaco Y, Wade MG, Bainbridge SA. Microplastics exposure: implications for human fertility, pregnancy and child health. Front Endocrinol (Lausanne). 2023;14:1330396.
54. Sharma RK, Kumari U, Kumar S. Impact of microplastics on pregnancy and fetal development: a systematic review. Cureus. 2024;16:e60712.
55. Thomason ME, Hect JL, Waller R, Curtin P. Interactive relations between maternal prenatal stress, fetal brain connectivity, and gestational age at delivery. Neuropsychopharmacology. 2021;46:1839–47.
56. Sookoian S, Gianotti TF, Burgueño AL, Pirola CJ. Fetal metabolic programming and epigenetic modifications: a systems biology approach. Pediatr Res. 2013;73:531–42.
57. Collins JM, Keane JM, Deady C, Khashan AS, McCarthy FP, O'Keeffe GW, Clarke G, Cryan JF, Caputi V, O'Mahony SM. Prenatal stress impacts foetal neurodevelopment: temporal windows of gestational vulnerability. Neurosci Biobehav Rev. 2024;164:105793.
58. Sutherland S, Brunwasser SM. Sex differences in vulnerability to prenatal stress: a review of the recent literature. Curr Psychiatry Rep. 2018;20:102.
59. Bernard N, Giguère Y, Mélançon J, Tessier R, Tarabulsy GM, Forest J-C. Sex-specific association of high maternal psychological stress during pregnancy on newborn birthweight. PLoS One. 2022;17:e0262641.
60. Giussani DA. The fetal brain sparing response to hypoxia: physiological mechanisms. J Physiol. 2016;594:1215–30.
61. Virani SS, Alonso A, Aparicio HJ, et al. Heart disease and stroke statistics-2021 update: a report from the American Heart Association. Circulation. 2021;143:e254–743.
62. Benjamin EJ, Muntner P, Alonso A, et al. Heart disease and stroke statistics-2019 update: a report from the American Heart Association. Circulation. 2019;139:e56–e528.
63. Gallucci G, Tartarone A, Lerose R, Lalinga AV, Capobianco AM. Cardiovascular risk of smoking and benefits of smoking cessation. J Thorac Dis. 2020;12:3866–76.
64. Gonna H, Ray KK. The importance of dyslipidaemia in the pathogenesis of cardiovascular disease in people with diabetes. Diabetes Obes Metab. 2019;21(Suppl 1):6–16.
65. Borén J, Öörni K, Catapano AL. The link between diabetes and cardiovascular disease. Atherosclerosis. 2024;394:117607.
66. Heath D, Reid Williams D. Fetal and placental size and risk of hypertension in adult life. BMJ. 1990;301:551–2.

67. Huang R-C, Mori TA, Beilin LJ. Early life programming of cardiometabolic disease in the Western Australian pregnancy cohort (Raine) study. Clin Exp Pharmacol Physiol. 2012;39:973–8.
68. Eriksson JG, Forsén T, Tuomilehto J, Osmond C, Barker DJ. Early growth and coronary heart disease in later life: longitudinal study. BMJ. 2001;322:949–53.
69. Yang F, Janszky I, Roos N, Li J, László KD. Prenatal exposure to severe stress and risks of ischemic heart disease and stroke in offspring. JAMA Netw Open. 2023;6:e2349463.
70. Plana-Ripoll O, Liu X, Momen NC, Parner E, Olsen J, Li J. Prenatal exposure to maternal stress following bereavement and cardiovascular disease: a nationwide population-based and sibling-matched cohort study. Eur J Prev Cardiol. 2016;23:1018–28.
71. Li J, Du Y, Liu Y, Du J, Zhang R, Qu P, Yan H, Wang D, Dang S. Maternal exposure to life events during pregnancy and congenital heart disease in offspring: a case-control study in a Chinese population. BMC Pregnancy Childbirth. 2021;21:677.
72. Semeia L, Bauer I, Sippel K, Hartkopf J, Schaal NK, Preissl H. Impact of maternal emotional state during pregnancy on fetal heart rate variability. Compr Psychoneuroendocrinol. 2023;14:100181.
73. Czarzasta K, Sztechman D, Zera T, Wojciechowska M, Segiet-Swiecicka A, Puchalska L, Momot K, Joniec-Maciejak I, Machaj E, Sajdel-Sulkowska EM. Age- and sex-dependent cardiovascular impact of maternal perinatal stress and altered dopaminergic metabolism in the medulla oblongata of the offspring. Am J Physiol Heart Circ Physiol. 2024;327:H614–30.
74. Lang RM, Bierig M, Devereux RB, et al. Recommendations for chamber quantification: a report from the American Society of Echocardiography's Guidelines and Standards Committee and the Chamber Quantification Writing Group, developed in conjunction with the European Association of Echocardiography, a branch of the European Society of Cardiology. J Am Soc Echocardiogr. 2005;18:1440–63.
75. Fulgenzi G, Tomassoni-Ardori F, Babini L, Becker J, Barrick C, Puverel S, Tessarollo L. BDNF modulates heart contraction force and long-term homeostasis through truncated TrkB.T1 receptor activation. J Cell Biol. 2015;210:1003–12.
76. Antolic A, Richards EM, Wood CE, Keller-Wood M. A transcriptomic model of postnatal cardiac effects of prenatal maternal cortisol excess in sheep. Front Physiol. 2019;10:816.
77. Hales CN, Barker DJ, Clark PM, Cox LJ, Fall C, Osmond C, Winter PD. Fetal and infant growth and impaired glucose tolerance at age 64. BMJ. 1991;303:1019–22.
78. Phipps K, Barker DJ, Hales CN, Fall CH, Osmond C, Clark PM. Fetal growth and impaired glucose tolerance in men and women. Diabetologia. 1993;36:225–8.
79. Li J, Olsen J, Vestergaard M, Obel C, Baker JL, Sørensen TIA. Prenatal stress exposure related to maternal bereavement and risk of childhood overweight. PLoS One. 2010;5:e11896.
80. Li J, Olsen J, Vestergaard M, Obel C, Baker JL, Sørensen TIA. Bereavement in early life and later childhood overweight. Obes Facts. 2012;5:881–9.
81. Ertel KA, Koenen KC, Rich-Edwards JW, Gillman MW. Antenatal and postpartum depressive symptoms are differentially associated with early childhood weight and adiposity. Paediatr Perinat Epidemiol. 2010;24:179–89.
82. van Dijk AE, van Eijsden M, Stronks K, Gemke RJBJ, Vrijkotte TGM. No associations of prenatal maternal psychosocial stress with fasting glucose metabolism in offspring at 5-6 years of age. J Dev Orig Health Dis. 2014;5:361–9.
83. Entringer S, Wüst S, Kumsta R, Layes IM, Nelson EL, Hellhammer DH, Wadhwa PD. Prenatal psychosocial stress exposure is associated with insulin resistance in young adults. Am J Obstet Gynecol. 2008;199:498.e1–7.
84. Vaughan OR, Sferruzzi-Perri AN, Fowden AL. Maternal corticosterone regulates nutrient allocation to fetal growth in mice. J Physiol. 2012;590:5529–40.
85. Phuthong S, Reyes-Hernández CG, Rodríguez-Rodríguez P, Ramiro-Cortijo D, Gil-Ortega M, González-Blázquez R, González MC, López de Pablo AL, Arribas SM. Sex differences in placental protein expression and efficiency in a rat model of fetal programming induced by maternal undernutrition. Int J Mol Sci. 2020;22:237. https://doi.org/10.3390/ijms22010237.

86. de Vries A, Holmes MC, Heijnis A, Seier JV, Heerden J, Louw J, Wolfe-Coote S, Meaney MJ, Levitt NS, Seckl JR. Prenatal dexamethasone exposure induces changes in nonhuman primate offspring cardiometabolic and hypothalamic-pituitary-adrenal axis function. J Clin Invest. 2007;117:1058–67.
87. Namburete AIL, Papież BW, Fernandes M, et al. Normative spatiotemporal fetal brain maturation with satisfactory development at 2 years. Nature. 2023;623:106–14.
88. Buss C, Davis EP, Muftuler LT, Head K, Sandman CA. High pregnancy anxiety during mid-gestation is associated with decreased gray matter density in 6-9-year-old children. Psychoneuroendocrinology. 2010;35:141–53.
89. Marecková K, Klasnja A, Bencurova P, Andrýsková L, Brázdil M, Paus T. Prenatal stress, mood, and gray matter volume in young adulthood. Cereb Cortex. 2019;29:1244–50.
90. Su X, Xu B, Liang H, Olsen J, Yuan W, Cnattingius S, László KD, Li J. Prenatal maternal bereavement and risk of eating disorders in infants and toddlers: a population-based cohort study. BMC Psychiatry. 2015;15:229.
91. Henry C, Kabbaj M, Simon H, Le Moal M, Maccari S. Prenatal stress increases the hypothalamo-pituitary-adrenal axis response in young and adult rats. J Neuroendocrinol. 1994;6:341–5.
92. Salaria S, Chana G, Caldara F, Feltrin E, Altieri M, Faggioni F, Domenici E, Merlo-Pich E, Everall IP. Microarray analysis of cultured human brain aggregates following cortisol exposure: implications for cellular functions relevant to mood disorders. Neurobiol Dis. 2006;23:630–6.
93. Welberg LA, Seckl JR, Holmes MC. Inhibition of 11beta-hydroxysteroid dehydrogenase, the foeto-placental barrier to maternal glucocorticoids, permanently programs amygdala GR mRNA expression and anxiety-like behaviour in the offspring. Eur J Neurosci. 2000;12:1047–54.
94. Babenko O, Kovalchuk I, Metz GAS. Stress-induced perinatal and transgenerational epigenetic programming of brain development and mental health. Neurosci Biobehav Rev. 2015;48:70–91.
95. Klose RJ, Bird AP. Genomic DNA methylation: the mark and its mediators. Trends Biochem Sci. 2006;31:89–97.
96. Kundakovic M, Jaric I. The epigenetic link between prenatal adverse environments and neurodevelopmental disorders. Genes (Basel). 2017;8:104. https://doi.org/10.3390/genes8030104.
97. Miller FD, Gauthier AS. Timing is everything: making neurons versus glia in the developing cortex. Neuron. 2007;54:357–69.
98. Cao-Lei L, van den Heuvel MI, Huse K, Platzer M, Elgbeili G, Braeken MAKA, Otte RA, Witte OW, Schwab M, Van den Bergh BRH. Epigenetic modifications associated with maternal anxiety during pregnancy and children's behavioral measures. Cells. 2021;10:2421. https://doi.org/10.3390/cells10092421.
99. Oberlander TF, Weinberg J, Papsdorf M, Grunau R, Misri S, Devlin AM. Prenatal exposure to maternal depression, neonatal methylation of human glucocorticoid receptor gene (NR3C1) and infant cortisol stress responses. Epigenetics. 2008;3:97–106.
100. Jensen Peña C, Monk C, Champagne FA. Epigenetic effects of prenatal stress on 11β-hydroxysteroid dehydrogenase-2 in the placenta and fetal brain. PLoS One. 2012;7:e39791.
101. Monk C, Feng T, Lee S, Krupska I, Champagne FA, Tycko B. Distress during pregnancy: epigenetic regulation of placenta glucocorticoid-related genes and fetal neurobehavior. Am J Psychiatry. 2016;173:705–13.
102. Dong E, Dzitoyeva SG, Matrisciano F, Tueting P, Grayson DR, Guidotti A. Brain-derived neurotrophic factor epigenetic modifications associated with schizophrenia-like phenotype induced by prenatal stress in mice. Biol Psychiatry. 2015;77:589–96.
103. Matrisciano F, Tueting P, Dalal I, Kadriu B, Grayson DR, Davis JM, Nicoletti F, Guidotti A. Epigenetic modifications of GABAergic interneurons are associated with the schizophrenia-like phenotype induced by prenatal stress in mice. Neuropharmacology. 2013;68:184–94.

104. Blaze J, Asok A, Borrelli K, Tulbert C, Bollinger J, Ronca AE, Roth TL. Intrauterine exposure to maternal stress alters Bdnf IV DNA methylation and telomere length in the brain of adult rat offspring. Int J Dev Neurosci. 2017;62:56–62.
105. Fuchikami M, Morinobu S, Segawa M, et al. DNA methylation profiles of the brain-derived neurotrophic factor (BDNF) gene as a potent diagnostic biomarker in major depression. PLoS One. 2011;6:e23881.
106. Zheng Y, Fan W, Zhang X, Dong E. Gestational stress induces depressive-like and anxiety-like phenotypes through epigenetic regulation of BDNF expression in offspring hippocampus. Epigenetics. 2016;11:150–62.
107. Davis EP, Hankin BL, Glynn LM, Head K, Kim DJ, Sandman CA. Prenatal maternal stress, child cortical thickness, and adolescent depressive symptoms. Child Dev. 2020;91:e432–50.
108. Mareckova K, Marecek R, Andryskova L, Brazdil M, Nikolova YS. Maternal depressive symptoms during pregnancy and brain age in young adult offspring: findings from a prenatal birth cohort. Cereb Cortex. 2020;30:3991–9.
109. Mareckova K, Miles A, Andryskova L, Brazdil M, Nikolova YS. Temporally and sex-specific effects of maternal perinatal stress on offspring cortical gyrification and mood in young adulthood. Hum Brain Mapp. 2020;41:4866–75.
110. Khashan AS, Abel KM, McNamee R, Pedersen MG, Webb RT, Baker PN, Kenny LC, Mortensen PB. Higher risk of offspring schizophrenia following antenatal maternal exposure to severe adverse life events. Arch Gen Psychiatry. 2008;65:146–52.
111. Mawson ER, Morris BJ. A consideration of the increased risk of schizophrenia due to prenatal maternal stress, and the possible role of microglia. Prog Neuro-Psychopharmacol Biol Psychiatry. 2023;125:110773.
112. Schmidt M, Rossetti AC, Brandwein C, Riva MA, Gass P, Elsner P, Hesse-Macabata J, Hipler U-C, Smesny S, Milleit B. Brain derived neurotrophic factor deficiency is associated with cognitive impairment and elevated phospholipase A2 activity in plasma of mice. Neuroscience. 2022;480:167–77.
113. Manzari N, Matvienko-Sikar K, Baldoni F, O'Keeffe GW, Khashan AS. Prenatal maternal stress and risk of neurodevelopmental disorders in the offspring: a systematic review and meta-analysis. Soc Psychiatry Psychiatr Epidemiol. 2019;54:1299–309.
114. Kinney DK, Miller AM, Crowley DJ, Huang E, Gerber E. Autism prevalence following prenatal exposure to hurricanes and tropical storms in Louisiana. J Autism Dev Disord. 2008;38:481–8.
115. Class QA, Abel KM, Khashan AS, Rickert ME, Dalman C, Larsson H, Hultman CM, Långström N, Lichtenstein P, D'Onofrio BM. Offspring psychopathology following preconception, prenatal and postnatal maternal bereavement stress. Psychol Med. 2014;44:71–84.
116. Mill J, Petronis A. Pre- and peri-natal environmental risks for attention-deficit hyperactivity disorder (ADHD): the potential role of epigenetic processes in mediating susceptibility. J Child Psychol Psychiatry. 2008;49:1020–30.
117. Schanen NC. Epigenetics of autism spectrum disorders. Hum Mol Genet. 2006;15 Spec No 2:R138–50.
118. Yao S, Lopez-Tello J, Sferruzzi-Perri AN. Developmental programming of the female reproductive system – a review. Biol Reprod. 2021;104:745–70.
119. Nguyen T-V, Jones SL, Elgbeili G, Monnier P, Yu C, Laplante DP, King S. Testosterone-cortisol dissociation in children exposed to prenatal maternal stress, and relationship with aggression: Project Ice Storm. Dev Psychopathol. 2018;30:981–94.
120. Bräuner EV, Koch T, Doherty DA, Dickinson JE, Juul A, Hart R, Hickey M. The association between in utero exposure to maternal psychological stress and female reproductive function in adolescence: a prospective cohort study. Compr Psychoneuroendocrinol. 2021;5:100026.
121. Bräuner EV, Koch T, Juul A, Doherty DA, Hart R, Hickey M. Prenatal exposure to maternal stressful life events and earlier age at menarche: the Raine Study. Hum Reprod. 2021;36:1959–69.
122. Guarneri AM, Kamboj MK. Physiology of pubertal development in females. Pediatr Med. 2019;2:1–8.

123. Yehuda R, Engel SM, Brand SR, Seckl J, Marcus SM, Berkowitz GS. Transgenerational effects of posttraumatic stress disorder in babies of mothers exposed to the World Trade Center attacks during pregnancy. J Clin Endocrinol Metab. 2005;90:4115–8.
124. Stonawski V, Frey S, Golub Y, et al. Associations of prenatal depressive symptoms with DNA methylation of HPA axis-related genes and diurnal cortisol profiles in primary school-aged children. Dev Psychopathol. 2019;31:419–31.
125. Laurent HK, Leve LD, Neiderhiser JM, Natsuaki MN, Shaw DS, Harold GT, Reiss D. Effects of prenatal and postnatal parent depressive symptoms on adopted child HPA regulation: independent and moderated influences. Dev Psychol. 2013;49:876–86.
126. Huizink AC, Bartels M, Rose RJ, Pulkkinen L, Eriksson CJP, Kaprio J. Chernobyl exposure as stressor during pregnancy and hormone levels in adolescent offspring. J Epidemiol Community Health (1978). 2008;62:e5.
127. Bräuner EV, Hansen ÅM, Doherty DA, Dickinson JE, Handelsman DJ, Hickey M, Skakkebæk NE, Juul A, Hart R. The association between in-utero exposure to stressful life events during pregnancy and male reproductive function in a cohort of 20-year-old offspring: the Raine Study. Hum Reprod. 2019;34:1345–55.
128. Plana-Ripoll O, Li J, Kesmodel US, Parner E, Olsen J, Basso O. Reproductive function in the sons of women who experienced stress due to bereavement before and during pregnancy: a nationwide population-based cohort study. Fertil Steril. 2017;107:189–197.e8.
129. Vargas Aguilar VM, Beltrán Beltrán KM, Arroyo Álvarez K. Pathophysiology of fetal programming and its impact on the future health. Ginecol Obstet Mex. 2023;91:588–99.
130. Li J, Vestergaard M, Obel C, Cnattingus S, Gissler M, Ahrensberg J, Olsen J. Antenatal maternal bereavement and childhood cancer in the offspring: a population-based cohort study in 6 million children. Br J Cancer. 2012;107:544–8.
131. Benavent N, Cañete A, Moreno L, Gros L, Verdú-Amorós J, Salinas JA, Navarro S, Álvaro T, Carbonell-Asins JA, Noguera R. Risk of developing neuroblastoma influenced by maternal stressful life events during pregnancy and congenital pathologies. Pediatr Blood Cancer. 2025;72:e31402.
132. Bermejo JL, Sundquist J, Hemminki K. Risk of cancer among the offspring of women who experienced parental death during pregnancy. Cancer Epidemiol Biomarkers Prev. 2007;16:2204–6.
133. Spector LG, Pankratz N, Marcotte EL. Genetic and nongenetic risk factors for childhood cancer. Pediatr Clin N Am. 2015;62:11–25.
134. Gapp K, Jawaid A, Sarkies P, Bohacek J, Pelczar P, Prados J, Farinelli L, Miska E, Mansuy IM. Implication of sperm RNAs in transgenerational inheritance of the effects of early trauma in mice. Nat Neurosci. 2014;17:667–9.
135. Bisgaard H, Li N, Bonnelykke K, Chawes BLK, Skov T, Paludan-Müller G, Stokholm J, Smith B, Krogfelt KA. Reduced diversity of the intestinal microbiota during infancy is associated with increased risk of allergic disease at school age. J Allergy Clin Immunol. 2011;128:646–52.e1–5.
136. Ismail IH, Oppedisano F, Joseph SJ, Boyle RJ, Licciardi PV, Robins-Browne RM, Tang MLK. Reduced gut microbial diversity in early life is associated with later development of eczema but not atopy in high-risk infants. Pediatr Allergy Immunol. 2012;23:674–81.
137. Abrahamsson TR, Jakobsson HE, Andersson AF, Björkstén B, Engstrand L, Jenmalm MC. Low diversity of the gut microbiota in infants with atopic eczema. J Allergy Clin Immunol. 2012;129:434–40, 440.e1–2.
138. Stewart CJ, Ajami NJ, O'Brien JL, et al. Temporal development of the gut microbiome in early childhood from the TEDDY study. Nature. 2018;562:583–8.
139. Gorczyca K, Obuchowska A, Kimber-Trojnar Ż, Wierzchowska-Opoka M, Leszczyńska-Gorzelak B. Changes in the gut microbiome and pathologies in pregnancy. Int J Environ Res Public Health. 2022;19:9961. https://doi.org/10.3390/ijerph19169961.
140. Agusti A, Lamers F, Tamayo M, Benito-Amat C, Molina-Mendoza GV, Penninx BWJH, Sanz Y. The gut microbiome in early life stress: a systematic review. Nutrients. 2023;15:2566. https://doi.org/10.3390/nu15112566.

141. Panzer JJ, Romero R, Greenberg JM, Winters AD, Galaz J, Gomez-Lopez N, Theis KR. Is there a placental microbiota? A critical review and re-analysis of published placental microbiota datasets. BMC Microbiol. 2023;23:76.
142. Theis KR, Romero R, Winters AD, et al. Does the human placenta delivered at term have a microbiota? Results of cultivation, quantitative real-time PCR, 16S rRNA gene sequencing, and metagenomics. Am J Obstet Gynecol. 2019;220:267.e1–267.e39.
143. de Goffau MC, Lager S, Sovio U, Gaccioli F, Cook E, Peacock SJ, Parkhill J, Charnock-Jones DS, Smith GCS. Human placenta has no microbiome but can contain potential pathogens. Nature. 2019;572:329–34.
144. Lopez-Tello J, Schofield Z, Kiu R, Dalby MJ, van Sinderen D, Le Gall G, Sferruzzi-Perri AN, Hall LJ. Maternal gut microbiota Bifidobacterium promotes placental morphogenesis, nutrient transport and fetal growth in mice. Cell Mol Life Sci. 2022;79:386.
145. Haq SU, Bhat UA, Kumar A. Prenatal stress effects on offspring brain and behavior: mediators, alterations and dysregulated epigenetic mechanisms. J Biosci. 2021;46:34.
146. Dutton CL, Maisha FM, Quinn EB, Morales KL, Moore JM, Mulligan CJ. Maternal psychosocial stress is associated with reduced diversity in the early infant gut microbiome. Microorganisms. 2023;11:975. https://doi.org/10.3390/microorganisms11040975.
147. Zijlmans MAC, Korpela K, Riksen-Walraven JM, de Vos WM, de Weerth C. Maternal prenatal stress is associated with the infant intestinal microbiota. Psychoneuroendocrinology. 2015;53:233–45.
148. Zhang A, de Ángel Solá D, Acevedo Flores M, Cao L, Wang L, Kim JG, Tarr PI, Warner BB, Rosario Matos N, Wang L. Infants exposed in utero to Hurricane Maria have gut microbiomes with reduced diversity and altered metabolic capacity. mSphere. 2023;8:e0013423.
149. Le K, Nguyen M. Armed conflict and birth weight. Econ Hum Biol. 2020;39:100921.
150. Li C, Gráda CÓ, Lumey LH. Famine mortality and contributions to later-life type 2 diabetes at the population level: a synthesis of findings from Ukrainian, Dutch and Chinese famines. BMJ Glob Health. 2024;9:e015355. https://doi.org/10.1136/bmjgh-2024-015355.
151. Roseboom TJ, van der Meulen JH, Osmond C, Barker DJ, Ravelli AC, Schroeder-Tanka JM, van Montfrans GA, Michels RP, Bleker OP. Coronary heart disease after prenatal exposure to the Dutch famine, 1944-45. Heart. 2000;84:595–8.
152. González Zapata LI, Alvarez-Dardet Díaz C, Nolasco Bonmatí A, Pina Romero JA, Medrano MJ. Famine in the Spanish civil war and mortality from coronary heart disease: a perspective from Barker's hypothesis. Gac Sanit. 2006;20:360–7.
153. Painter RC, De Rooij SR, Bossuyt PMM, Osmond C, Barker DJP, Bleker OP, Roseboom TJ. A possible link between prenatal exposure to famine and breast cancer: a preliminary study. Am J Hum Biol. 2006;18:853–6.
154. Lopuhaä CE, Roseboom TJ, Osmond C, Barker DJ, Ravelli AC, Bleker OP, van der Zee JS, van der Meulen JH. Atopy, lung function, and obstructive airways disease after prenatal exposure to famine. Thorax. 2000;55:555–61.
155. Lumey LH, Ekamper P, Bijwaard G, Conti G, van Poppel F. Overweight and obesity at age 19 after pre-natal famine exposure. Int J Obes. 2021;45:1668–76.
156. Lumey LH, Stein AD, Kahn HS, Romijn JA. Lipid profiles in middle-aged men and women after famine exposure during gestation: the Dutch Hunger Winter Families Study. Am J Clin Nutr. 2009;89:1737–43.
157. Yarde F, Broekmans FJM, van der Pal-de Bruin KM, Schönbeck Y, te Velde ER, Stein AD, Lumey LH. Prenatal famine, birthweight, reproductive performance and age at menopause: the Dutch Hunger Winter Families Study. Hum Reprod. 2013;28:3328–36.
158. Stanner SA, Yudkin JS. Fetal programming and the Leningrad Siege study. Twin Res. 2001;4:287–92.
159. Stanner SA, Bulmer K, Andrès C, Lantseva OE, Borodina V, Poteen VV, Yudkin JS. Does malnutrition in utero determine diabetes and coronary heart disease in adulthood? Results from the Leningrad siege study, a cross sectional study. BMJ. 1997;315:1342–8.

160. Tolkunova K, Usoltsev D, Moguchaia E, et al. Transgenerational and intergenerational effects of early childhood famine exposure in the cohort of offspring of Leningrad siege survivors. Sci Rep. 2023;13:11188.
161. Rotar O, Moguchaia E, Boyarinova M, et al. Seventy years after the siege of Leningrad: does early life famine still affect cardiovascular risk and aging? J Hypertens. 2015;33:1772–9; discussion 1779.
162. Rich-Edwards JW, Gillman MW. Commentary: a hypothesis challenged. BMJ. 1997;315:1348–9.
163. Eriksson JG, Forsén T, Tuomilehto J, Winter PD, Osmond C, Barker DJ. Catch-up growth in childhood and death from coronary heart disease: longitudinal study. BMJ. 1999;318:427–31.
164. Li J, Yang Q, An R, et al. Famine and trajectories of body mass index, waist circumference, and blood pressure in two generations: results from the CHNS from 1993-2015. Hypertension. 2022;79:518–31.
165. Zhang X, Wang G, Forman MR, Fu Q, Rogers CJ, Wu S, Gao X. In utero and childhood exposure to the Great Chinese famine and risk of cancer in adulthood: the Kailuan Study. Am J Clin Nutr. 2021;114:2017–24.
166. Tan Y, Jiang X, Ding X, Wei Z, Song Z, Chen S, Yang P, Zhao D, Wu S, Li Y. Early life exposure to Chinese famine and risk of digestive system cancer in midlife. Appl Physiol Nutr Metab. 2024;49:751–61.
167. Ma T, Hao X-M, Zhang X, Liu X-Y, Wang Y-M, Zhang Q-S, Zhang J. In utero and childhood exposure to the great Chinese famine and risk of aging in adulthood. Sci Rep. 2024;14:25089.
168. Srichaikul K, Hegele RA, Jenkins DJA. Great Chinese famine and the effects on cardiometabolic health for future generations. Hypertension. 2022;79:532–5.
169. Ogah OS, Oguntade AS, Chukwuonye II, et al. Childhood and infant exposure to famine in the Biafran war is associated with hypertension in later life: the Abia NCDS study. J Hum Hypertens. 2023;37:936–43.
170. Hult M, Tornhammar P, Ueda P, Chima C, Bonamy A-KE, Ozumba B, Norman M. Hypertension, diabetes and overweight: looming legacies of the Biafran famine. PLoS One. 2010;5:e13582.
171. Arage G, Belachew T, Hassen H, Abera M, Abdulhay F, Abdulahi M, Hassen Abate K. Effects of prenatal exposure to the 1983-1985 Ethiopian great famine on the metabolic syndrome in adults: a historical cohort study. Br J Nutr. 2020;124:1052–60.
172. Abate KH, Abdulahi M, Abdulhay F, Arage G, Mecha M, Yenuss M, Hassen H, Belachew T. Consequences of exposure to prenatal famine on estimated glomerular filtration rate and risk of chronic kidney disease among survivors of the great Ethiopian famine (1983-85): a historical cohort study. Nutr J. 2021;20:19.
173. Harville E, Xiong X, Buekens P. Disasters and perinatal health: a systematic review. Obstet Gynecol Surv. 2010;65:713–28.
174. Sherrieb K, Norris FH. Public health consequences of terrorism on maternal-child health in New York City and Madrid. J Urban Health. 2013;90:369–87.
175. Brown R. The intergenerational impact of terror: did the 9/11 tragedy impact the initial human capital of the next generation? Demography. 2020;57:1459–81.
176. Nugent JL, Khashan AS, Baker PN. Reduced infant birth weight in the North West of England consequent upon "maternal exposure" to 7/7 terrorist attacks on central London. J Obstet Gynaecol. 2011;31:118–21.
177. Quintana-Domeque C, Ródenas-Serrano P. The hidden costs of terrorism: the effects on health at birth. J Health Econ. 2017;56:47–60.
178. Schmitz LL, Duque V. In utero exposure to the Great Depression is reflected in late-life epigenetic aging signatures. Proc Natl Acad Sci. 2022;119:e2208530119. https://doi.org/10.1073/pnas.2208530119.
179. King S, Laplante DP. The effects of prenatal maternal stress on children's cognitive development: Project Ice Storm. Stress. 2005;8:35–45.
180. Moss KM, Simcock G, Cobham V, Kildea S, Elgbeili G, Laplante DP, King S. A potential psychological mechanism linking disaster-related prenatal maternal stress with child

cognitive and motor development at 16 months: the QF2011 Queensland Flood Study. Dev Psychol. 2017;53:629–41.
181. Mazumder B, Almond D, Park K, Crimmins EM, Finch CE. Lingering prenatal effects of the 1918 influenza pandemic on cardiovascular disease. J Dev Orig Health Dis. 2010;1:26–34.
182. Schoenmakers S, Verweij EJJ, Beijers R, Bijma HH, Been JV, Steegers-Theunissen RPM, Koopmans MPG, Reiss IKM, Steegers EAP. The impact of maternal prenatal stress related to the COVID-19 pandemic during the first 1000 days: a historical perspective. Int J Environ Res Public Health. 2022;19:4710. https://doi.org/10.3390/ijerph19084710.
183. Wei SQ, Bilodeau-Bertrand M, Liu S, Auger N. The impact of COVID-19 on pregnancy outcomes: a systematic review and meta-analysis. CMAJ. 2021;193:E540–8.
184. Villar-Alises O, Martinez-Miranda P, Martinez-Calderon J. Prenatal yoga-based interventions may improve mental health during pregnancy: an overview of systematic reviews with meta-analysis. Int J Environ Res Public Health. 2023;20:1556. https://doi.org/10.3390/ijerph20021556.
185. Crovetto F, Nakaki A, Arranz A, et al. Effect of a Mediterranean diet or mindfulness-based stress reduction during pregnancy on child neurodevelopment. JAMA Netw Open. 2023;6:e2330255.
186. Camacho-Morales A, Caba M, García-Juárez M, Caba-Flores MD, Viveros-Contreras R, Martínez-Valenzuela C. Breastfeeding contributes to physiological immune programming in the newborn. Front Pediatr. 2021;9:744104.
187. Center for Disease Control and Prevention (CDC). Breastfeeding benefits both baby and mom. In: Breastfeeding. CDC; 2023. https://www.cdc.gov/breastfeeding/features/breastfeeding-benefits.html. Accessed 16 Jan 2025.
188. Ames SR, Lotoski LC, Azad MB. Comparing early life nutritional sources and human milk feeding practices: personalized and dynamic nutrition supports infant gut microbiome development and immune system maturation. Gut Microbes. 2023;15:2190305. https://doi.org/10.1080/19490976.2023.2190305.
189. Dawod B, Marshall JS, Azad MB. Breastfeeding and the developmental origins of mucosal immunity: how human milk shapes the innate and adaptive mucosal immune systems. Curr Opin Gastroenterol. 2021;37:547–56.
190. Riskin A, Almog M, Peri R, Halasz K, Srugo I, Kessel A. Changes in immunomodulatory constituents of human milk in response to active infection in the nursing infant. Pediatr Res. 2012;71:220–5.
191. Fernández-Tuñas MDC, Pérez-Muñuzuri A, Trastoy-Pena R, Pérez Del Molino ML, Couce ML. Effects of maternal stress on breast milk production and the microbiota of very premature infants. Nutrients. 2023;15:4006. https://doi.org/10.3390/nu15184006.
192. Juncker HG, Jakobsen RR, Naninck EFG, Davids M, Herrema H, van Goudoever JB, de Rooij SR, Korosi A. Maternal stress in the early postpartum period is associated with alterations in human milk microbiome composition. Brain Behav Immun. 2025;124:74–84.
193. Wu Y, Zhang Q, Xiao X. The effect and potential mechanism of maternal micronutrient intake on offspring glucose metabolism: an emerging field. Front Nutr. 2021;8:763809. https://doi.org/10.3389/fnut.2021.763809.
194. Eberle C, Fasig T, Brüseke F, Stichling S. Impact of maternal prenatal stress by glucocorticoids on metabolic and cardiovascular outcomes in their offspring: a systematic scoping review. PLoS One. 2021;16:e0245386.
195. Ng R, Sutradhar R, Yao Z, Wodchis WP, Rosella LC. Smoking, drinking, diet and physical activity-modifiable lifestyle risk factors and their associations with age to first chronic disease. Int J Epidemiol. 2020;49:113–30.
196. Department of Health and Human Services. Healthy habits can lengthen life. National Institute of Health (NIH); 2018. https://newsinhealth.nih.gov/2018/06/healthy-habits-can-lengthen-life. Accessed 16 Jan 2025.

Scientific Interventions to Reduce Maternal Stress: Improvement of Maternal and Fetal Outcomes

14

Ling Li Leng, Wenhan Xiao, and Xiye He

Abstract

Maternal stress during pregnancy and postpartum poses significant risks to both maternal and fetal health. This chapter synthesizes empirical evidence on the efficacy of four non-pharmacological interventions—mindfulness-based interventions (MBIs), cognitive-behavioral therapy (CBT), interpersonal psychotherapy (IPT), and relaxation training—in reducing maternal stress and improving maternal-fetal outcomes.

MBIs demonstrate robust effects on psychological outcomes and physiological stress markers, such as reduced cortisol levels and improved autonomic regulation, while also enhancing childbirth experiences. CBT effectively mitigates perinatal depression and anxiety, benefits offspring neurodevelopment, and now enhances its accessibility and adaptability through partner-inclusive and digital formats. IPT addresses interpersonal stressors and role transitions, showing rapid symptom relief, though long-term efficacy requires further validation. Relaxation training, including yoga and guided imagery, reduces physiological stress and may lower preterm birth risks. Despite their promise, challenges such as adherence disparities and cultural adaptability persist.

The chapter underscores the need for longitudinal studies, comparative effectiveness research, and scalable implementations, especially in low-resource settings. Integrating these interventions into perinatal care offers a holistic approach to breaking the cycle of intergenerational stress transmission and promoting equitable maternal and child health outcomes.

L. L. Leng (✉) · W. Xiao · X. He
The Department of Sociology, Zhejiang University, Hangzhou, China
e-mail: linglileng@zju.edu.cn

R. A. Caparros-Gonzalez (ed.), *Maternal Stress during Pregnancy and Postpartum*, https://doi.org/10.1007/978-3-032-09245-8_14

Keywords

Maternal stress · Mindfulness · Cognitive-behavioral therapy · Interpersonal therapy · Relaxation training · Fetal outcomes

14.1 Introduction

Maternal stress during pregnancy and postpartum represents a significant public health concern with far-reaching implications for both maternal and offspring well-being. Elevated stress levels during these critical times can impair maternal mental health, obstetric outcomes, and parenting capacity, while simultaneously influencing fetal health and development. To address these challenges, scientific interventions aimed at reducing maternal stress have become integral to perinatal care, offering holistic solutions that bridge psychological and physiological domains.

This chapter provides an overview of current research on scientific interventions to reduce maternal stress, emphasizing their effectiveness in improving maternal outcomes and optimizing fetal development. It examines diverse approaches—such as mindfulness-based interventions (MBIs), cognitive-behavioral therapy (CBT), interpersonal psychotherapy (IPT), and relaxation training—tailored to address the unique challenges faced by perinatal women. By reviewing empirical evidence, long-term benefits, and the mechanisms through which these interventions operate, this chapter synthesizes strategies that are available to healthcare providers and expectant mothers. Additionally, the chapter highlights the role of these interventions in breaking the cycle of intergenerational stress transmission by elucidating the transformative potential in enhancing maternal and fetal health outcomes in clinical and community settings.

14.2 Scientific Stress-Reducing Interventions on Maternal Outcomes

The evidence base for psychological interventions in reducing maternal stress is extensive and robust. Such evidence reflects a strong preference among perinatal women for non-pharmaceutical approaches due to safety concerns about psychotropic medication during pregnancy and breastfeeding. Among these, MBIs, CBT, IPT, and relaxation training are most extensively studied and prioritized for their efficacy. This section examines these interventions, focusing on applications to maternal stress-related issues and the strength of supporting evidence.

14.2.1 Mindfulness-Based Interventions

MBIs are well-established psychological approaches designed to cultivate mindfulness, defined as nonjudgmental, present-moment awareness characterized by openness, curiosity, and acceptance. These interventions are grounded in nine foundational attitudes: nonjudgment, patience, beginner's mind, trust, non-striving, acceptance, letting go, gratitude, and generosity [1]. MBIs employ structured group programs incorporating techniques such as mindful breathing, body scanning, loving-kindness meditation, and mindful eating. The core principles of mindfulness include regulating attention and adopting a specific attitude toward one's experiences [2].

Rooted in ancient Eastern Buddhist traditions, the scientific engagement with meditation can be traced back to the 1930s, while Wallace's seminal work in the 1970s, which examined its impact on stress, brought significant attention to the field [3]. A further significant milestone was the development of the *Mindfulness-Based Stress Reduction* (MBSR) program by Jon Kabat-Zinn in the 1990s, which was designed to reduce chronic pain and stress and has since become a cornerstone of mindfulness-based approaches [4]. Another influential MBI is *Mindfulness-Based Cognitive Therapy* (MBCT), which was specifically developed to prevent relapse in individuals with recurrent depression [5]. These programs have established MBIs as evidence-based practices with broad applications in mental and physical health.

14.2.1.1 Effects of MBIs on Maternal Stress

Over the past decade, MBIs have demonstrated significant efficacy in alleviating perinatal psychological stress. Meta-analyses of randomized controlled trials (RCTs) have shown that MBIs significantly reduce maternal stress, depression, and anxiety during the perinatal period [6–9]. A synthesis of 25 RCTs found that MBIs were effective in reducing maternal depression with medium effect sizes compared to the control group [8]. The effect was even more pronounced in treating perinatal depression among women with depression or anxiety disorders, exhibiting a large effect size in this subgroup.

Another meta-analysis of 21 RCTs confirmed the significant impact of MBIs in treating maternal stress disorders among perinatal women experiencing elevated maternal stress, depression, anxiety, and fear of childbirth [9]. Supporting these results, a clinical trial evaluating the *Mindful Self-Compassion* intervention for 314 pregnant women with heightened depressive symptoms demonstrated significant reductions in postpartum depressive symptoms and parenting stress compared to the control group [10]. Additionally, pregnant women with comorbid depression and anxiety disorders who participated in MBCT exhibited significantly greater reductions in both depressive and anxiety symptoms relative to the control group [11]. Moreover, an 8-week mindful parenting program significantly reduced perinatal depression, stress, and anxiety among pregnant women at risk for psychological distress [12]. These studies suggest the efficacy of MBIs in addressing a transdiagnostic spectrum of perinatal psychological stress, particularly among women with mental health risks.

Long-Term Benefits of MBIs on Psychological Stress

Meta-analytic evidence indicates that the benefits of prenatal MBIs on maternal psychological stress are sustainable, with significantly greater improvements maintained into the postpartum period compared to control conditions [8]. For example, the *Mindfulness-Based Cognitive Therapy adapted for perinatal depression* (MBCT-PD) has effectively prevented depression relapse in pregnant women with a history of depression [13]. Likewise, an electronic mindfulness-based intervention also produced a preventive effect on depression in women with elevated antenatal depressive symptoms. In both trials, the benefits were sustained for 6 months post-intervention [14].

Similarly, the evidence of *Mindfulness-Based Childbirth and Parenting* (MBCP) intervention revealed its effects in reducing maternal stress, depression, and anxiety up to 4 months postpartum among low-risk pregnant women, compared to those receiving standard antenatal care [15]. Another RCT evaluating MBCP among pregnant women at high risk for depression documented significant improvements in maternal stress and depressive symptoms compared to an active control condition [16]. However, these effects were not sustained during longer-term follow-ups at 3, 9, and 12 months postpartum [17]. This discrepancy may be attributed to differences in adherence to mindfulness practices post-childbirth; approximately 30% of women discontinued formal mindfulness practice due to time constraints, whereas those receiving online support maintained the engagement [15, 17]. Building on these findings, continued practice and post-intervention support may play a crucial role in sustaining the benefits of MBIs.

Effects of MBIs on Physiological Stress

Emerging empirical evidence suggests that MBIs can positively impact physiological indices of maternal stress by modulating biological systems involved in stress adaptation. For example, Zhang and Emory (2020) found that an MBI significantly reduced pregnancy-related stress and lowered salivary cortisol levels—a key biomarker of hypothalamic-pituitary-adrenal (HPA) axis activity—in low-income pregnant African-American women [18]. In addition, a pilot RCT by Matvienko-Sikar and Dockray (2017) reported significant reductions in both waking and evening cortisol levels among pregnant women participating in an MBI [19].

Beyond cortisol regulation, MBIs may also enhance parasympathetic nervous system function, as demonstrated by increased heart rate variability (HRV) in pregnant women practicing mindfulness meditation compared to controls [20]. This finding suggested that MBIs have contributed to improved autonomic regulation and greater stress resilience. Additionally, a pilot trial by Bublitz et al. (2023) demonstrated significant improvements in systolic and diastolic blood pressure among pregnant women at risk for hypertensive disorders who engaged in an MBI, highlighting its potential to mitigate cardiovascular stress [21].

Narratives of Perinatal Women Participating in MBIs

Qualitative evaluations revealed that MBIs were particularly well-suited to address the unique stressors encountered by perinatal women, including physical discomfort, body image problems, heightened health concerns, fears related to childbirth and breastfeeding [22], and rapid shift in roles, responsibilities, and self-identity [23]. Participants reported that cultivating nonjudgmental awareness through mindfulness enhances self-regulation and emotional resilience, enabling them to navigate challenges with greater adaptability [24, 25]. For example, women participating in MBIs describe an improved capacity to manage pain during labor and reduced anxiety, along with greater tolerance for maternal stress and discomfort. Furthermore, MBIs have been shown to enhance positive affect and self-compassion which are critical for mitigating self-critical thoughts common in perinatal populations [24]. Transformative shifts in self-perspective were also reported, with women describing heightened acceptance of their evolving roles as mothers and increased confidence in their parenting abilities [25]. This re-framing perception was especially beneficial during the transformative periods of childbirth and early parenting.

14.2.1.2 Effects of MBIs on Childbirth Outcomes

Emerging evidence suggests that MBIs can improve childbirth outcomes by mitigating maternal stress and its physiological sequelae. Empirical studies indicated that MBIs are associated with decreased utilization of medical interventions during labor, including cesarean sections and epidural analgesia [26–28]. For instance, an RCT evaluating the *Mindful Thrive Pregnancy* program demonstrated a 50% reduction in the likelihood of emergent cesarean delivery among participants compared to controls, an effect partially mediated by reductions in antenatal depressive symptoms [28].

While the difference in labor length between the *Mindful Thrive Pregnancy* group and the control group was not statistically significant, the direct regulation of sensory pain processing observed in the MBI cohort suggests that reducing maternal stress may facilitate the labor process by improving pain tolerance and coping mechanisms [29]. Further support for MBIs' role in optimizing childbirth experiences comes from studies on MBCP. Participants in MBCP reported enhanced coping skills during labor and more positive evaluations of their birth experiences compared to non-intervention groups, underscoring the dual psychological and obstetric benefits of mindfulness training [24].

14.2.2 Cognitive-Behavioral Therapy

Since its development by Aaron Beck in the 1960s, CBT has been an evidence-based psychological intervention that integrates cognitive and behavioral principles. CBT posits that emotional distress and maladaptive behaviors arise from distorted thought patterns, termed "cognitive distortions," which reinforce negative emotional states [30]. This structured, goal-oriented approach emphasizes two core components: cognitive restructuring, which targets the identification and modification of irrational or harmful thoughts [31], and behavioral activation, which encourages engagement in meaningful activities to counteract avoidance behaviors linked to depression and stress [32]. By systematically addressing these cognitive and behavioral factors, CBT fosters psychological resilience and empowers individuals to manage stressors effectively [33, 34].

CBT has shown robust efficacy in treating and preventing major depression across diverse populations [35, 36]. While interventions may vary in emphasis, ranging from cognitive reconstruction to behavioral activation's action-oriented focus, the synergy of cognitive and behavioral components underpins their success. This integrative approach ensures adaptability to individual needs, particularly in the perinatal period, where dynamic stressors require flexible, skill-based strategies.

For perinatal populations, CBT often adopts a multimodal approach, tailored to address the unique challenges of pregnancy and postpartum. These elements include psychoeducation on emotion management, problem-solving training, cognitive strategies, behavioral activation, and assertiveness training. Some interventions extend beyond these core elements to address perinatal-specific demands, including sleep management [37], planning for parenthood [38], and relationship management to improve partner dynamics and support [39].

14.2.2.1 Effects of CBT on Maternal Stress

CBT is the most extensively utilized and empirically validated intervention for alleviating maternal stress during the perinatal period [40]. Meta-analyses of RCTs consistently demonstrated that CBT produces moderate to large effect sizes in reducing maternal stress, depression, and anxiety during pregnancy, postpartum, and across both the pregnancy and postpartum period [41–44]. For example, a synthesis of 79 RCTs and quasi-RCTs demonstrated CBT's superior efficacy over control conditions in alleviating stress, depressive symptoms, and anxiety across culturally and socio-economically diverse perinatal populations, including those in low- and middle-income countries (LMICs) [42]. CBT has shown effectiveness not only in treating existing symptoms but also in preventing the onset of stress-related disorders, with amplified benefits observed among interventions initiated during pregnancy, possibly because it equips women with stress-management skills before the challenges of the postpartum period arise [43, 44]. These findings reinforce CBT's utility as a frontline intervention for perinatal women with moderate to severe psychological distress.

The adaptability of CBT is evident in its successful implementation across multiple delivery formats, including individual, group, and Internet-based modalities [45]. Partner-inclusive CBT, which integrates couples into therapeutic processes, has emerged as a relatively more effective approach. Meta-analytic evidence indicates that CBT involving partners in group or individual settings significantly improved perinatal stress and depression, emphasizing the value of leveraging relational dynamics and partner-derived social support [46]. Moreover, 3-h prenatal CBT sessions incorporating partners, but not those involving women alone, yielded superior reductions in maternal stress compared to controls at 6 weeks postpartum, likely due to enhanced conflict mitigation and emotional support [47].

Internet-delivered CBT (i-CBT) also shows promising efficacy, even without specialist facilitation. The *MUMentum Postnatal Program*, a 6-week i-CBT intervention designed for postpartum women with limited access to traditional services, achieved significant reductions in depression, anxiety, and distress compared to treatment-as-usual among individuals with elevated symptoms [48]. This program also provided preliminary evidence that clinician guidance may not be necessary to achieve large treatment benefits, making it a promising, scalable, and cost-effective intervention approach [48].

In LMICs, CBT adaptations often integrate resource allocation with skill-building to address systemic barriers. For example, the *Thinking Healthy Program*, which embeds CBT into community clinicians' routines, exemplifies this approach. Costing under $16 per woman for each unit improvement on the depression scale annually, the program achieved recovery in 50% of participants, demonstrating its remarkable cost-effectiveness [49]. Its success has prompted adoption by the World Health Organization for global dissemination, underscoring its scalability and relevance in resource-constrained settings.

Long-Term Benefits of CBT on Psychological Stress

CBT has also demonstrated sustained efficacy in alleviating perinatal stress, depression, and anxiety, with therapeutic benefits lasting from 3 to 12 months post-intervention [42]. This finding is echoed in another review, which showed that CBT has long-term efficacy in reducing maternal depression during both pregnancy and the postpartum period [40]. Its benefits for perinatal stress are more pronounced during pregnancy, with limited sustained effects postnatally [43]. This discrepancy of effect duration may reflect the complex interplay of postpartum hormonal fluctuations and evolving stressors, such as sleep deprivation and caregiving demands, which can exacerbate depressive symptoms and diminish the durability of CBT's therapeutic gains [50].

Preliminary evidence also suggests CBT's effect in preventing perinatal post-traumatic stress disorder (PTSD). According to the meta-analysis by Li et al. (2022), although one trial reported no significant short-term efficacy for PTSD, CBT demonstrated substantial long-term reductions in PTSD symptoms across two trials [42]. These outcomes may suggest a delayed therapeutic effect for PTSD, suggesting that sustained application and consolidation of acquired cognitive-behavioral techniques beyond the formal intervention period are essential for long-term efficacy [42].

Guided i-CBT also shows promising long-term efficacy. As evident in general population, guided i-CBT had stable long-term efficacy in reducing maternal stress, anxiety, and depression, with benefits persisting up to 12 months post-intervention [51]. Specifically, meta-analyses of 17 RCTs with the follow-up data ≥12 months post-randomization found that guided i-CBT outperforms treatment-as-usual and waitlist controls in terms of remission and response rates [51]. However, evidence for i-CBT among perinatal populations remains inconclusive. Considering that perinatal stress can persist for up to a year postpartum, there is a critical need for future research to explore i-CBT support in sustaining therapeutic outcomes [51].

Effects of CBT on Physiological Stress

By improving overall stress resilience, CBT can modulate physiological stress responses, particularly within the HPA axis. Prenatal CBT interventions have demonstrated efficacy in restoring its balance among both high-risk and healthy perinatal populations. For instance, an 8-session *Cognitive Behavioral Stress Management* (CBSM) program significantly reduced waking salivary cortisol levels in pregnant women with elevated stress compared to controls [52]. Similar reductions in cortisol have been observed across diverse populations, including low-income cohorts [53] and healthy pregnant women [54], underscoring CBT's broad applicability.

Beyond cortisol, CBT also enhances levels of dehydroepiandrosterone, an endogenous "anti-stress" hormone that counteracts cortisol's deleterious effects. Baranov et al. (2022) found that the *Thinking Healthy Program*, a prenatal CBT-based intervention, increased DHEA concentrations in mothers and their infants at 1 year postpartum compared to enhanced usual care [55]. This intergenerational effect suggests that CBT's benefits may extend to offspring, potentially buffering against stress-related vulnerabilities early in life.

Empirical evidence also suggests that CBT can effectively alleviate stress-related complications in high-risk pregnancies, such as gestational diabetes mellitus (GDM). An RCT evaluating the CBSM program in pregnant women with GDM demonstrated significant reductions in psychological stress and fasting plasma glucose levels compared to routine care, suggesting CBT is a dual-purpose intervention, addressing both metabolic and psychological health in high-risk obstetric populations [56].

Narratives of Perinatal Women Participating in CBT

Women participating in CBT reported that the therapy equipped them with effective coping strategies, such as cognitive restructuring, to challenge negative thoughts and improve emotional adjustment [57, 58]. The structured approach provided tangible exercises that helped women navigate the challenges of the perinatal period. Furthermore, these therapeutic experiences fostered a more positive outlook on life and the future, enhancing their sense of control and self-esteem [59, 60].

CBT has also enabled women to develop better relationships with their babies and gain a deeper understanding of postnatal depression [60]. Women described how they had gained knowledge about infants' development and their importance in their child's development [61]. Many felt that their improved mood had led to a better relationship with their children, helping them become more relaxed, patient, and secure in their parental roles [62].

The support and social interaction provided through group-based CBT sessions were often cited as beneficial, fostering a sense of community and reducing feelings of isolation. The group format contributes to normalization as participants realized they shared similar experiences and were not alone. However, some women have expressed concerns about not feeling safe disclosing their feelings within the group, leading them to censor what they share [63].

14.2.2.2 Effects of CBT on Childbirth Outcomes

Emerging evidence suggests that CBT may positively influence childbirth outcomes. One study found that perinatal CBT significantly increased rates of spontaneous vaginal delivery compared to routine care, suggesting its potential to reduce reliance on medical interventions such as cesarean sections [64]. The study further reported that CBT participants experienced lower intraoperative blood loss and reduced pain intensity during labor, as measured by the visual analog scale [64].

Participants reported comparable levels of. These findings imply that CBT's stress reduction mechanisms may mitigate physiological stress responses, decreasing complications such as excessive bleeding and hyperalgesia.

However, the efficacy of CBT in improving childbirth outcomes appears to vary by population. Burger et al. (2020) conducted a trial among women with antenatal depression or anxiety and found that CBT did not improve childbirth outcomes or maternal symptoms compared to usual care [65]. This discrepancy suggests that CBT's impact on childbirth outcomes may be limited in populations with pre-existing mental health conditions, where biological and psychosocial complexities could attenuate treatment effects.

14.2.3 Interpersonal Therapy

IPT is a time-limited, empirically validated approach originally developed to treat depression [66]. It is grounded in the belief that interpersonal relationships are central to mental health, and psychological distress often arises from difficulties in social functioning. Drawing on attachment and interpersonal theories, IPT focuses on how past relationships impact current interactions and emphasizes the improvement of interpersonal skills to alleviate distress [67]. In this regard, the four primary problem areas addressed by IPT are typically summarized as grief, role transitions, interpersonal disputes, and interpersonal deficits [68].

IPT works by improving communication patterns, enhancing attachment security, and strengthening social support networks, which play a crucial role in coping with stress [68]. Social support in IPT is multifaceted, including emotional support, practical help, social companionship, and motivational support [69]. By improving these support systems, IPT aims to increase resilience and facilitate better coping mechanisms, ultimately improving psychological well-being and interpersonal functioning. As a manualized and easily taught intervention, IPT can be conducted by multi-professionals (e.g., psychologists, clinic nurses, and family social workers) working in clinical or primary healthcare settings, regardless of socioeconomic levels [70].

IPT has also been adapted for various populations. In the context of perinatal mental health, IPT's focus on role transitions, interpersonal disputes, grief, and interpersonal deficits directly targets common challenges faced by women during pregnancy and the postpartum period. By addressing stressors such as low social support, marital dissatisfaction, and role transitions associated with parenthood, IPT helps to reduce symptoms of maternal stress, depression, and anxiety while enhancing relationship quality and social support [71].

14.2.3.1 Effects of IPT on Maternal Stress

The efficacy of IPT in reducing psychological distress among perinatal women has been supported by extensive empirical evidence. Three available meta-analytic reviews consistently endorsed IPT's efficacy in both preventing and treating psychological distress among pregnant and postpartum women [71–73].

As a preventive measure, IPT effectively reduces symptoms of maternal depression and anxiety, particularly among high-risk populations with subthreshold symptoms or psychosocial risk factors. For instance, an RCT evaluating the MomCare program—an individually delivered IPT intervention—demonstrated significant improvements in depressive symptoms among 234 pregnant women with elevated depressive symptoms, compared to those who received enhanced usual care [74]. By focusing on interpersonal challenges such as role transitions and social support deficits, IPT equips women with strategies to navigate stressors inherent to pregnancy and early motherhood, thereby mitigating the onset of depression.

As a treatment, IPT not only reduces psychological distress but also enhances relational functioning, social support, and grief processing [72]. A pilot RCT comparing IPT to CBT for major depressive disorder following perinatal loss highlighted IPT's superior acceptability and preliminary efficacy [75]. IPT participants experienced greater improvements in social functioning. This advantage may stem from IPT's emphasis on emotional expression and processing of loss, with sessions dedicated more time to discussing perinatal loss, facilitating mourning, and addressing communication challenges compared to CBT's cognitive restructuring focus [75].

Evidence synthesis also suggests that group-delivered IPT demonstrated greater effectiveness in reducing maternal psychological distress relative to individual formats [72]. The additional benefit of group intervention may lie in the fact that group setting fosters therapeutic factors such as universality, vicarious learning, and peer support, which normalize women's experiences and enhance coping strategies [76]. Participants gain insight into shared challenges, reducing feelings of isolation, while opportunities to support peers bolster self-efficacy [77]. Additionally, group IPT cultivates social skills that directly address relationship difficulties—a key stressor in the perinatal period—thereby preventing symptom escalation [72].

Long-Term Benefits of IPT on Psychological Stress

IPT also demonstrates potential long-term benefits for perinatal women, particularly in mitigating depressive symptoms. An RCT evaluating group-based IPT found that mothers receiving the intervention exhibited rapid short-term improvements in depressive symptoms and interpersonal functioning compared to control groups. Additionally, 57% of IPT participants maintained symptom remission over a 2-year follow-up period, and fewer of them experienced persistent depression compared to controls [78]. Similarly, Posmontier et al. (2019) reported sustained reductions in depressive symptoms compared to baseline among postpartum women with depression up to 4 weeks post-intervention following 8 sessions of group IPT [79].

However, evidence for IPT's long-term efficacy remains mixed. An RCT of 12 weekly, 60-minute telephone-IPT sessions delivered by nurses to 241 postpartum women with major depression found that the difference in self-reported depressive symptoms compared to standard care was no longer significant at the 36-week follow-up [80]. This inconsistency is echoed in a study by Leung and Lam (2012), where brief IPT administered to 156 pregnant women yielded short-term improvements in maternal stress but no lasting effects compared to usual care [81].

Discrepancies in long-term outcomes may be attributed to variability in study design, participant characteristics, and intervention protocols. For instance, Nylen et al. identified baseline depression severity, personal history of depression, and treatment duration during follow-up as significant predictors of symptom trajectories [82]. This finding suggests that tailored continued or boosted IPT sessions may enhance long-term efficacy, particularly for individuals with residual symptoms or recurrent depression.

Narratives of Perinatal Women Participating in IPT

Qualitative insights from perinatal women participating in IPT reveal transformative experiences in managing interpersonal stress and emotional processing. A study comparing IPT to enhanced maternity support services found that participants in the IPT group experienced significant improvements in interpersonal stress management and interpersonal skills. Specifically, women in the IPT group demonstrated significantly greater success in mitigating interpersonal stress through adaptive strategies, such as accepting relational limitations and cognitive reframing of conflicts [83]. Another study also suggested that IPT enhanced social support in perinatal women by enabling them to rebuild their social support networks. Tools such as asking for help and relationship mapping are particularly effective [84].

Another distinctive theme in IPT narratives was the centrality of the therapist-client relationship. Participants frequently characterized their therapist as a "transitional anchor"—a temporary yet critical source of validation and guidance during periods of social isolation or role transition. This bond appeared to compensate for gaps in external support systems, fostering psychological resilience even when tangible social resources were scarce [83]. Importantly, the emotional interaction of IPT was perceived as more responsive compared to the therapist-guided approach used in a CBT-based study [84].

Related to this, IPT was also reported to be useful in reframing women's emotional experiences through fostering adaptive coping strategies, such as recording emotional timelines [84]. Moreover, IPT participants also exhibited enhanced emotional literacy, with marked progress in identifying, reflecting on, and regulating emotions [83]. Despite these gains, IPT did not enhance engagement with broader social networks. Participants reported comparable levels of support from family, friends, or colleagues to those in the control group [83]. This suggests that while IPT equips perinatal women with intrapersonal and dyadic skills, it may not directly address systemic or environmental barriers to social connectedness during this vulnerable period.

14.2.4 Relaxation Training

Relaxation training is a systematic and structured approach aimed at reducing physiological arousal and psychological stress through evidence-based techniques. Grounded in psychophysiological theories, it employs methods such as progressive muscle relaxation (PMR), diaphragmatic breathing, and guided imagery to activate the parasympathetic nervous system. Thus, it counteracts the "fight-or-flight" response and reduces corresponding stress reactivity, such as cortisol levels and heart rate variability [85, 86].

Relaxation training encompasses a diverse range of approaches. Traditional methods, such as PMR, focus on systematically reducing muscle tension to alleviate physical stress, and diaphragmatic breathing techniques emphasize regulating autonomic nervous system activity through controlled respiration [86]. In addition to the isolated relaxation techniques, an increasing number of relaxation interventions have incorporated strategies from other therapeutic approaches. For instance, modern adaptations integrate mindfulness principles, emphasizing nonjudgmental awareness to break cognitive-emotional stress cycles [87]. Yoga also functions as a multimodal relaxation strategy by combining physical postures, breath regulation, and mindfulness [88].

14.2.4.1 Effects of Relaxation Training on Maternal Stress

Meta-analytic evidence underscores relaxation training's effectiveness in alleviating perinatal psychological distress. A synthesis of 6 RCTs involving 410 pregnant women found that traditional techniques (e.g., PMR, deep breathing) significantly reduced maternal stress, with effects comparable to CBT and mindfulness [89]. A broader meta-analysis of 32 RCTs and quasi-RCTs highlighted significant reductions in maternal stress, depression, and anxiety across diverse relaxation interventions among perinatal women, including yoga, music therapy, and mindfulness, with durations ranging from 10 min to 6 months [90].

Characterized by its accessibility and inclusivity, relaxation training can be suitable for both general and high-risk perinatal populations. For instance, a 6-week *Stress Management Program* combining PMR and diaphragmatic breathing (twice daily) significantly reduced maternal stress and enhanced feelings of control among pregnant women [91]. Similarly, an 8-week yoga program with weekly group sessions and home practice markedly decreased stress levels in pregnant participants [92].

For high-risk subgroups, such as women with prior psychological disorders or adverse socio-environmental conditions, relaxation training remains effective. For example, a 6-session PMR and guided imagery intervention significantly reduced stress and anxiety in psychologically distressed pregnant women compared to usual care [93]. However, while immediate benefits are well-documented, the long-term impact on maternal stress remains understudied, which may be attributed to the emphasis on short-term goals in study design and the challenges of maintaining long-term adherence.

Effects of Relaxation Training on Physiological Stress

Technological advancements, including biofeedback devices and mobile apps, have enabled real-time monitoring of physiological markers (e.g., HRV), enhancing the precision of relaxation interventions. For example, in a study of healthy pregnant women in the third trimester, a brief guided yogic relaxation consisting of 2-h sessions and 3 days/week increased parasympathetic activity (measured by the high-frequency band of HRV) by 64% at 20 weeks and 150% at 36 weeks, outperforming standard prenatal exercises [94].

Empirical evidence also suggests the efficacy of relaxation techniques in enhancing both maternal and fetal cardiovascular parameters. A large RCT of music therapy and virtual reality interventions ($N = 343$) during the third trimester and labor significantly reduced systolic and diastolic blood pressure and maternal heart rate. Moreover, fetuses in the experiment group also exhibited lower rates of non-reassuring fetal heart rate tracings [95]. Additionally, high-risk populations, such as perinatal women with hypertension or asthma, also benefit from relaxation training. Evidence showed that systematic relaxation training alone or with biofeedback effectively reduced blood pressure in hypertensive pregnancies [96], while PMR positively regulated the blood improved pressure, lung parameters and heart rate, as well as diminished anger levels in pregnancies with bronchial asthma symptoms [97].

Emerging evidence highlights relaxation training's potential role in regulating the HPA axis. For instance, PMR and guided imagery significantly reduced cortisol levels immediately and suppressed adrenocorticotropin hormone within 10 min after relaxation, with both effects maintained throughout the study period [98]. Similarly, a 12-week yoga program for prenatally depressed women ($N = 92$) lowered cortisol levels, with additional reductions in estriol and progesterone post-intervention [99].

Narratives of Perinatal Women Participating in Relaxation Training

Qualitative studies exploring antenatal relaxation classes demonstrate that structured interventions can significantly enhance perinatal psychological well-being by reframing childbirth expectations. Participants described these sessions as "recognition of an inner resource," exemplified by the relaxation therapeutic experiences, such as the guided imagery technique, which reduced fear of labor [100].

Even brief exposures to relaxation training hold value: a study on expectant parents' perspectives found that a single antenatal relaxation class helped couples develop shared coping strategies, fostering mutual support and reducing pregnancy-related anxiety. Moreover, participating in antenatal relaxation classes could also lead to a positive outlook on childbirth experiences. Specifically, understanding the physiological impact of fear versus calmness during labor fosters a new mindset, encouraging women to practice relaxation techniques that enhance their sense of calm and motivation, ultimately shaping a more positive childbirth experience [101].

14.2.4.2 Effects of Relaxation Training on Childbirth Outcomes

Empirical evidence has shown a significant correlation between relaxation training and improved childbirth outcomes, particularly in low-risk pregnant women. A meta-analysis of 4816 pregnant women suggested that the combination of relaxation interventions, such as yoga, music, and education, significantly reduced the incidence of preterm birth in healthy women [102].

Among varied types of relaxation, music-based relaxation offers multifaceted benefits during childbirth. In the RCT involving 490 women in the late stage of pregnancy, participants receiving music stimulation during non-stress tests experienced a shorter first-stage labor, a higher rate of spontaneous onset of labour and a lower use of induction/augmentation medication compared to controls [103]. In addition to this finding, another RCT involving 161 laboring women demonstrated that self-selected music significantly reduced postpartum pain [104]. These findings support music therapy as a noninvasive, cost-effective adjunct to standard perinatal care.

14.3 Scientific Maternal Stress-Reducing Interventions on Fetal Outcomes

The impact of stress-reducing intervention on fetal outcomes represents a burgeoning field of research, with growing interest in elucidating how these interventions shape fetal development and long-term health trajectories.

14.3.1 Effects of MBIs

Mindfulness practices that reduce maternal stress and promote emotional regulation are linked to healthier developmental trajectories for the fetus [105]. Empirical evidence has shown that by attenuating stress-related physiological responses (e.g., elevated cortisol levels), MBIs may improve neonatal health indicators, including preterm birth, brain structure, and Apgar scores—a critical measure of newborn vitality [28, 106–109]. A landmark RCT involving 1184 high-risk pregnant women compared MBSR with a *Mediterranean diet program* and standard prenatal care. The findings indicated that both MBSR and the *Mediterranean dietary intervention* significantly reduced the incidence of small-for-gestational-age newborns (birth weight <10th percentile) compared to usual care [108]. Longitudinal follow-up revealed that offspring in the MBSR group exhibited enhanced neurodevelopmental profiles, including larger volumes of the fetal left anterior cingulate gyrus (measured via MRI) during 36 to 39 gestational week and even superior scores on the Neonatal Neurobehavioral Assessment Scale for state regulation within 3 months after birth [109], suggesting MBIs may promote early brain development.

Emerging evidence also highlights MBIs' influence on infant gut microbiota. In an RCT by Zhang et al. (2022), a sample of 160 pregnant women with symptoms of depression or anxiety was randomized to either a MBI group or a control group receiving usual perinatal care [110]. Researchers collected meconium within 48 h of birth to analyze the infant gut microbiota, finding that maternal mindfulness practice positively altered microbial composition.

14.3.2 Effects of CBT

Overall, CBT shows promise in improving fetal and child neurodevelopmental outcomes following maternal intervention. A pioneering RCT by Bleker et al. (2019) evaluated the long-term effects of antenatal CBT for maternal depression on offspring brain structure. Neuroimaging of 16 6-year-old children born to mothers in the CBT group revealed enhanced cortical development, including thicker right lateral occipital cortices and lingual gyri, alongside increased gray matter concentration compared to controls [111]. These structural differences suggest that maternal psychological interventions during pregnancy may confer lasting benefits for offspring brain development.

However, evidence for CBT's influence on infant cognitive development is currently mixed. An integrative antenatal CBT program targeting maternal antenatal depression in Pakistan also improved infant cognitive performance in communication, motor skills, and problem-solving domains compared to controls [112]. Conversely, other CBT trials for prenatal depression have failed to replicate these benefits [65, 113].

Social-emotional development outcomes in infants also yield inconsistent findings. A pilot RCT by Milgrom et al. (2015) reported reduced infant negative affectivity and improved compliance at 9 months post-intervention [114]. In contrast, another trial found no significant behavioral improvements at 6 months, underscoring the need for standardized protocols and longer follow-up periods [113].

Lastly, CBT's impact on neonatal anthropometric outcomes (e.g., weight, length) remains limited [65, 112]. Trials involving 282 women with anxiety and depression found no significant improvements in neonatal weight, suggesting that relaxation-focused methods may be more effective for this outcome [65].

14.3.3 Effects of Relaxation Training

Current evidence on relaxation training's impact on fetal growth is inconclusive. Birth weight remains the most studied outcome to date, recent meta-analyses of pregnancy relaxation training revealed traditional relaxation techniques, especially PMR have demonstrated benefits in reducing the risk of low birth weight among included 8 RCTs [90]. For instance, PMR and breathing techniques for 7 weeks from the first to second trimester have modestly improved birth weight in 110 participants, and reduced low birth weight incidence in the experimental group below both control values and the average for developing and developed countries [115]. Further evidence of an RCT involving 88 and 239 pregnant women, respectively, demonstrated that daily or twice a week PMR both significantly lowered maternal depressive levels and incidence of low birth weight [116, 117].

However, yoga and music therapy, which have also emerged as common components of relaxation programs, show limited effects on fetal growth [90]. Specifically, mid-to-late pregnancy yoga practices conducted over a 6-week failed to significantly alter birth weights or Apgar scores [118]. Similarly, neither short-term music therapy during labor nor long-term music relaxation over a 2-week improved fetal birth weight [119, 120].

Moreover, single-session relaxation interventions may also contribute to enhanced fetal cardiovascular stability. For instance, a study involving 33 healthy pregnant women in late pregnancy found that a 2-h training session of PMR or guided imagery significantly increased fetal HRV and reduced fetal heart rate acceleration—both of which are markers of a stable intrauterine environment [121].

14.4 Clinical and Research Implications

The evidence synthesized in this chapter underscores the transformative potential of scientific interventions in reducing maternal stress and enhancing fetal outcomes. However, translating these findings into clinical practice and advancing research requires addressing key implications across multiple domains.

14.4.1 Clinical Implications

The integration of evidence-based, non-pharmaceutical interventions into perinatal care is critical for addressing maternal stress and optimizing outcomes for both mothers and infants. Non-pharmaceutical interventions, including MBIs, CBT, IPT, and relaxation training (e.g., progressive muscle relaxation, guided imagery, and prenatal yoga), should be systematically incorporated into standard care protocols. These interventions demonstrate robust efficacy in enhancing maternal psychological well-being, reducing stress-related physiological markers, and promoting healthier fetal development.

A risk-stratified stepped-care model is essential to tailor interventions to individual needs and resource availability. Universal prevention strategies, such as routine prenatal yoga or psychoeducational apps, should be offered to all pregnant individuals during standard prenatal visits. For those with subclinical symptoms or psychosocial vulnerabilities (e.g., financial instability, social isolation), targeted interventions like group IPT, internet-delivered MBIs, or partner-inclusive CBT can mitigate escalating distress. Women diagnosed with anxiety, depression, or PTSD require specialized, high-intensity care, such as trauma-informed MBIs or intensive CBT. Postpartum continuity of care is equally vital, as the transition to motherhood often exacerbates stress; telehealth platforms, support groups, and booster sessions can sustain therapeutic gains and reduce relapse risks.

Healthcare providers, including obstetricians, midwives, and mental health professionals, require specialized training to deliver these interventions with fidelity. Crucially, to address the stark perinatal care gap for maternal stress, particularly among LMICs where disparities in care are pervasive, task-sharing models should be prioritized to bridge workforce shortages. Nonspecialist providers, such as community health workers or nurses trained in manualized psychotherapies, have proven effective in delivering manualized psychotherapies under supervision [122]. Meta-analytic evidence supports their role in reducing maternal depression and anxiety, offering a cost-effective solution to bridge care disparities in under-resourced settings. For example, programs like the *Thinking Healthy Programme* demonstrate how task-sharing can scale access to quality care while maintaining clinical rigor. These nonspecialist providers represent a critical human resource for addressing maternal stress due to their widespread availability, cost-effectiveness, and frequent contact with mothers.

Technology-enhanced solutions, such as mobile apps, Internet-based platforms, and biofeedback devices, expand access to personalized, real-time interventions.

Emerging evidence highlights the efficacy of digital CBT and MBIs in reducing perinatal stress, depression, and anxiety, particularly when combined with therapist-guided support [123]. Hybrid models, blending in-person sessions with bio-feedback devices for stress monitoring, offer scalable solutions for under-served regions. Digital platforms also enable the training and supervision of non-specialists, ensuring quality assurance while addressing systemic workforce shortages.

Family-centered approaches, such as partner-inclusive CBT and IPT, should be expanded to amplify intervention effects by strengthening relational support systems. Involving partners and families in interventions can enhance relational support and communal resilience, addressing stressors rooted in interpersonal dynamics. These strategies not only improve maternal mental health but also foster supportive environments that are critical for long-term family well-being.

14.4.2 Research Implications

The current evidence base on maternal stress interventions reveals critical gaps that necessitate a comprehensive research agenda to advance clinical practice and inform policy decisions.

First, longitudinal studies are urgently required to evaluate the sustained efficacy of stress reduction strategies beyond the first postpartum year. These studies should focus on the sustained impact of interventions on maternal mental health trajectories as well as on offspring psychosomatic development underpinned by the mechanisms of stress intergenerational transmission. Additionally, mechanistic investigations are essential to elucidate biological pathways, such as HPA axis regulation, inflammatory marker dynamics, and gut microbiota modulation, to understand how interventions disrupt intergenerational stress transmission.

Second, the comparative effectiveness of existing interventions remains understudied, limiting evidence-based decision-making for relative efficacy and resource allocation. While recent network meta-analyses suggest that MBIs may outperform other evidence-based interventions in reducing perinatal depression and anxiety, these findings are largely confined to high-risk cohorts [124]. Further rigorous trials comparing active interventions, including hybrid models combining MBIs with CBT, are also necessary to identify synergistic strategies and optimize outcomes across diverse symptom presentations.

Third, larger-scale effectiveness trials are required to assess the scalability and feasibility of existing evidence-based interventions in diverse settings, including lower-risk primary care populations. Further research may consider whether interventions tailored to overall symptom reduction are sensitive enough to account for the broad range of presentations of maternal stress.

Fourth, research in LMICs should prioritize scalable, low-cost programs (e.g., task-shared CBT delivered by community health workers) while addressing structural determinants of maternal stress, such as poverty and gender inequality, to ensure interventions align with local socioeconomic and cultural realities. Cultural adaptation and equity-focused research are imperative. Empirical validation of interventions for underrepresented groups, including racially diverse communities and economically marginalized perinatal populations, is essential. Co-design frameworks that integrate local traditions, values, and context-specific stressors (e.g., systemic racism, and economic marginalization) must be prioritized to enhance accessibility and efficacy.

Fifth, despite the promise of digital interventions, such as Internet-based CBT and Internet-based MBIs, suboptimal engagement and adherence limit their real-world efficacy [125]. Future studies must identify barriers and enablers for the delivery and sustainability of digital interventions and test strategies to enhance retention. Previous qualitative interviews with perinatal individuals experiencing depression or anxiety revealed the importance of considering specific aspects of digital interventions for perinatal mental health, including personalized content, access to support resources, and transparent data-sharing options [126].

14.5 Conclusion

Maternal stress during the perinatal period represents a critical public health challenge with far-reaching consequences for maternal well-being and fetal development. This chapter synthesizes available empirical evidence on the efficacy of non-pharmaceutical interventions—mindfulness-based interventions (MBIs), cognitive-behavioral therapy (CBT), interpersonal therapy (IPT), and relaxation training—in alleviating maternal stress, depression, and anxiety. These evidence-based interventions demonstrate significant potential to address the biological, psychological, and social dimensions of maternal distress, offering pathways to healthier outcomes for both mothers and their children. By integrating findings from clinical trials, meta-analyses, and qualitative studies, this chapter reveals the transformative potential of these interventions in clinical and community settings, while highlighting gaps that warrant further exploration.

14.5.1 Summary of Key Findings

The evidence presented demonstrates that MBIs, CBT, IPT, and relaxation training are effective in reducing maternal stress and improving psychological and physiological outcomes. MBIs excel in cultivating nonjudgmental awareness, reducing cortisol levels, and enhancing autonomic regulation, which mitigate maternal stress and improve childbirth experiences. For instance, MBIs like *Mindfulness-Based Stress Reduction* and *Mindfulness-Based Childbirth and Parenting* have been associated with reduced cortisol levels, sustained reductions in perinatal depressive symptoms, lower rates of cesarean sections, and improved pain tolerance. However, long-term adherence remains a challenge, necessitating post-intervention support to maintain benefits.

CBT emerges as a versatile, evidence-based tool for addressing cross-diagnostic stress presentations (e.g., perinatal anxiety and depression), particularly in with elevated symptoms. Its structured approach—combining cognitive restructuring and behavioral activation—equips women with skills to manage stressors adaptively. Partner-inclusive CBT models further enhance outcomes by improving relational dynamics and social support. In low-resource settings, task-shared CBT programs, such as the *Thinking Healthy Programme*, demonstrate remarkable cost-effectiveness, underscoring its scalability.

IPT uniquely targets role transitions, grief, and social isolation, fostering emotional resilience through enhanced communication and relational support. Group IPT, in particular, leverages peer solidarity to normalize stressors and reduce feelings of isolation. While IPT shows rapid short-term efficacy, its long-term benefits require further validation, particularly in diverse treatment contexts.

Relaxation training, including progressive muscle relaxation, guided imagery, and prenatal yoga, is effective for reducing real-time physiological stress markers (e.g., blood pressure, cortisol) and preterm birth risks. Its accessibility makes it suitable for both general and high-risk populations. However, standardized protocols are needed to ensure consistent and sustained benefits. Digital adaptations, such as music therapy and biofeedback apps, further enhance its reach and practicality.

Intergenerational and Holistic Benefits

Beyond maternal mental health, evidence-based interventions confer significant benefits for fetal and child development. These maternal stress-reducing interventions, such as MBI and relaxation training correlate with higher Apgar scores, improved neonatal neurobehavioral profiles, and healthier infant gut microbiota, likely mediated by reduced maternal cortisol exposure. Evidence also indicate the intergenerational effects including enhanced cortical development in offspring, as evidenced by neuroimaging studies. Such findings suggest the importance of maternal stress reduction as a preventive measure against long-term neurodevelopmental and metabolic disorders in children. However, the impact on neonatal anthropometry such as weight and length appears relatively limited, with only PMR-based relaxation training showing promise in reducing the risk of low birth weight. In addition, the long-term infant cognitive and social-emotional benefits of CBT remain encouraging yet inconsistent, the gains in communication, motor, and problem-solving domains still await replication.

14.5.2 Clinical Implications

Universal prevention strategies, such as prenatal yoga and psychoeducational apps, should be integrated into routine prenatal care to address broad populations. Targeted interventions, including group IPT or digital MBIs, can mitigate escalating distress in high-risk groups, while specialized care—such as trauma-informed MBIs or intensive CBT—is critical for women diagnosed with anxiety, depression, or PTSD. Postpartum continuity of care, facilitated by telehealth platforms and support groups, is essential to sustain therapeutic gains during the transition to motherhood, a period marked by hormonal fluctuations and caregiving demands. Task-sharing models, which train nonspecialists like community health workers to deliver manualized interventions, are indispensable for bridging care gaps in low- and middle-income countries (LMICs). Technology-enhanced hybrid models, blending in-person sessions with AI-driven tools for stress monitoring or virtual reality for pain management, offer scalable solutions for underserved regions. Family-centered approaches, such as partner-inclusive CBT and multigenerational mindfulness programs, strengthen relational support systems, addressing stressors rooted in interpersonal dynamics and intergenerational trauma.

14.5.3 Research Implications

Despite the compelling evidence, critical research gaps persist. Longitudinal studies are urgently needed to evaluate the sustained efficacy of interventions beyond the first postpartum year and elucidate biological pathways, such as HPA axis regulation and epigenetic changes. Comparative effectiveness research must clarify the optimal use of MBIs, CBT, IPT, and relaxation training across diverse populations, while hybrid models combining these approaches could unlock synergistic benefits. Implementation science should prioritize scalable, low-cost programs in LMICs, addressing structural determinants like poverty and gender inequality to ensure contextual relevance. Cultural adaptations require co-design frameworks that integrate local traditions and address context-specific stressors. Digital interventions, though promising, need optimization to enhance engagement through personalized content, transparent data policies, and therapist-guided support.

14.5.4 A Call to Action

The integration of these interventions into perinatal care represents a paradigm shift toward preventive, holistic medicine. By addressing the multifaceted nature of maternal stress, spanning psychological, physiological, and social realms, we can disrupt cycles of intergenerational disadvantage and foster resilient families. This vision demands interdisciplinary collaboration, community engagement, and sustained investment in research and practice. Healthcare providers, researchers, and policymakers must unite to ensure maternal well-being becomes a universal priority, laying the foundation for thriving generations.

In conclusion, the transformative potential of scientific interventions, such as MBIs, CBT, IPT, and relaxation training, lies not only in their capacity to alleviate maternal distress but also in their ripple effects on societal health. By prioritizing equitable access, cultural humility, and innovation, we can transform perinatal care into a cornerstone of global health equity—one mother, one child, and one community at a time.

References

1. Kabat-Zinn J. The Foundations of Mindfulness Practice. In: *Full Catastrophe Living: Using the Wisdom of Your Body and Mind to Face Stress, Pain, and Illness*. Rev ed. New York: Bantam Books; 2013: 31–46.
2. Chiesa A, Anselmi R, Serretti A. Psychological mechanisms of mindfulness-based interventions: what do we know? Holist Nurs Pract. 2014(2);28:124–148.
3. Wallace BA. *Mind in the balance: meditation in science, Buddhism, and Christianity*. New York: Columbia University Press; 2014: 37–200.
4. Kabat-Zinn J. An outpatient program in behavioral medicine for chronic pain patients based on the practice of mindfulness meditation: theoretical considerations and preliminary results. Gen Hosp Psychiatry. 1982;4(1):33–47.
5. Teasdale JD, Segal Z, Williams JMG. How does cognitive therapy prevent depressive relapse and why should attentional control (mindfulness) training help? Behav Res Ther. 1995;33(1):25–39.
6. Corbally L, Wilkinson M. The effect of mindfulness-based interventions on stress, depression and anxiety during the perinatal period in women without pre-existing stress, depressive or anxiety disorders: a systematic review and meta-analysis of controlled trials. Mindfulness. 2021;12(10):2357–2370.
7. Reangsing C, Rittiwong T, Schneider JK. Effects of mindfulness meditation interventions on depression in older adults: a meta-analysis. Aging Ment Health. 2021;25(7):1181–1190.
8. Leng LL, Yin XC, Ng SM. Mindfulness-based intervention for clinical and subthreshold perinatal depression and anxiety: a systematic review and meta-analysis of randomized controlled trial. Compr Psychiatry. 2023;122:152375.
9. Yan H, Wu Y, Li H. Effect of mindfulness-based interventions on mental health of perinatal women with or without current mental health issues: a systematic review and meta-analysis of randomized controlled trials. J Affect Disord. 2022;305:102–114.
10. Guo L, Zhang J, Mu L, Ye Z. Preventing postpartum depression with mindful self-compassion intervention: a randomized control study. J Nerv Ment Dis. 2020;208(2):101–107.
11. Zemestani M, Fazeli Nikoo Z. Effectiveness of mindfulness-based cognitive therapy for comorbid depression and anxiety in pregnancy: a randomized controlled trial. Arch Womens Ment Health. 2020;23(2):207–214.
12. Townshend K, Caltabiano NJ, Powrie R, O'Grady H. A preliminary study investigating the effectiveness of the caring for body and mind in pregnancy (CBMP) in reducing perinatal depression, anxiety and stress. J Child Fam Stud. 2018;27(5):1556–1566.
13. Dimidjian S, Goodman SH, Felder JN, Gallop R, Brown AP, Beck A. Staying well during pregnancy and the postpartum: a pilot randomized trial of mindfulness-based cognitive therapy for the prevention of depressive relapse/recurrence. J Consult Clin Psychol. 2016;84:134–145.
14. Hassdenteufel K, Müller M, Abele H, Brucker SY. Graf J, Zipfel S, et al. Using an electronic mindfulness-based intervention (eMBI) to improve maternal mental health during pregnancy: results from a randomized controlled trial. Psychiatry Res, 2023, 330: 115599.
15. Pan WL, Lin LC, Kuo LY, Chiu MJ, Ling PY. Effects of a prenatal mindfulness program on longitudinal changes in stress, anxiety, depression, and mother–infant bonding of women with a tendency to perinatal mood and anxiety disorder: a randomized controlled trial. BMC Pregnancy Childbirth. 2023;23(1):547.
16. Lönnberg G, Jonas W, Unternaehrer E, Bränström R, Nissen E, Niemi M. Effects of a mindfulness based childbirth and parenting program on pregnant women's perceived stress and risk of perinatal depression–results from a randomized controlled trial. J Affect Disord. 2020;262:133–142.
17. Lönnberg G, Jonas W, Bränström R, Nissen E, Niemi M. Long-term effects of a mindfulness-based childbirth and parenting program—a randomized controlled trial. Mindfulness. 2021;12(2):476–488.

18. Zhang H, Emory EK. A mindfulness-based intervention for pregnant African-American women. Mindfulness. 2015;6(3):663–674.
19. Matvienko-Sikar K, Dockray S. Effects of a novel positive psychological intervention on prenatal stress and well-being: a pilot randomised controlled trial. Women Birth. 2017;30(2):e111–e118.
20. Muthukrishnan S, Jain R, Kohli S, Batra S. Effect of mindfulness meditation on perceived stress scores and autonomic function tests of pregnant Indian women. J Clin Diagn Res. 2016;10(4):CC05–CC08.
21. Bublitz MH, Salmoirago-Blotcher E, Sanapo L, Ayala N, Mehta N, Bourjeily G. Feasibility, acceptability, and preliminary effects of mindfulness training on antenatal blood pressure. J Psychosom Res. 2023;165:111146.
22. Kantrowitz-Gordon I, Abbott S, Hoehn R. Experiences of postpartum women after mindfulness childbirth classes: a qualitative study. J Midwifery Womens Health, 2018, 63(4): 462-469.
23. Hennekam S. Identity transition during pregnancy: the importance of role models. Hum Relat. 2016;69(9):1765–1790.
24. Duncan LG, Bardacke N. Mindfulness-based childbirth and parenting education: promoting family mindfulness during the perinatal period. J Child Fam Stud. 2010;19(2):190–202.
25. Lönnberg G, Nissen E, Niemi M. What is learned from mindfulness based childbirth and parenting education? – participants' experiences. BMC Pregnancy Childbirth. 2018;18(1):1–9.
26. Duncan LG, Cohn MA, Chao MT, Cook JG, Riccobono J, Bardacke N. Benefits of preparing for childbirth with mindfulness training: a randomized controlled trial with active comparison. BMC Pregnancy Childbirth, 2017, 17(1): 140
27. Mackinnon AL, Madsen JW, Giesbrecht GF, Campbell T, Carlson LE, Dimidjian S, et al. Effects of mindfulness-based cognitive therapy in pregnancy on psychological distress and gestational age: outcomes of a randomized controlled trial. Mindfulness. 2021;12(5):1173–1184.
28. Leng LL, Yin XC, Chan CLW, Ng SM. Antenatal mobile-delivered mindfulness-based intervention to reduce perinatal depression risk and improve obstetric and neonatal outcomes: a randomized controlled trial. J Affect Disord. 2023;335:216–227.
29. Gillespie A, Harmer CJ. Can you feel the burn? Using neuroimaging to illuminate the mechanisms of mindfulness interventions for pain. Am J Psychiatry. 2022;179(10):705–707.
30. Beck AT, Haigh EA. Advances in cognitive theory and therapy: the generic cognitive model. Annu Rev Clin Psychol. 2014;10(1):1–24.
31. Hope DA, Burns JA, Hayes SA, Herbert JD, Warner MD. Automatic thoughts and cognitive restructuring in cognitive behavioral group therapy for social anxiety disorder. Cognit Ther Res. 2010;34(1):1–12.
32. Cuijpers P, Van Straten A, Smit F, Mihalopoulos C, Beekman A. Preventing the onset of depressive disorders: a meta-analytic review of psychological interventions. Am J Psychiatry. 2008;165(10):1272–1280.
33. Johansson R, Andersson G. Internet-based psychological treatments for depression. Expert Rev Neurother. 2012;12(7):861–870.
34. Steel Z, Marnane C, Iranpour C, Chey T, Jackson JW, Patel V, et al. The global prevalence of common mental disorders: a systematic review and meta-analysis 1980–2013. Int J Epidemiol. 2014;43(2):476–493.
35. Cuijpers P, Berking M, Andersson G, Quigley L, Kleiboer A, Dobson KS. A meta-analysis of cognitive-behavioural therapy for adult depression, alone and in comparison with other treatments. Can J Psychiatr. 2013;58(7):376–385.
36. van Zoonen K, Buntrock C, Ebert DD, Smit F, Reynolds CF III, Beekman AT, et al. Preventing the onset of major depressive disorder: a meta-analytic review of psychological interventions. Int J Epidemiol. 2014;43(2):318–329.
37. Forsell E, Bendix M, Holländare F, von Schultz BS, Nasiell J, Blomdahl-Wetterholm M, et al. Internet delivered cognitive behavior therapy for antenatal depression: a randomised controlled trial. J Affect Disord. 2017;221:56–64.

38. Trevillion K, Ryan EG, Pickles A, Heslin M, Byford S, Nath S, et al. An exploratory parallel-group randomised controlled trial of antenatal guided self-help (plus usual care) versus usual care alone for pregnant women with depression: dawn trial. J Affect Disord. 2020;261:187–197.
39. O'Mahen H, Himle JA, Fedock G, Henshaw E, Flynn H. A pilot randomized controlled trial of cognitive behavioral therapy for perinatal depression adapted for women with low incomes. Depress Anxiety. 2013;30(7):679–687.
40. Nillni YI, Mehralizade A, Mayer L, Milanovic S. Treatment of depression, anxiety, and trauma-related disorders during the perinatal period: a systematic review. Clin Psychol Rev. 2018;66:136–148.
41. Dooley RL, Mcaloon J. The efficacy of antenatal cognitive behavioural therapy for antenatal and postnatal depression: a PRISMA based systematic review and meta-analysis. J Affect Disord. 2025;376:225–240.
42. Li X, Laplante DP, Paquin V, Lafortune S, Elgbeili G, King S. Effectiveness of cognitive behavioral therapy for perinatal maternal depression, anxiety and stress: a systematic review and meta-analysis of randomized controlled trials. Clin Psychol Rev. 2022;92:102129.
43. Pettman D, Mahen OH, Blomberg O, Svanberg AS, von Essen L, Woodford J. Effectiveness of cognitive behavioural therapy-based interventions for maternal perinatal depression: a systematic review and meta-analysis. BMC Psychiatry. 2023;23(1):208.
44. Sockol LE. A systematic review of the efficacy of cognitive behavioral therapy for treating and preventing perinatal depression. J Affect Disord. 2015;177:7–21.
45. Matvienko-Sikar K, Redsell S, Flannery C. Effects of maternal stress and/or anxiety interventions in the first 1000 days: systematic review of reviews. J Reprod Infant Psychol. 2023;41(2):114–151.
46. Epstein NB, Zheng L. Cognitive-behavioral couple therapy. Curr Opin Psychol. 2017;13:142–147.
47. Ngai FW, Wong PC, Chung KF, Chau PH, Hui PW. Effect of couple-based cognitive behavioural intervention on prevention of postnatal depression: multisite randomised controlled trial. BJOG. 2020;127(4):500–507.
48. Loughnan SA, Butler C, Sie AA, Grierson AB, Chen AZ, Hobbs MJ, et al. A randomised controlled trial of "MUMentum postnatal": internet-delivered cognitive behavioural therapy for anxiety and depression in postpartum women. Behav Res Ther. 2019;116:94–103.
49. Sikander S, Ahmad I, Atif N, Zaidi A, Vanobberghen F, Weiss HA, et al. Delivering the thinking healthy programme for perinatal depression through volunteer peers: a cluster randomised controlled trial in Pakistan. Lancet Psychiatry. 2019;6(2):128–139.
50. Seth AK, Friston KJ. Active interoceptive inference and the emotional brain. Philos Trans R Soc B. 2016;371(1708):20160007.
51. Zainal NH, Soh CP, Van Doren N, Benjet C. Do the effects of internet-delivered cognitive-behavioral therapy (i-CBT) last after a year and beyond? A meta-analysis of 154 randomized controlled trials (RCTs). Clin Psychol Rev. 2024;114:102518.
52. Richter J, Bittner A, Petrowski K, Junge-Hoffmeister J, Bergmann S, Joraschky P, et al. Effects of an early intervention on perceived stress and diurnal cortisol in pregnant women with elevated stress, anxiety, and depressive symptomatology. J Psychosom Obstet Gynaecol. 2012;33(4):162–170.
53. Urizar GG Jr, Yim IS, Rodriguez A, Schetter CD. The smart moms program: a randomized trial of the impact of stress management on perceived stress and cortisol in low-income pregnant women. Psychoneuroendocrinology. 2019;104:174–184.
54. Romero-Gonzalez B, Puertas-Gonzalez JA, Strivens-Vilchez H, Gonzalez-Perez R, Peralta-Ramirez MI. Effects of cognitive-behavioural therapy for stress management on stress and hair cortisol levels in pregnant women: a randomised controlled trial. J Psychosom Res. 2020;135:110162.
55. Baranov V, Frost A, Hagaman A, Simmons JG, Manzoor MS, Biroli P, et al. Effects of a maternal psychosocial intervention on hair derived biomarkers of HPA axis function in mothers and children in rural Pakistan. SSM Ment Health. 2022;2:100082.

56. Zaheri H, Najar S, Abbaspoor Z. Effectiveness of cognitive-behavioral stress management on psychological stress and glycemic control in gestational diabetes: a randomized controlled trial. J Matern Fetal Neonatal Med. 2017;30(11):1378–1382.
57. Varambally M, Layton H, Jack SM, Van Lieshout RJ. Mothers' and birthing parents' experiences with 1-day cognitive behavioural therapy-based workshops for postpartum depression: a descriptive qualitative study. J Psychiatr Ment Health Nurs. 2024;31(4):507–514.
58. Masood Y, Lovell K, Lunat F, Atif N, Waheed W, Rahman A, et al. Group psychological intervention for postnatal depression: a nested qualitative study with British South Asian women. BMC Womens Health. 2015;15(1):109.
59. Massoudi P, Strömwall LA, Åhlen J, Kärrman Fredriksson M, Dencker A, Andersson E. Women's experiences of psychological treatment and psychosocial interventions for postpartum depression: a qualitative systematic review and meta-synthesis. BMC Womens Health. 2023;23(1):604.
60. Hadfield H, Glendenning S, Bee P, Wittkowski A. Psychological therapy for postnatal depression in UK primary care mental health services: a qualitative investigation using framework analysis. J Child Fam Stud. 2019;28(12):3519–3532.
61. Rossiter C, Fowler C, Mcmahon C, Kowalenko N. Supporting depressed mothers at home: their views on an innovative relationship-based intervention. Contemp Nurse. 2012;41(1):90–100.
62. Pugh NE, Hadjistavropoulos HD, Hampton AJ, Bowen A, Williams J. Client experiences of guided internet cognitive behavior therapy for postpartum depression: a qualitative study. Arch Womens Ment Health. 2015;18(2):209–219.
63. Scope A, Booth A, Sutcliffe P. Women's perceptions and experiences of group cognitive behaviour therapy and other group interventions for postnatal depression: a qualitative synthesis. J Adv Nurs. 2012;68(9):1909–1919.
64. Guo X, Guo X, Wang R, Zhang Y. Effects of perinatal cognitive behavioral therapy on delivery mode, fetal outcome, and postpartum depression and anxiety in women. Comput Math Methods Med. 2022;2022(1):8304405.
65. Burger H, Verbeek T, Aris-Meijer JL, Beijers C, Mol BW, Hollon SD, et al. Effects of psychological treatment of mental health problems in pregnant women to protect their offspring: randomised controlled trial. Br J Psychol. 2020;216(4):182–188.
66. Klerman GL, Weissman MM, Rounsaville BJ, Chevron ES. *Interpersonal psychotherapy of depression: a brief, focused, specific strategy*. Lanham: Rowman & Littlefield; 1994:15.
67. Stuart S, Schultz J, Molina AP, Siber-Sanderowitz S. Interpersonal psychotherapy: a review of theory, history, and evidence of efficacy. Psychodyn Psychiatry. 2024;52(3):370–407.
68. Weissman MM, Markowitz JC, Klerman G. Chapter 1: An outline of IPT. In: *Comprehensive guide to interpersonal psychotherapy*. New York: Basic Books; 2008.
69. Stuart S, Robertson M. Chapter 6. Interpersonal Fomulation. In: *Interpersonal psychotherapy 2E a clinician's guide*. 2nd ed. London: CRC Press; 2012: 84–95.
70. Cooper PJ, Tomlinson M, Swartz L, Landman M, Molteno C, Stein A, et al. Improving quality of mother-infant relationship and infant attachment in socioeconomically deprived community in South Africa: randomised controlled trial. BMJ. 2009;338:b974.
71. Sockol LE. A systematic review and meta-analysis of interpersonal psychotherapy for perinatal women. J Affect Disord. 2018;232:316–328.
72. Bright KS, Charrois EM, Mughal MK, Wajid A, McNeil D, Stuart S, et al. Interpersonal psychotherapy to reduce psychological distress in perinatal women: a systematic review. Int J Environ Res Public Health. 2020;17(22):8421.
73. Claridge AM. Efficacy of systemically oriented psychotherapies in the treatment of perinatal depression: a meta-analysis. Arch Womens Ment Health. 2014;17(1):3–15.
74. Hankin BL, Demers CH, Hennessey EP, Perzow SE, Curran MC, Gallop RJ, et al. Effect of brief interpersonal therapy on depression during pregnancy: a randomized clinical trial. JAMA Psychiatr. 2023;80(6):539–547.
75. Johnson JE, Price AB, Kao JC, Fernandes K, Stout R, Gobin RL, et al. Interpersonal psychotherapy (IPT) for major depression following perinatal loss: a pilot randomized controlled trial. Arch Womens Ment Health. 2016;19(5):845–859.

76. Marmarosh C, Holtz A, Schottenbauer M. Group cohesiveness, group-derived collective self-esteem, group-derived hope, and the well-being of group therapy members. Group Dyn Theory Res Pract. 2005;9(1):32-44.
77. Reay RE, Mulcahy R, Wilkinson RB, Owen C, Shadbolt B, Raphael B. The development and content of an interpersonal psychotherapy group for postnatal depression. Int J Group Psychother, 2012; 62(2): 221-251.
78. Reay RE, Owen C, Shadbolt B, Raphael B, Mulcahy R, Wilkinson RB. Trajectories of long-term outcomes for postnatally depressed mothers treated with group interpersonal psychotherapy. Arch Womens Ment Health. 2012;15:217–228.
79. Posmontier B, Bina R, Glasser S, Cinamon T, Styr B, Sammarco T. Incorporating interpersonal psychotherapy for postpartum depression into social work practice in Israel. Res Soc Work Pract. 2019;29(1):61–68.
80. Dennis CL, Grigoriadis S, Zupancic J, Kiss A, Ravitz P. Telephone-based nurse-delivered interpersonal psychotherapy for postpartum depression: nationwide randomised controlled trial. Br J Psychiatry, 2020, 216(4): 189-196.
81. Leung SS, Lam TH. Group antenatal intervention to reduce perinatal stress and depressive symptoms related to intergenerational conflicts: a randomized controlled trial. Int J Nurs Stud. 2012;49(11):1391–1402.
82. Nylen KJ, O'Hara MW, Brock R, Moel J, Gorman L, Stuart S. Predictors of the longitudinal course of postpartum depression following interpersonal psychotherapy. J Consult Clin Psychol. 2010;78(5):757.
83. Grote NK, Lohr MJ, Curran MC, Cristofalo M. Change mechanisms in brief interpersonal psychotherapy for women with perinatal depression: qualitative study. Am J Psychother. 2021;74(3):112–118.
84. Ingram J, Johnson D, O'Mahen HA, Law R, Culpin I, Kessler D, et al. "Asking for help": a qualitative interview study exploring the experiences of interpersonal counselling (IPC) compared to low-intensity cognitive behavioural therapy (CBT) for women with depression during pregnancy. BMC Pregnancy Childbirth. 2021;21(1):1–8.
85. Hazlett-Stevens H. Chapter 5: Relaxation strategies. In: *Psychological approaches to generalized anxiety disorder: a clinician's guide to assessment and treatment*. New York: Springer Science & Business Media; 2008: 81–106.
86. Perciavalle V, Blandini M, Fecarotta P, Buscemi A, Di Corrado D, Bertolo L, et al. The role of deep breathing on stress. Neurol Sci. 2017;38(3):451–458.
87. Kabat-Zinn J. Mindfulness-based interventions in context: past, present, and future. Clin Psychol Sci Pract. 2003;10(2):144–156.
88. Khajuria A, Kumar A, Joshi D, Kumaran SS. Reducing stress with yoga: a systematic review based on multimodal biosignals. Int J Yoga. 2023;16(3):156–170.
89. Guo P, Zhang X, Liu N, Wang J, Chen D, Sun W, et al. Mind-body interventions on stress management in pregnant women: a systematic review and meta-analysis of randomized controlled trials. J Adv Nurs. 2021;77(1):125–146.
90. Abera M, Hanlon C, Daniel B, Tesfaye M, Workicho A, Girma T, et al. Effects of relaxation interventions during pregnancy on maternal mental health, and pregnancy and newborn outcomes: a systematic review and meta-analysis. PLoS One. 2024;19(1):e278432.
91. Tragea C, Chrousos GP, Alexopoulos EC, Darviri C. A randomized controlled trial of the effects of a stress management programme during pregnancy. Complement Ther Med. 2014;22(2):203–211.
92. Davis K, Goodman SH, Leiferman J, Taylor M, Dimidjian S. A randomized controlled trial of yoga for pregnant women with symptoms of depression and anxiety. Complement Ther Clin Pract. 2015;21(3):166–172.
93. Nasiri S, Akbari H, Tagharrobi L, Tabatabaee AS. The effect of progressive muscle relaxation and guided imagery on stress, anxiety, and depression of pregnant women referred to health centers. J Educ Health Promot. 2018;7:41.
94. Satyapriya M, Nagendra HR, Nagarathna R, Padmalatha V. Effect of integrated yoga on stress and heart rate variability in pregnant women. Int J Gynaecol Obstet. 2009;104(3):218–222.

95. Estrella-Juarez F, Requena-Mullor M, Garcia-Gonzalez J, Lopez-Villen A, Alarcon-Rodriguez R. Effect of virtual reality and music therapy on the physiologic parameters of pregnant women and fetuses and on anxiety levels: a randomized controlled trial. J Midwifery Womens Health. 2023;68(1):35–43.
96. Little BC, Hayworth J, Benson P, Hall F, Beard RW, Dewhurst J, et al. Treatment of hypertension in pregnancy by relaxation and biofeedback. Lancet. 1984;323(8382):865–867.
97. Nickel C, Lahmann C, Muehlbacher M, Pedrosa Gil F, Kaplan P, Buschmann W, et al. Pregnant women with bronchial asthma benefit from progressive muscle relaxation: a randomized, prospective, controlled trial. Psychother Psychosom. 2006;75(4):237–243.
98. Urech C, Fink NS, Hoesli I, Wilhelm FH, Bitzer J, Alder J. Effects of relaxation on psychobiological wellbeing during pregnancy: a randomized controlled trial. Psychoneuroendocrinology. 2010;35(9):1348–1355.
99. Field T, Diego M, Delgado J, Medina L. Yoga and social support reduce prenatal depression, anxiety and cortisol. J Bodyw Mov Ther. 2013;17(4):397–403.
100. Tabib M, Humphrey T, Forbes-Mckay K. The influence of antenatal relaxation classes on perinatal psychological wellbeing and childbirth experiences: a qualitative study. J Reprod Infant Psychol. 2024:1–19.
101. Tabib M, Humphrey T, Forbes-McKay K, Lau A. Expectant parents' perspectives on the influence of a single antenatal relaxation class: a qualitative study. Complement Ther Clin Pract. 2021;43:101341.
102. Janssen LE, Gieskes AA, Kok M, de Groot CJM, Oudijk MA, de Boer MA. Stress-reducing interventions in pregnancy for the prevention of preterm birth: a systematic review and meta-analysis. J Psychosom Obstet Gynaecol. 2023;44(1):2281238.
103. García González J, Ventura Miranda MI, Requena Mullor M, Parron Carreño T, Alarcón Rodriguez R. Effects of prenatal music stimulation on state/trait anxiety in full-term pregnancy and its influence on childbirth: a randomized controlled trial. J Matern Fetal Neonatal Med. 2018;31(8):1058–1065.
104. Simavli S, Kaygusuz I, Gumus I, Usluogulları B, Yildirim M, Kafali H. Effect of music therapy during vaginal delivery on postpartum pain relief and mental health. J Affect Disord. 2014;156:194–199.
105. Field T. Prenatal depression effects on early development: a review. Infant Behav Dev. 2011;34(1):1–14.
106. Sriboonpimsuay W. Meditation for preterm birth prevention: a randomized controlled trial in Udonthani, Thailand. Int J Public Health Res. 2011;1(1):31–39.
107. Xie W, Wang M, Ng S, Lu S, Yeung A, Chan KP, et al. Effects of a mindfulness-based intervention delivered by mobile phone on perinatal-specific stress and neonatal outcomes: a randomized controlled trial. Mindfulness. 2024;15:2595–2608.
108. Crovetto F, Crispi F, Casas R, Martín-Asuero A, Borràs R, Vieta E, et al. Effects of Mediterranean diet or mindfulness-based stress reduction on prevention of small-for-gestational age birth weights in newborns born to at-risk pregnant individuals: the impact BCN randomized clinical trial. JAMA. 2021;326(21):2150–2160.
109. Nakaki A, Crovetto F, Urru A, Piella G, Borras R, Comte V, et al. Effects of Mediterranean diet or mindfulness-based stress reduction on fetal and neonatal brain development: a secondary analysis of a randomized clinical trial. Am J Obstet Gynecol MFM. 2023;5(12):101188.
110. Zhang X, Mao F, Li Y, Wang J, Wu L, Sun J, et al. Effects of a maternal mindfulness intervention targeting prenatal psychological distress on infants' meconium microbiota: a randomized controlled trial. Psychoneuroendocrinology. 2022;145:105913.
111. Bleker LS, Milgrom J, Parker D, Gemmill AW, Holt CJ, Connelly A, et al. Brain magnetic resonance imaging findings in children after antenatal maternal depression treatment, a longitudinal study built on a pilot randomized controlled trial. Int J Environ Res Public Health. 2019;16(10):1816.
112. Husain N, Kiran T, Fatima B, Chaudhry IB, Husain M, Shah S, et al. An integrated parenting intervention for maternal depression and child development in a low-resource setting: cluster randomized controlled trial. Depress Anxiety. 2021;38(9):925–939.

113. Holt C, Gentilleau C, Gemmill AW, Milgrom J. Improving the mother-infant relationship following postnatal depression: a randomised controlled trial of a brief intervention (HUGS). Arch Womens Ment Health. 2021; 24(6): 913-923.
114. Milgrom J, Holt C, Holt CJ, Ross J, Ericksen J, Gemmill AW. Feasibility study and pilot randomised trial of an antenatal depression treatment with infant follow-up. Arch Womens Ment Health. 2015;18(5):717–730.
115. Bastani F, Hidarnia A, Montgomery KS, Aguilar-Vafaei ME, Kazemnejad A. Does relaxation education in anxious primigravid Iranian women influence adverse pregnancy outcomes?: a randomized controlled trial. J Perinat Neonatal Nurs. 2006;20(2):138–146.
116. Ghorbannejad S, MehdizadehTourzani Z, Kabir K. The effectiveness of Jacobson's progressive muscle relaxation technique on maternal, fetal and neonatal outcomes in women with non-severe preeclampsia: a randomized clinical trial. Heliyon. 2022;8(6).
117. Rajeswari S, Sanjeevareddy N. Efficacy of progressive muscle relaxation on pregnancy outcome among anxious Indian primi mothers. Iran J Nurs Midwifery Res. 2020;25(1):23–30.
118. Chuntharapat S, Petpichetchian W, Hatthakit U. Yoga during pregnancy: effects on maternal comfort, labor pain and birth outcomes. Complement Ther Clin Pract. 2008;14(2):105–115.
119. Simavli S, Gumus I, Kaygusuz I, Yildirim M, Usluogullari B, Kafali H. Effect of music on labor pain relief, anxiety level and postpartum analgesic requirement: a randomized controlled clinical trial. Gynecol Obstet Investig. 2014;78(4):244–250.
120. García González J, Ventura Miranda MI, Manchon García F, Pallarés Ruiz TI, Marin Gascón ML, Requena Mullor M, et al. Effects of prenatal music stimulation on fetal cardiac state, newborn anthropometric measurements and vital signs of pregnant women: a randomized controlled trial. Complement Ther Clin Pract. 2017;27:61–67.
121. Fink NS, Urech C, Isabel F, Meyer A, Hoesli I, Bitzer J, et al. Fetal response to abbreviated relaxation techniques. A randomized controlled study. Early Hum Dev. 2011;87(2):121–127.
122. Singla DR, Lawson A, Kohrt BA, Jung JW, Meng Z, Ratjen C, et al. Implementation and effectiveness of nonspecialist-delivered interventions for perinatal mental health in high-income countries: a systematic review and meta-analysis. JAMA Psychiatry. 2021;78(5):498–509.
123. Lau Y, Cheng JY, Wong SH, Yen KY, Cheng LJ. Effectiveness of digital psychotherapeutic intervention among perinatal women: a systematic review and meta-analysis of randomized controlled trials. World J Psychiatry. 2021;11(4):133.
124. Zeng G, Niu J, Zhu K, Li F, Li L, Gao K, et al. Effects of non-pharmacological interventions on depressive and anxiety symptoms in pregnant women: a systematic review and network meta-analysis. EClinicalMedicine. 2025;79:103011.
125. Davis JA, Ohan JL, Gibson LY, Prescott SL, Finlay-Jones AL. Understanding engagement in digital mental health and well-being programs for women in the perinatal period: systematic review without meta-analysis. J Med Internet Res. 2022;24(8):e36620.
126. Zimmermann M, Yonkers KA, Tabb KM, Schaefer A, Peacock-Chambers E, Clare CA, et al. Developing personas to inform the design of digital interventions for perinatal mental health. JAMIA Open. 2024;7(4):ooae112.

Index

R. A. Caparros-Gonzalez (ed.), *Maternal Stress during Pregnancy and Postpartum*, https://doi.org/10.1007/978-3-032-09245-8

MIX
Papier aus verantwortungsvollen Quellen
Paper from responsible sources
FSC® C105338

If you have any concerns about our products,
you can contact us on
ProductSafety@springernature.com

In case Publisher is established outside the EU,
the EU authorized representative is:
Springer Nature Customer Service Center GmbH
Europaplatz 3, 69115 Heidelberg, Germany

Printed by Libri Plureos GmbH
in Hamburg, Germany